Experimental Approaches to Diabetic Retinopathy

Frontiers in Diabetes

Vol. 20

Series Editors

M. Porta Turin
F.M. Matschinsky Philadelphia, Pa.

Experimental Approaches to Diabetic Retinopathy

Volume Editors

H.-P. Hammes Mannheim
M. Porta Turin

47 figures, 25 in color, and 7 tables, 2010

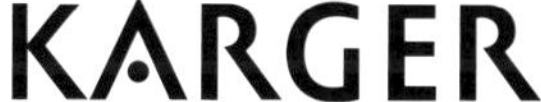

Basel · Freiburg · Paris · London · New York · Bangalore · Bangkok · Shanghai · Singapore · Tokyo · Sydney

Frontiers in Diabetes
Founded 1981 by F. Belfiore, Catania

Prof. Hans-Peter Hammes
Section of Endocrinology
5th Medical Department
Mannheim Medical Faculty
University Hospital Mannheim
Ruprechts-Karls University Heidelberg
Mannheim, Germany

Prof. Massimo Porta
Department of Medicine
University of Turin
Turin, Italy

Library of Congress Cataloging-in-Publication Data

Experimental approaches to diabetic retinopathy / volume editors, H.-P. Hammes, M. Porta.
p. ; cm. – (Frontiers in diabetes, ISSN 0251-5342; v. 20)
Includes bibliographical references and indexes.
ISBN 978-3-8055-9275-8 (hard cover: alk. paper)
1. Diabetic retinopathy – Research – Methodology. I. Hammes, H.-P. II. Porta, M.
III. Series: Frontiers in diabetes, v. 20. 0251-5342;
[DNLM: 1. Diabetic Retinopathy – physiopathology. 2. Retina – physiopathology.
W1 FR945X v.20 2010 / WK 835 E96 2010]
RE661.D5E68 2010
362.197'735–dc22
2009033409

Bibliographic Indices. This publication is listed in bibliographic services.

Disclaimer. The statements, opinions and data contained in this publication are solely those of the individual authors and contributors and not of the publisher and the editor(s). The appearance of advertisements in the book is not a warranty, endorsement, or approval of the products or services advertised or of their effectiveness, quality or safety. The publisher and the editor(s) disclaim responsibility for any injury to persons or property resulting from any ideas, methods, instructions or products referred to in the content or advertisements.

Drug Dosage. The authors and the publisher have exerted every effort to ensure that drug selection and dosage set forth in this text are in accord with current recommendations and practice at the time of publication. However, in view of ongoing research, changes in government regulations, and the constant flow of information relating to drug therapy and drug reactions, the reader is urged to check the package insert for each drug for any change in indications and dosage and for added warnings and precautions. This is particularly important when the recommended agent is a new and/or infrequently employed drug.

www.karger.com
Printed in Switzerland on acid-free and non-aging paper (ISO 9706) by Reinhardt Druck, Basel
ISSN 0251–5342
ISBN 978–3–8055–9275–8
e-ISBN 978–3–8055–9276–5

Contents

Preface

It is almost commonplace to state that diabetic retinopathy is the leading cause of visual loss in the working age population of industrialized countries and, as can be expected, the statement contains some elements of truth and some that are no longer tenable. As a matter of fact, proliferative diabetic retinopathy remains a severe sight-threatening condition for people with type 1 diabetes, who become diabetic early in life and will still be in working age when it develops. However, the most dangerous condition today is not retinal angiogenesis but the development of macular edema following breakdown of the blood-retinal barrier and that affects with equally vicious consequences patients with type 1 and 2 diabetes. Since the latter is at least 10 times more prevalent than the former, visual loss is becoming more and more the problem of elderly patients, all the more so because we lack effective, definitive treatments for macular edema. Worse, we do not know why retinal capillaries become leaky at some stage of the disease.

Another widely held opinion is that retinopathy can be prevented by optimizing blood glucose and blood pressure control. Try that in the real world and you will be shocked by the number of patients who do not reach therapeutic targets and, more so, by those who develop retinopathy in spite of attaining the goals. Yet, the incidence of severe retinopathy is decreasing among people who developed type 1 diabetes in more recent years, as attention and facilities focus more and more on day to day management of glycemia and hypertension. At any rate, the hypotheses we have on the pathways leading to glucose-induced damage will not explain why edema and/or new vessels develop at some stage, in certain areas of the retina, and only in some patients.

The search for pathogenic mechanisms that entirely explain the natural history of retinopathy and indicate a clear-cut therapeutic target (like, say, iron deficiency and replacement in iron-deficient anemia) is still unsuccessful. Laboratories around the world, with few exceptions, pursue separate lines of research on distinct substrates. Experimental work aiming at a sufficient mechanistic explanation of retinopathy genesis is often carried out by using representative cells cultured in high glucose, or in rodents which have, at best, approximate applicability to human pathology. Basic scientists may not be fully aware of the sequence and the way retinopathy presents itself in the patients' eyes, apart from archetypical fundus photographs of new vessels and hard exudates. Conversely, clinicians, when they manage to devote some preciously earned time to research, stick mostly to clinical issues and may be daunted by the rapid pace of basic science progress.

If researcher segregation and want of experimental models are some of the reasons why retinopathy remains a silent morbidity condition at large, we felt that a volume that includes the anatomoclinical correlates of retinopathy and which overviews some of the hottest issues in basic research could benefit both scientists and physicians involved in the quest for a solution.

Hans-Peter Hammes, Mannheim
Massimo Porta, Turin

Hammes H-P, Porta M (eds): Experimental Approaches to Diabetic Retinopathy.
Front Diabetes. Basel, Karger, 2010, vol 20, pp 1–19

Clinical Presentations and Pathological Correlates of Retinopathy

Toke Bek

Department of Ophthalmology, Århus University Hospital, Århus, Denmark

Abstract

Diabetic retinopathy consists of a variety of morphological lesions in the retinal fundus related to disturbances in retinal blood flow. In this chapter, these clinical manifestations of diabetic retinopathy will be described, and the background and development of each individual lesion type and combinations of different lesion types will be discussed in relation to relevant theories and working hypotheses for the pathophysiology of the disease. Finally, the implications for central and peripheral vision of each lesion type occurring as part of diabetic retinopathy will be discussed.

Diabetic retinopathy is a frequent cause of blindness among young adults in the industrialised countries, and with the current epidemic of especially type 2 diabetes mellitus sweeping the Western world, diabetic complications including retinopathy can be expected to become even more frequent in the future [1].

The initial sign of diabetic complications in the retina is disturbances in visual function as evidenced by changes in the oscillatory potential of the electroretinogram [2], and these early functional changes constitute a risk factor for later development of central visual loss. However, paradoxically diabetic retinopathy is not diagnosed and monitored on the basis of functional changes in the retina, but on the basis of its morphological appearance as studied by ophthalmoscopy or fundus photography.

This appearance can be divided into:

1. Early changes that are reversible and do not threaten central vision. These changes are termed simplex retinopathy or background retinopathy, alluding to the fact that the lesions remain in the eye background.
2. Later vision-threatening changes that may assume one or both of two forms:
   a. Diabetic maculopathy with retinal exudation and oedema that extends to the foveal region and threatens central vision.
   b. Proliferative diabetic retinopathy which is growth of new vessels from the larger retinal venules. These new vessels may cause visual loss by spontaneous haemorrhage into the vitreous body or by inducing retinal detachment due to traction from connective tissue in the new vessels.

It is the detection of morphological lesions not appreciated by the patient that renders diabetic retinopathy suitable for screening by funduscopic inspection [3]. The clinical appearance of diabetic retinopathy has inspired a number of working

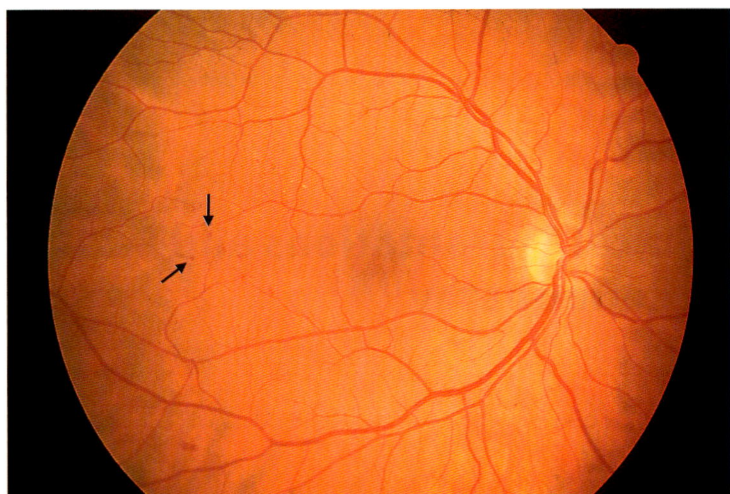

Fig. 1. Microaneurysms and haemorrhages temporal from the fovea (arrows).

hypotheses and methodological approaches for understanding the disease, based on the fact that the observed morphological lesions are related to disturbances in retinal blood flow. These disturbances include both hyperperfusion as a consequence of reduced tone in the retinal resistance vessels, which is most prominent in the macular area, and hypoperfusion as a consequence of capillary occlusion, which is most pronounced in the peripheral retina. The experimental approaches for studying these mechanisms are diverse and will be treated in more detail in other chapters of this volume.

In this chapter, the clinical manifestations of diabetic retinopathy will be described, and the background and development of each individual lesion type and combinations of different lesion types will be discussed in relation to relevant theories and working hypotheses for the pathophysiology of diabetic retinopathy.

Morphological Lesions

Microaneurysms and Haemorrhages

The initial sign of diabetic retinopathy is small red dots in the fundus background, typically located temporally from the foveal area [4], from where the lesion may spread to other parts of the macular area and the retinal periphery (fig. 1). Generally, the density of red dots reflects the density of the retinal capillary system which is highest in the macular area apart from the foveal avascular zone, and decreases towards the retinal periphery. The red dots occur together with retinal hyperperfusion and may represent microaneurysmatic dilations of the retinal capillaries or small haemorrhages resulting from localised ruptures of the retinal capillaries. By definition, the diameter of a microaneurysm is less than 100 μm, but most frequently the diameter of the lesion is not larger than 10–20 μm [5]. The differentiation of a microaneurysm from a small well-defined dot haemorrhage cannot be done on the basis of ophthalmoscopy alone, but requires fluorescein angiography by which a microaneurysm fills with fluorescein, whereas a haemorrhage remains dark [6]. The appearance of a haemorrhage often differs from that of a microaneurysm because the haemorrhage distributes around the surrounding anatomical structures. This is most clearly observed near the optic disk where haemorrhages may be arranged in flame-shaped lines

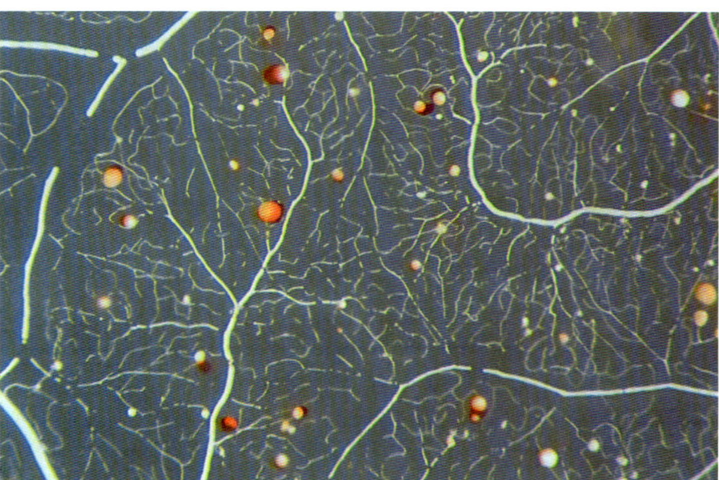

Fig. 2. Cast of human diabetic retinal capillary bed with organising microaneurysms. The red cap seen around the white casting material in the microaneurysms represents erythrocytes trapped in the thrombotic tissue growing from the cap of the lesions.

around the retinal nerve fibres. Furthermore, haemorrhages often become larger than microaneurysms or display an unsharp delimitation due to partial resorption. However, a differentiation of microaneurysms from dot haemorrhages does not have any practical implications since the two lesion types share a common pathophysiological background and have the same clinical significance.

The number of microaneurysms and haemorrhages is an indicator of the risk of further progression of diabetic retinopathy. Thus, it has been shown that the presence of a few red dots implies the same risk of progression of diabetic retinopathy as no lesions, and the risk of developing retinopathy increases with the number of red dots in the fundus [7–10]. Similarly, it has been shown that the visual prognosis after retinal photocoagulation is better when the treatment results in a reduction in the number of red dots to ≤4, than when this goal is not reached [11]. The number of microaneurysms and haemorrhages increases in parallel with the development of diabetic retinopathy, typically over years to decades [9]. However, the presence of a certain number of lesions covers a dynamic pattern with considerable turnover of lesions. Thus, fundus photographs taken repeatedly with 1-week intervals may often show the same number of lesions; however located at a new position from one examination to another, indicating a continuous new formation and resorption of the lesions [12].

The pathophysiology underlying the turnover of microaneurysms and haemorrhages is different. Thus, the formation of a microaneurysm starts with a localised dilation of a retinal capillary, probably secondary to both an increased hydrostatic pressure in the vessels and weakening of the structure of the capillary wall [5, 6, 13]. Subsequently, the microaneurysm gradually fills with thrombotic material (fig. 2) and undergoes organisation [14], during which the haemoglobin in the erythrocytes that have become trapped in the microaneurysm will be resorbed and the thrombotic mass will become invisible. The vascular wall remains thickened at the location of an organised microaneurysm, which implies that new microaneurysms are not formed at the same position. Therefore, it is a misconception of the natural history of diabetic retinopathy when it is recommended to eliminate microaneurysm by focal photocoagulation. The lesion will disappear

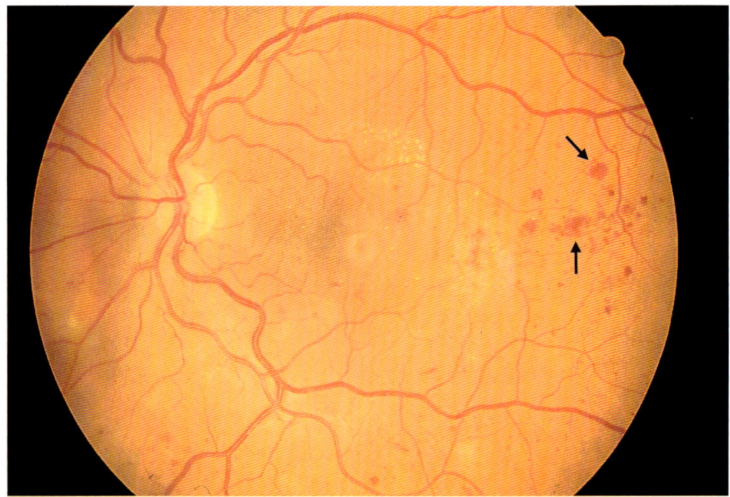

Fig. 3. Larger blot haemorrhages temporal from the fovea (arrows).

anyway. A possible positive effect on retinopathy is not due to the elimination of the microaneurysm, but to the more unspecific effect of outer retinal damage which is seen after photocoagulation in general. An organised whitish microaneurysm located in the centre of a haemorrhage may have an appearance similar to the hat batch named a cocarde. However, cocarde lesions may also develop secondary to other systemic and retinal diseases and do not play a specific diagnostic or prognostic role in diabetic retinopathy.

Retinal haemorrhages display a dynamic pattern of development which has two forms. One pattern is the formation and resorption of haemorrhages at the same location from time to time in so-called hot spots, indicating repetitive stress on the same retinal vessel. The other pattern consists of haemorrhages that develop at different locations from time to time in the retina, indicating that the areas where the capillary network is stressed varies from place to place.

Smaller dot haemorrhages are differentiated from larger blot haemorrhages on the basis of whether the diameter is smaller or larger than the diameter of the temporal arterioles at the crossing of the optic disk (fig. 3). The presence of a few blot haemorrhages alone is not a risk factor for progression of retinopathy. However, the presence of many blot haemorrhages distributed in clusters temporally in the macular area indicates severe peripheral ischaemia and that retinopathy has progressed to a pre-proliferative stage [15]. A special type of blot haemorrhage with the same prognostic significance as cluster haemorrhages develops from the perifoveal capillaries to extend over the foveal area and reduce visual acuity. Foveal haemorrhages always resolve spontaneously and result in an almost normalisation of central vision. These lesions are one of the few manifestations of diabetic retinopathy where a subjective symptom of a potentially vision-threatening retinopathy may encourage the patient to seek an ophthalmologist [15].

Exudates, Blood-Retina Barrier Leakage and Retinal Oedema

Retinal exudates are precipitations of plasma protein that have leaked from the retinal vessels [16, 17]. The typical 'hard' exudate appears as a sharply delimited whitish lesion in the surrounding reddish retina. The typical exudate has approximately the size of a microaneurysm, but the

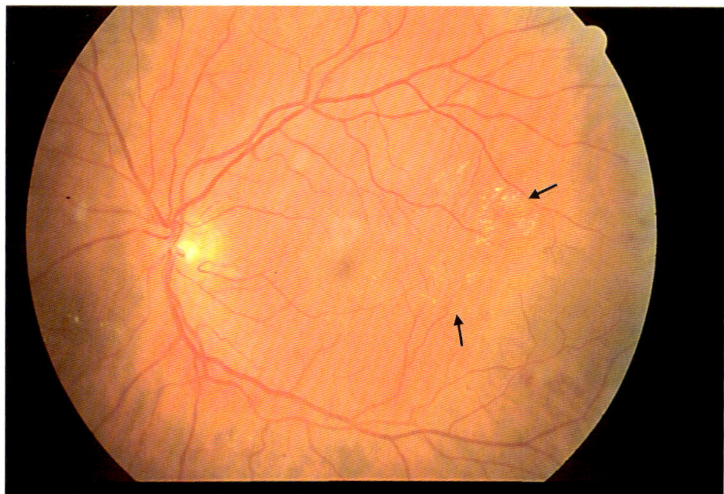

Fig. 4. Hard exudates in the macular area, some of which are forming exudate rings (arrows).

lesion may expand and merge with neighbouring lesions to form larger conglomerates of exudates. Exudates may occur as solitary lesions, in groups, or arranged in a circinate pattern concentrically around a single leakage point to form so-called exudate rings (fig. 4). Frequently, the first indication of a weakness of the microvasculature leading to leakage will be the occurrence of a dot haemorrhage that may have resorbed totally or partially when the exudate ring is observed concentrically around the haemorrhage.

Due to the occurrence of exudate rings around single leakage points, it is assumed that exudates represent precipitation lines located at a distance from the leakage point where the concentration of plasma proteins in the plasma ultrafiltrate is sufficiently high. This balance is determined by the local ultrafiltration and resorption of plasma proteins and fluid. An increased ultrafiltration of plasma is caused by the breakdown of the normal barrier properties of the retinal vessels. This breakdown may be due to both structural changes in the capillary walls and an increase in the hydrostatic pressure of the vessels secondary to hyperperfusion. Breakdown of the blood-retina barrier can by studied by fluorescein angiography where intravenously injected fluorescein can be seen to leak out of the blood vessels, either corresponding to focal leakage points or more diffusely [18]. However, the fluorescein molecule is small, corresponding to about the size of a hydrated potassium ion, which implies that leakage of fluorescein does not necessarily reflect the presence of larger leakage points that would allow the leakage of plasma proteins [19].

It is a widely promulgated misconception that leakage of fluorescein per se reflects retinal oedema. Oedema is due to abnormal accumulation of fluid in the tissue because of a disturbance in the balance between hydrostatic, electric and osmotic forces across the vascular wall [20]. These variables are not fully described by studying the transport of fluorescein across the blood-retina barrier, and fluorescein leakage itself does not indicate that the retinal sensory function is disturbed [21]. Most of the variables involved in the formation of diabetic retinal oedema such as changes in the active transport of fluid over the retinal pigment epithelium and dynamic variations in the distribution of hard exudates, have only been sparsely studied. Therefore, fluorescein leakage is still a widely used marker

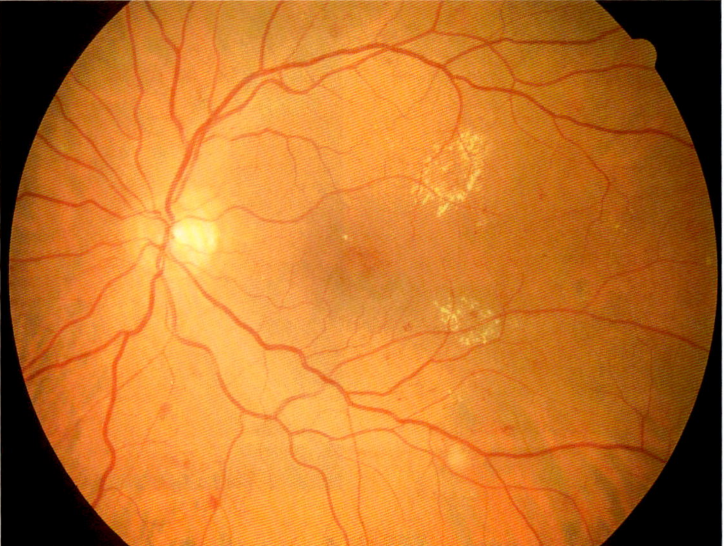

Fig. 5. Clinically significant macular oedema with hard exudates in the foveal region in addition to hard exudate rings.

of the mechanisms leading to diabetic retinal oedema.

Hard exudates develop later than microaneurysms and haemorrhages, but typically show the same spatial pattern of distribution with the lesions starting temporally from the fovea from where they may spread to other parts of the macular area. The density of hard exudates decreases from the vascular arcades and the lesion is typically absent from the retinal periphery. When exudate rings extend on each side of a temporal vascular arcade, the exudates located peripheral from the arcade will typically be much thinner than the segment located central from the arcade. In most cases, exudates are accompanied by retinal oedema which has a destructive effect on the neuronal tissue in the retina. Therefore, the presence of exudates and retinal oedema in the macular area is an indication that diabetic retinopathy has entered a potentially vision-threatening stage, so-called *diabetic maculopathy*. When an area with exudates and/or retinal oedema is either larger than one disk diameter and a part of this area is within one disk diameter from the fovea, or if these lesions develop within ½ disk diameter from the fovea, there is a high risk of visual damage, and the condition is termed *clinically significant macular oedema* (fig. 5). This advanced stage of diabetic maculopathy is treated with retinal photocoagulation which may halve the risk of developing visual loss [22]. Larger conglomerates of hard exudates that extend to the foveal area may block the light from reaching the photoreceptors and consequently induce visual loss and extrafoveal fixation. These visual disturbances may to some extent improve if retinal photocoagulation induces changes in retinal fluid dynamics so that the central exudates are resorbed [23]. However, visual impairment induced by retinal oedema will most often be irreversible. Retinal oedema is diagnosed semiquantitatively by binocular inspection [24] or quantitatively by optical coherence tomography scanning [25].

In younger diabetic patients, the initial sign of macular oedema may be reflections from the posterior hyaloid membrane in the macular area (fig. 6). These reflections are normal in younger persons because the light used to illuminate

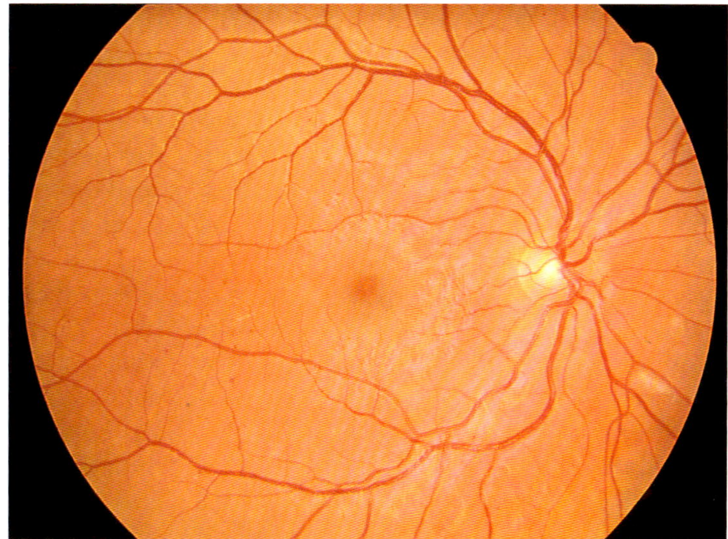

Fig. 6. Reflections from the posterior hyaloid membrane representing subclinical retinal oedema.

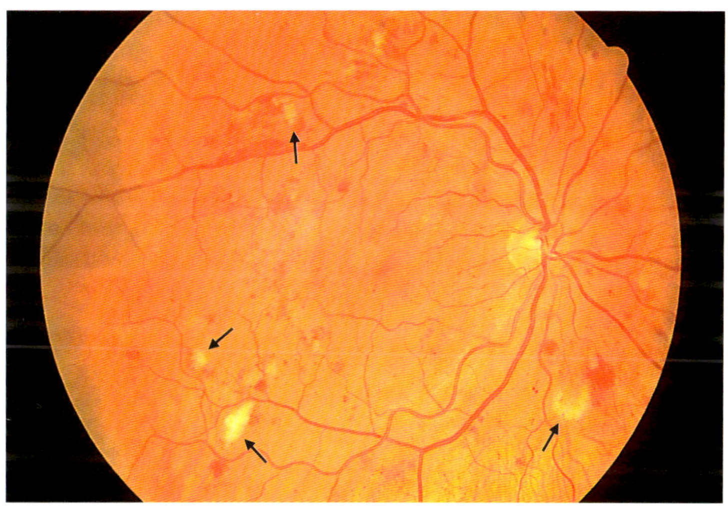

Fig. 7. Retinal cotton wool spots (arrows).

the retina is reflected from the posterior hyaloid membrane where it rides over the larger vessels or corresponding to the perifoveal thickening of the retinal ganglion cell layer. However, the reflections secondary to incipient retinal oedema appear more irregularly distributed in the macular area.

Cotton Wool Spots

Retinal cotton wool spots are unsharply delimited whitish lesions located in the superficial retinal layers with a diameter of one third to a half disk diameter (fig. 7). The cotton wool spot is unfortunately often referred to as a 'soft exudate', although the lesion does not involve exudation and it has not been verified what 'soft' means. Another misconception is that the cotton wool spot per se represents a retinal infarction.

Cotton wool spots are caused by localised disturbances in the axoplasmic transport of the retinal nerve fibres [26], which *may* be due to an infarction, but which may also have other causes, especially in diabetic retinopathy. An arrest of the axoplasmic transport will result in an accumulation of intracellular organelles [16] that are transported retrogradely from the terminal end of the axon in the lateral geniculate body. This results in a swelling of the retinal nerve fibres in the affected area, and the resulting thickening of the inner retinal layers will diffuse light and give the lesion its typical whitish and unsharply delimited appearance. In rare cases, one can also observe accumulation of intracellular organelles that are transported anterogradely the shorter distance from the nerve fibre somata in the retinal ganglion cells. In these cases, the cotton wool spot will appear as a double lesion with one part on each side of the area where the axoplasmic transport has stopped.

Cotton wool spots may result in localised relative microscotomas as a consequence of diffusion of the light impinging on the retina [27, 28]. Most often, the lesion will not be accompanied by arcuate scotomas, which indicates that, in spite of the disturbance in the axoplasmic transport, the conduction of axon potentials in the retinal nerve fibres in the affected area has remained intact. However, if cotton wool spots persist for a longer time, the nervous conduction may also be affected with consequent arcuate scotomas in the visual field.

Cotton wool spots that occur solitarily without any other signs of diabetic retinopathy are not a particular risk factor for progression of the disease [29]. In diabetic retinopathy, the number of cotton wool spots is often seen to increase transiently during periods with larger oscillations in the blood glucose [30], which is probably due to metabolic disturbances in the retinal nerve fibre layer secondary to the changes in the blood glucose. However, an increase in the number of cotton wool spots may also indicate that diabetic retinopathy is progressing, and this pattern is part of the definition of advanced non-proliferative diabetic retinopathy that may potentially progress to a treatment-requiring stage [29].

The distribution of retinal cotton wool spots reflects the thickness of the retinal nerve fibre layer. Therefore, the preponderance of cotton wool spots around the larger vascular arcades is not due to the close relationship with these vessels, but is due to the fact that the vessels course through the area where the retinal nerve fibre layer is thickest. Accordingly, the prevalence of cotton wool spots decreases towards the retinal periphery in parallel with the thickness of the retinal nerve fibre layer, and cotton wool spots are absent from the foveal area which is devoid of retinal nerve fibres. Cotton wool spots develop within days by a gradual uniform whitening of the affected area, and regress over months depending on the underlying cause of the lesion [31]. During the regression of a cotton wool spot, the size of the lesion will gradually diminish and assume an irregular grainy shape until it disappears totally.

Arteriolar Changes

In the early stages of diabetic retinopathy, retinal arterioles dilate and lengthen. This results in increased tortuosity of the vessels [20, 32, 33], which is assumed to be due to the early hyperperfusion observed in the disease. Additionally, in areas with retinal hyperperfusion, the perivascular glial cells can be seen to express increasing immunoreactivity to S-100 protein [34]. The generalised macrovascular complications observed in diabetic patients, such as arterial hypertension and atherosclerosis, can also be observed funduscopically as accentuated sclerosing of the retinal arterioles [35, 36], but generally the arteriolar changes observed in diabetic patients are not specific for diabetic retinopathy, and therefore play

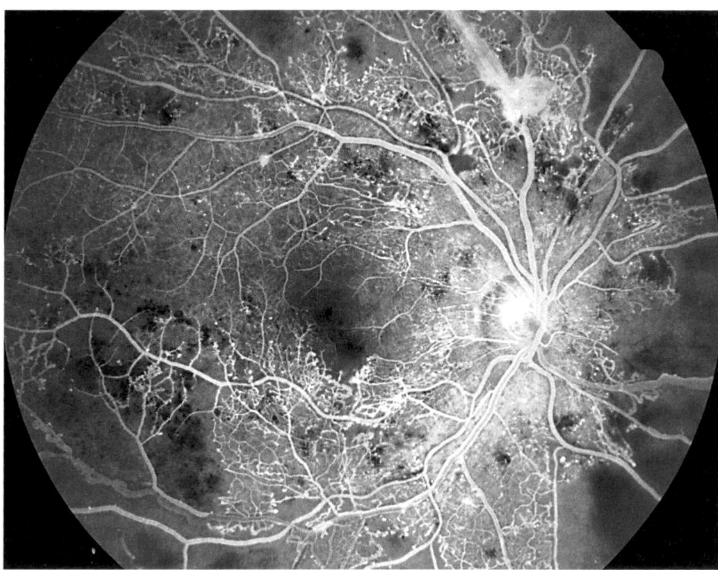

Fig. 8. Fluorescein angiography showing multiple areas of lack of fluorescein filling due to capillary occlusion.

no practical role for the diagnosis and management of the disease.

Capillary Occlusion

Occlusion of the retinal capillaries may occur in the more advanced stages of diabetic retinopathy. The occlusion process starts in the retinal mid-periphery and extends towards the retinal periphery [37], whereas the macular area is only rarely affected. In the rare cases of ischaemic maculopathy, the capillary occlusion extends from the temporal area and the vascular arcades towards the foveal region, whereas the papillomacular bundle is most resistant and is only affected in extremely rare cases [38, 39] (fig. 8). Retinal ischaemia may develop in older diabetic patients after cataract surgery, but for some unknown reasons the neovascular response often develops from the chamber angle instead of the retinal vessels in these patients. Therefore, this condition may start with symptoms of increased intraocular pressure and neovascular glaucoma. To the skilled clinician, ischaemic diabetic maculopathy may present with a typical yellowish appearance. A similar appearance may also be due to a nuclear cataract, and consequently among older patients an ischaemic fundus is much easier to diagnose in pseudophakic patients.

Capillary occlusion is demonstrated by fluorescein angiography where the capillary-free areas appear as well delimited dark non-perfused areas where the contours of the choroidal background fluorescence are blurred. This blurring is probably due to diffusion of light in an amorphous material that has accumulated between the photoreceptor outer segments and the pigment epithelium corresponding to the ischaemic areas [40].

Capillary occlusion starts on the arteriolar side of the microvascular units and expands towards their venolar side [41]. The pathophysiology of capillary occlusion is unknown, but the condition is irreversible and histological studies have shown ingrowth of retinal Müller cells in the occluded vessels [42]. An angiographic appearance similar to that of occluded capillaries is seen corresponding to retinal cotton wool spots. However, in these lesions the lack of capillary filling may be due to compression of the capillary from the tissue oedema, since the non-perfusion may disappear together with the cotton wool spot [43]. Microaneurysms often occur abundantly on the capillaries bordering areas of capillary occlusion, and the interdependence between these two lesion types is a matter of continued debate in the literature [44].

Areas of capillary occlusion result in localised scotomas in the visual field [45]. This indicates that the functional loss is most pronounced in the middle retinal layers, since it can be assumed that the choroidal supply to the outer retinal layers is preserved and the lack of arcuate scotomas indicates that the function of the retinal nerve fibre layer is preserved.

Intra-Retinal Microvascular Abnormalities

Intra-retinal microvascular abnormalities (IRMA vessels) are pre-existing retinal capillaries that have adapted to changes in the distribution of the retinal blood flow (fig. 9). These changes develop because of dilation of retinal resistance vessels in order to bypass areas of capillary occlusion. IRMA vessels are often observed as vascular irregularities, and can often be seen as shunt vessels that connect the arterial and the venous part of the retinal vascular system [46]. The presence of IRMA vessels is a result of disturbances in the retinal blood flow, indicating that retinopathy has entered a pre-proliferative stage. Normally, the larger retinal vessels are located on the retinal surface with terminal arterioles branching to supply the deeper retinal layers. Histologically, IRMA vessels are observed as large-calibre vessels that are located abnormally deep in the retina [47].

In clinical practice, IRMA vessels are often confused with retinal neovascularisations. However, the two types of vascular abnormalities can be differentiated on the basis of the characteristics described in table 1.

Venous Changes

Dilatation of retinal venules may occur in the later stages of diabetic retinopathy [48]. A uniform dilatation of the retinal venules may be difficult to detect since the vascular diameter is assessed by comparison with the diameter of the adjoining arteriole which may also be changed. Normally, the calibre of a vessel tapers with increasing distance from the heart, and consequently segmental dilatation of a vessel with the diameter becoming larger peripherally along a vascular segment is definitely abnormal. In severe cases, this condition may present as a string of sausages or beads (fig. 10). Changes in the calibre of retinal venules indicate that diabetic retinopathy has entered a pre-proliferative stage. The background for venous dilation is unknown, but may be an adaptation to the increased blood flow. The more pronounced venous changes such as beading may be induced by metabolic acidosis as a result of the peripheral ischaemia secondary to the capillary occlusion.

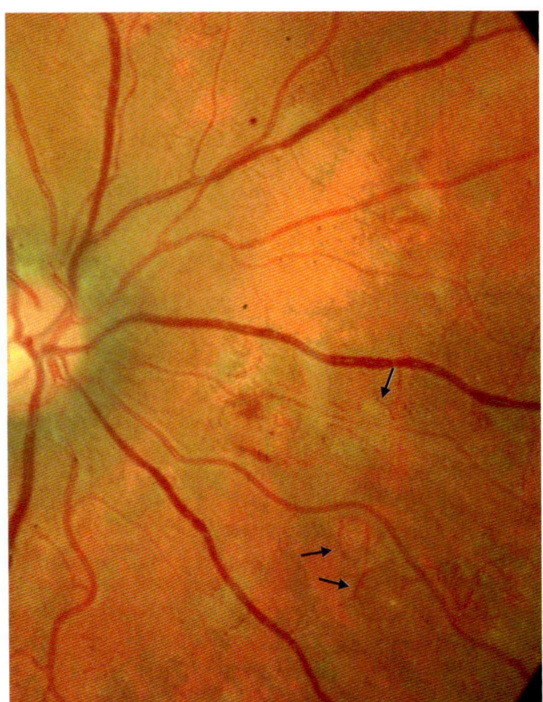

Fig. 9. IRMAs (arrows).

Table 1. Characteristics of IRMA vessels and retinal neovascularisations

IRMA	Neovascularisations
Connect arterioles with venules	Originate from larger venules and course back to their point of origin
Are usually tortuous with few side branches	Are usually heavily branched
Develop intra-retinally	Grow pre-retinally
Do not contain connective tissue	May contain connective tissue
Never cross their feeder vessel	May cross their feeder vessel

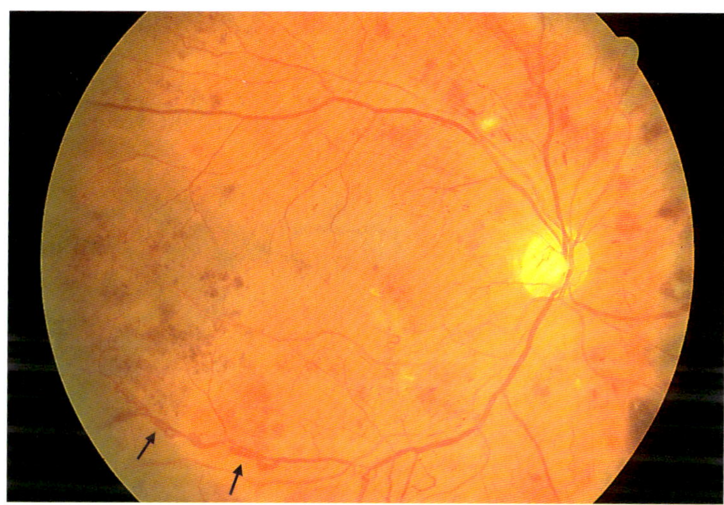

Fig. 10. Venous beading (arrows).

Neovascularisations

Retinal neovascularisations develop from the larger retinal venules and are stimulated by growth factors released from the peripheral retinal areas with ischaemia secondary to capillary occlusion. The neovascular growth pattern resembles that of foetal angiogenesis where new vessel formation is stimulated by the relative ischaemia that develops in parallel with the increasing number of metabolically active cells during retinal development [49]. The proliferation of endothelial cells from the larger venules forms vascular fronts that connect with the arteriolar counterparts to form the microcirculation. However, in the mature retina, the newly formed vessels are unable to grow inside the retinal tissue to replace the occluded vessels [50]. Therefore, the new vessels grow into the vitreous body where they may branch extensively and never get to connect with an arteriole to allow circulation of the blood. The resulting neovascularisation will appear as a fan of vessels spreading

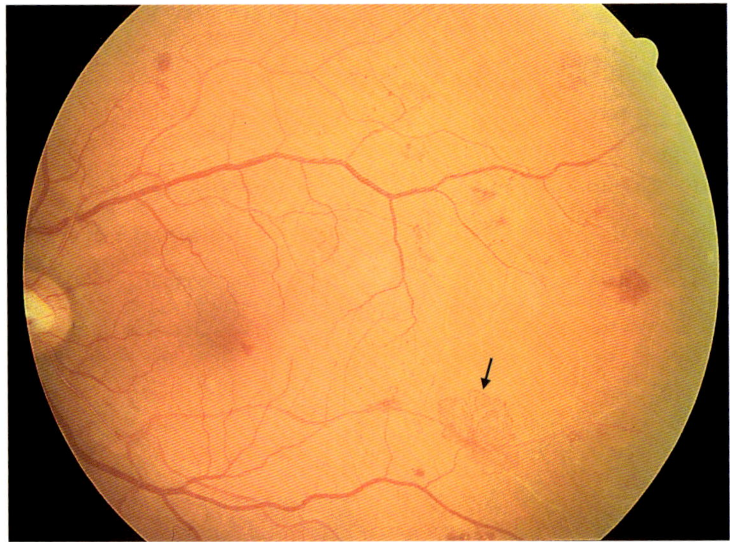

Fig. 11. Fan of new vessels growing from the lower temporal arcade venule (arrow).

from two feeder vessels that originate from the same location on the venule [14] (fig. 11). Since the pressure difference between these feeder vessels is negligible, there will be no circulation of blood in the neovascularisation. Pre-retinal new vessels may contain connective tissue that shrinks and results in tractional retinal detachment. Due to the lack of anatomical apposition to the retinal tissue, the neovascularisations will not mature and assume normal barrier properties. In the early stages, this can be visualised by leakage of fluorescein [51], and in the later stages by spontaneous ruptures of the new vessels resulting in vitreous haemorrhage. After retinal photocoagulation, the retinal ischaemia will be reduced, and the retinal neovascularisations will often regress, but not necessarily disappear. A neovascularisation which has reached an end stage may present with long thin feeder vessels to supply an unbranched front with broader lumen. These vessels form part of the clinical picture denoted as 'posttreatment quiescent retinopathy', and do not imply a risk of further progression of the disease (fig. 12).

Loops and Reduplications

These lesions are deviations of the larger venules to bypass a localised obstruction of the vascular lumen. The lesions may occur as single bypass channels (loops), typically with an appearance as a Greek omega, or as several shunt vessels (reduplications) bypassing the occlusion point [52] (fig. 13). Clinical studies have shown that the lesion is initiated by a localised narrowing of one of the larger retinal venules [46], which proceeds too slowly to result in a classical clinical picture of retinal vein occlusion, but rather stimulates the gradual development of shunt vessels that bypass the occlusion site. Histological studies have shown that the occlusion represents endothelial cells that have proliferated inside the vascular lumen. Venous loops and reduplications occur in less than 1% of diabetic patients in the general screening population, but in 7–8% of the patients with advanced diabetic retinopathy [53], and all patients with loops and reduplications have developed or will develop proliferative diabetic retinopathy within a few months after detection of the lesion. Consequently, loops and reduplications have been interpreted as a

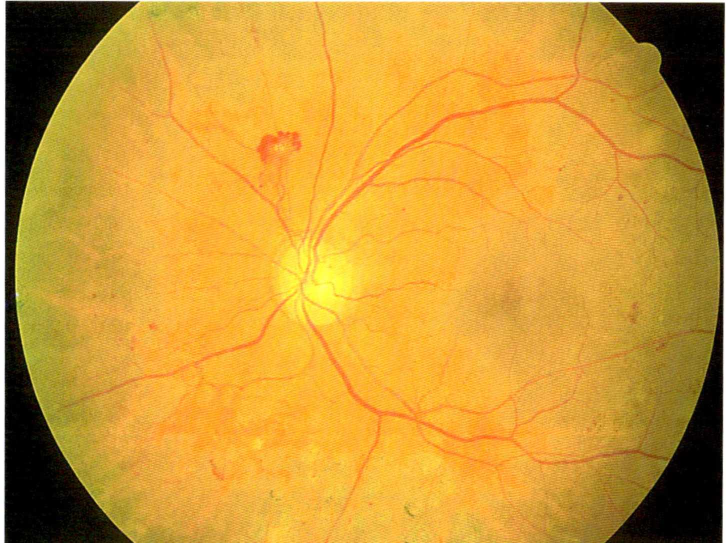

Fig. 12. Post-treatment quiescent retinopathy. Unbranching neovascularisation with dilated front emerging from the optic disk.

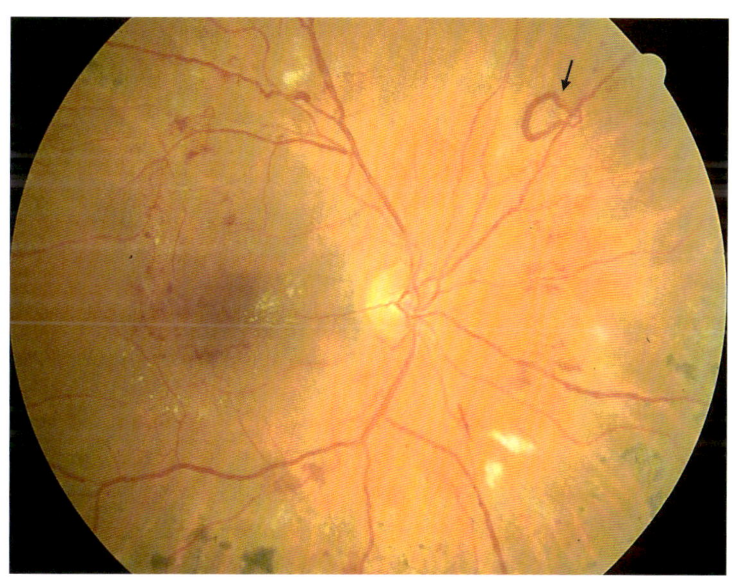

Fig. 13. Venous loop (arrow). The smaller loop on the right side of the vessel indicates that two shunts have developed to bypass the venule. This configuration with more than one loop is termed a reduplication.

special type of proliferative diabetic retinopathy where the endothelial cell proliferation occurs inside the larger venules rather than by growth out of the vessel to enter the vitreous body [47].

Diabetic Papillopathy

Diabetic papillopathy is optic disk swelling in diabetic patients that cannot be attributed to any other cause than the diabetic metabolism. The pathophysiology of the lesion is unknown, but it has been suggested that the condition may be a risk factor for progression of diabetic retinopathy [54].

Pattern of Distribution of Retinopathy Lesions

All the individual morphological lesions observed in diabetic retinopathy can be found in a number of other diseases of the retinal vascular system. Therefore, diabetic retinopathy is not diagnosed on the basis of these lesions alone, but rather on the basis of the pattern of distribution, the dynamics, and the combination of different retinopathy lesions.

Regional Differences in Vision-Threatening Complications

The regional distribution of diabetic retinopathy lesions to some extent reflects a different response pattern of vessels in different parts of the retina. Hyperperfusion develops in the macular area which results in the formation of microaneurysms, haemorrhages, exudates and oedema, whereas capillary occlusion develops in the retinal periphery which results in retinal ischaemia. The dividing line between these two response patterns is approximately around the temporal vascular arcades. This is similar to what is seen in other retinal vascular diseases that may affect both the central and peripheral parts of the retina, such as retinal vein thrombosis. This suggests the existence of different functional and anatomical properties of the retinal arterioles on each side of these vascular arcades. It has been suggested that the differences in response pattern might be due to age [55]. Thus, the predominance of diabetic maculopathy in patients with type 2 diabetes mellitus might be related to an age-related reduction in the capacity of the retinal arterioles to regulate the arteriolar diameter. Conversely, the predominance of proliferative diabetic retinopathy in patients with type 1 diabetes mellitus might be attributed to favourable conditions for neovascularisation in younger persons because the posterior hyaloid membrane is intact as a substrate for the neovascular growth. However, other studies suggest that this is not the whole explanation and that it is highly likely that other differences in the response pattern of the central and peripheral retinal arterioles than those related to age are predisposing to the regional differences of vision-threatening complications of diabetic retinopathy [56].

Regional Differences in Individual Retinopathy Lesions

It is characteristic for diabetic retinopathy that the morphological lesions do not correlate with the distribution area of single retinal arterioles, but develop simultaneously in different parts of the retinal microcirculation. The lesions secondary to hyperperfusion tend to start temporal from the foveal region and spread from here to the remaining part of the macular area [4]. This spreading pattern indicates that the disease is primarily related to changes in the retinal microcirculation and not to the increased intraluminal pressure in the larger retinal arterioles. This is supported by the observation that the presence of diabetic retinopathy lesions around the larger vascular arcades does not prognosticate later development of vision-threatening maculopathy, whereas the development of lesions distant from the vascular arcades, both in the macular area and in the retinal periphery, is such a prognostic sign [57]. Finally, diabetic patients with a low blood pressure may have lesions that are localised corresponding to the microcirculatory units temporal from the foveal area, whereas patients who have a blood pressure which is high within the normal limits may develop a distribution of retinopathy lesions around the optic nerve head and the larger arterioles that resembles hypertensive retinopathy [58] (fig. 14). This may be

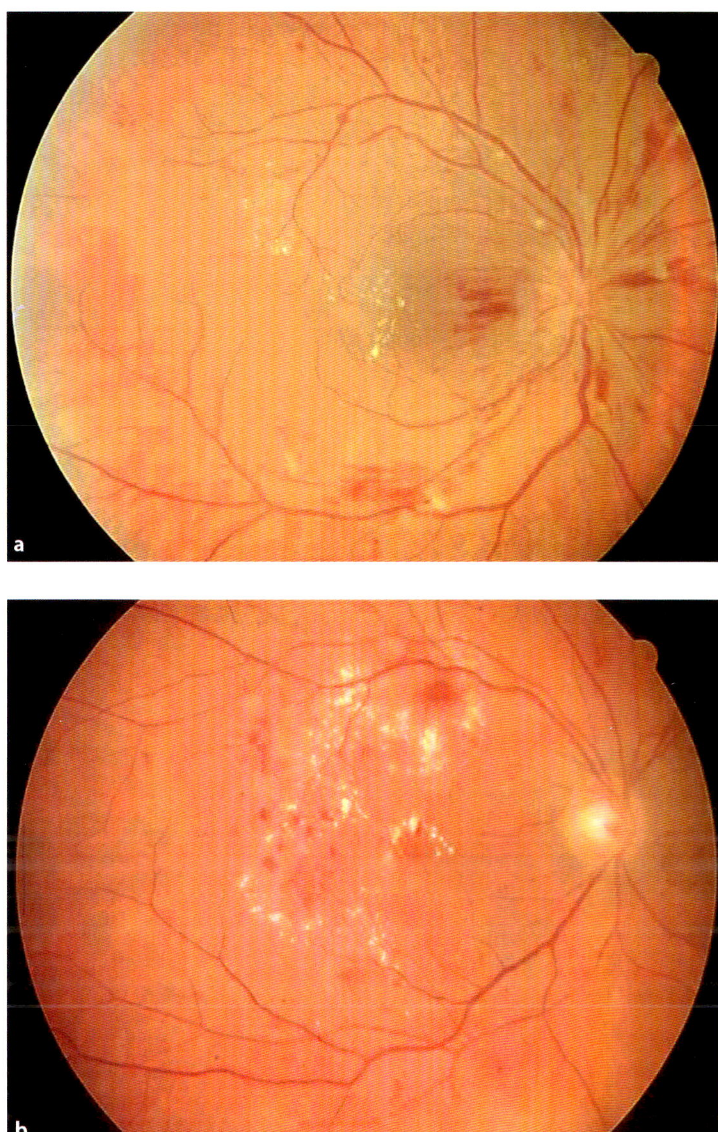

Fig. 14. a Retinopathy lesions predominating around the optic disk in diabetic patient with a blood pressure high in the normal range. **b** Retinopathy lesions predominating temporal from the fovea in diabetic patient with normal blood pressure.

due to impaired autoregulation [59, 60] and confirms that the arterial blood pressure is a risk factor for the development of diabetic retinopathy. However, blood pressure is not the whole explanation since the lesions do not primarily occur in the areas where the arterial pressure load is most pronounced.

Dynamics of Retinopathy Lesions

The initial sign of diabetic retinopathy is the occurrence of red dots which may represent both microaneurysms and dot haemorrhages, although there has been some controversy in the literature as to whether microaneurysms are preceded by capillary occlusion [44]. However, the fact that red dots is the initial funduscopically visible lesion implies that the presence of white lesions occuring alone are not hard exudates. This may be an important diagnostic parameter especially in older type 2 diabetic patients where white lesions may represent drusen secondary to age-related maculopathy. Small sharply delimited whitish drusen that are difficult to differentiate from exudates may also occur in younger persons. However, these lesions can be identified by repeating the examination after more than 1 month where drusen will be unchanged, whereas the dynamic nature of exudates implies that this lesion will always have a changed size, location or configuration.

The fact that exudates often arrange in rings around a leakage point with a microaneurysm and/or a haemorrhage in the centre demonstrates an interdependence between these two lesion types with the red dot being the immediate response and the hard exudate the more sustained response to a localised vascular abnormality. The radius of the exudate ring will represent the diffusion distance from the leakage point to the point of plasma protein precipitation.

The presence of haemorrhages and retinal oedema without exudates may be observed in diabetic maculopathy of the ischaemic type. Ischaemic maculopathy may be difficult to diagnose without fluorescein angiography to show the typical capillary occlusion.

Visual Impairment in Diabetic Retinopathy

The general purpose of the management of diabetic retinopathy is to prevent impairment of central vision secondary to the two complications diabetic maculopathy and proliferative diabetic retinopathy. However, several other types of visual impairment may occur in diabetic patients. Generalised changes such as subclinical perturbations in the electroretinogram [2] may not be appreciated by the patient, whereas changes in contrast sensitivity, dark adaptation and the peripheral visual field induced by retinal photocoagulation may be serious adverse effects that limit normal activities [61, 62]. However, the individual retinopathy lesions may also affect visual function, the severity of symptoms depending on the size and the location of the retinal area involved. Table 2 gives an overview of these different types of visual impairment in diabetic retinopathy [23, 63].

It appears that individual retinal lesions can affect visual function through a variety of mechanisms and may contribute to the visual dysfunction experienced by diabetic patients. The fact that the morphological lesions correlate with functional pathology in diabetic patients is important for understanding how the disease leads to visual loss.

Conclusions

The diagnosis and management of diabetic retinopathy depends on both the correct detection of morphological lesions related to impaired retinal vascular supply, and the correct interpretation of the dynamics, the relative occurrence, and the spatial distribution of these lesions in the ocular fundus. The pathological correlates of these changes include anatomical changes that can be studied by clinical inspection and by histopathological techniques, and functional changes that can be studied by electrophysiological or psychophysical examination techniques. Therefore, these approaches are necessary in order to distinguish the disease patterns that are unique for diabetic retinopathy from those seen in retinal vascular diseases in general. This is crucial for gaining a deeper insight into the pathophysiology of diabetic retinopathy and for improving screening, diagnosis and treatment of diabetic retinopathy in the future.

Table 2. Overview of different types of visual impairment in diabetic retinopathy

Lesion type	Visual impairment	Clinical course
Microaneurysms	none	
Haemorrhages	blocking of retinal photoreceptors, foveally and extrafoveally	partly reversible
Exudates	blocking of retinal photoreceptors, foveally and extrafoveally	partly reversible
Barrier leakage	none	
Retinal oedema	gradual reduction of visual function	almost always irreversible
Cotton wool spots	local relative scotoma that regresses partly; longer lasting lesions may result in arcuate scotoma	Partly reversible
Arterial changes	none	
Venous changes	none	
Retinal ischaemia	localised defects in visual field	irreversible
Neovascularisations	blocking of retinal photoreceptors	reversible
Vitreous haemorrhage	blocking of retinal photoreceptors	reversible
Tractional retinal detachment	retinal damage	almost always irreversible
Photocoagulation	retinal damage	irreversible

References

1 Diamant AL, Babey SH, Hasters TA, Brown ER: Diabetes: the growing epidemic. Policy Brief UCLA Cent Health Policy Res 2007;PB2007-9:1–12.
2 Simonsen SE: ERG in diabetics; in Francois (ed): The Clinical Value of Electroretinography. Fifth ISCERG Symp, Basel, Karger, pp 403–412.
3 Porta M: To screen or not to screen? High-tech responses to a not-so-hamletic question. Diabetes Metab 2008;34:189–191.
4 Dobree JH: Simple diabetic retinopathy. Evolution of the lesions and therapeutic considerations. Br J Ophthalmol 1970;54:1–10.
5 Stitt AW, Gardiner TA, Archer DB: Histological and ultrastructural investigation of retinal microaneurysm development in diabetic patients. Br J Ophthalmol 1995;70:362–367.
6 de Venecia G, Davis M, Engerman R: Clinicopathological correlations in diabetic retinopathy I. Histology and fluorescein angiography of microaneurysms. Arch Ophthalmol 1976;94:1766–1773.
7 Kohner E, Sleightholm M: Does microaneurysm count reflect severity of early diabetic retinopathy? Ophthalmology 1986;95:586–589.
8 Klein R, Meuer SM, Moss SE, Klein BE: The relationship of microaneurysm counts to the 4-year progression of diabetic retinopathy. Arch Ophthalmol 1989;107:1780–1785.
9 Klein R, Meuer SM, Moss SE, Klein BE: Retinal microaneurysm counts and 10-year progression of diabetic retinopathy. Arch Ophthalmol 1995;113:1386–1389.
10 Kohner EM, Stratton IM, Aldington SJ, Turner RC, Matthews DR: Microaneurysms in the development of diabetic retinopathy (UKPDS42). Diabetologia 1999;42:1107–1112.
11 Bek T, Kjaergaard J: The prognostic value of post-treatment retinopathy after panretinal laser photocoagulation for proliferative diabetic retinopathy in type 1 diabetes. Eur J Ophthalmol 2004;14:538–542.
12 Bek T: Diabetic retinopathy caused by changes in retinal vasomotion. A new hypothesis. Editorial. Acta Ophthalmol 1999;77:376–380.
13 Bloodworth JM, Molitor DL: Ultrastructural aspects of human and canine diabetic retinopathy. Invest Ophthalmol Vis Sci 1965;4:1037–1048.

14 Bek T: Histopathology and pathophysiology of diabetic retinopathy. In: van Beijsterveld OP. Diabetic Retinopathy. London, Dunitz, 2000, pp 169–187.
15 Lahrmann C, Bek T: Foveal haemorrhages in non-proliferative diabetic retinopathy. Clinical characteristics and visual outcome. Acta Ophthalmol 2000;78:169–172.
16 Diezel PB, Willert HG: Morphologie und Histochemie der harten und weichen Exsudate der Retina bei Diabetes mellitus und essentieller Hypertonie. Klin Monatsbl Augenheilk 1961;139:475–491.
17 Murata T, Ishibashi T, Inomata H: Immunohistochemical detection of extravasated fibrinogen (fibrin) in human diabetic retina. Graefes Arch Clin Exp Ophthalmol 1992;230:428–431.
18 Bresnick G: Diabetic maculopathy. A critical review highligting diffuse macular edema. Ophthalmology 1983;90:1301–1317.
19 Dalgaard P, Barker VA, Lund-Andersen H: Vitreous fluorophotometry: mathematical analysis of the effect of peripheral leakage on axial scans. Invest Ophthalmol Vis Sci 1989;30:1522–1526.
20 Stefansson E, Landers MB 3rd, Wolbarsht ML: Oxygenation and vasodilatation in relation to diabetic and other proliferative retinopathies. Ophthalmic Surg 1983;14:209–226.
21 Bek T, Lund-Andersen H: Localised Blood-Retinal Barrier Leakage and Retinal Light Sensitivity in Diabetic Retinopathy. Br J Ophthalmol 1990a;74:388-392.
22 Early Treatment for Diabetic Retinopathy Study Research Group (ETDRSRG): Photocoagulation for diabetic macular edema. Early treatment for diabetic retinopathy study report number 1. Arch Ophthalmol 1985;103:1796–1806.
23 Møller F, Bek T: The relation between visual acuity, fixation stability, and the size of foveal hard exudates after photocoagulation for diabetic maculopathy. A 1-year follow-up study. Graefe's Arch Clin Exp Ophthalmol 2003;241:458–462.
24 Wilkinson CP, Ferris FL 3rd, Klein RE, Lee PP, Agardh CD, Davis M, Dills D, Kampik A, Pararajasegaram R, Verdaguer JT, Global Diabetic Retinopathy Project Group: Proposed international clinical diabetic retinopathy and diabetic macular edema disease severity scales. Ophthalmology 2003;110:1677–1682.
25 Bolz M, Ritter M, Schneider M, Simader C, Scholda C, Schmidt-Erfurth U: A systematic correlation of angiography and high-resolution optical coherence tomography in diabetic macular edema. Ophthalmology 2009:166:66–72.
26 McLeod D, Marshall J, Kohner EM, Bird A: The role of axoplasmic transport in the pathogenesis of retinal cotton-wool spots. Br J Ophthalmol 1977;61:177–191.
27 Williams DK, Drance SM, Harris GS, Fairclough M: Diabetic cotton-wool spots: an evaluation using perimetric and angiographic techniques. Can J Ophthalmol 1970;5:68–77.
28 Bek T, Lund-Andersen H: Cotton-wool spots and retinal light sensitivity in diabetic retinopathy. Br J Ophthalmol 1991;75:13–17.
29 Grading diabetic retinopathy from stereoscopic color fundus photographs – an extension of the modified Airlie House classification. ETDRS report number 10. Early Treatment for Diabetic Retinopathy Study Group (ETDRS). Ophthalmology 1991;98(suppl 5):786–806.
30 Roy M, Rick ME, Higgins KE, McCulloch JC: Retinal cotton-wool spots: an early finding in diabetic retinopathy? Br J Ophthalmol 1986;70:772–778.
31 Kohner EM, Dollery CT, Bulpitt CK: Cotton-wool spots in diabetic retinopathy. Diabetes 1969;18:691–704.
32 Kristinsson JK, Gottfredsdottir MS, Stefansson E: Retinal vessel dilatation and elongation precedes diabetic macular oedema. Br J Ophthalmol 1997;81:274–278.
33 Kylstra JA, Wierzbicki T, Wolbarsht ML, Landers MB 3rd, Stefansson E: The relationship between retinal vessel tortuosity, diameter, and transmural pressure. Graefes Arch Clin Exp Ophthalmol 1986;224:477–480.
34 Bek T: Immunohistochemical characterisation of retinal glial cell changes in diabetic retinopathy. Acta Ophthalmol 1997b;75:388–392.
35 Ashton N: Arteriolar involvement in diabetic retinopathy. Br J Ophthalmol 1953;37:282–292.
36 Yamagishi S, Nakamura K, Imaizumi T: Advanced glycation end products (AGEs) and diabetic vascular complications. Curr Diabetes Rev 2005;1:93–106.
37 Shimizu K, Muraoka K: Diabetic retinopathy. Is it a maculopathy? A superwide fluorescein angiographic evaluation. Dev Ophthalmol 1981;2:235–242.
38 Bresnick G, Engerman R, Davis MD, de Venecia G, Myers FL: Patterns of ischemia in diabetic retinopathy. Trans Am Acad Ophthalmol Otolaryngol 1976;81:694–709.
39 Bloodworth JMB: Diabetic retinopathy. Diabetes 1962;11:1–22.
40 Bek T: Transretinal histopathological changes in capillary-free areas of diabetic retinopathy. Acta Ophthalmol 1994;72:409–415.
41 Ashton N: Studies of the retinal capillaries in relation to diabetic and other retinopathies. Br J Ophthalmol 1963;47:625–630.
42 Bek T: Glial cell involvement in vascular occlusion of diabetic retinopathy. Acta Ophthalmol 1997a;75:239–243.
43 Kohner E, Henkind P: Correlation of fluorescein angiogram and retinal digest in diabetic retinopathy. Am J Ophthalmol 1970;69:403–414.
44 Chibber R, Ben-Mahmoud BM, Chibber S, Kohner EM: Leucocytes in diabetic retinopathy. Curr Diabetes Rev 2007;3:3–14. Review.
45 Bek T: Localised scotomata and types of vascular occlusion in diabetic retinopathy. Acta Ophthalmol 1991;69:11-18.
46 Imesch PD, Bindley CD, Wallow IHL: Clinicopathological correlation of intraretinal microvascular abnormalities. Retina 1997;17:321–329.
47 Bek T: A clinicopathological study of venous loops and reduplications in diabetic retinopathy. Acta Ophthalmol 2002;80:69–75.
48 Philps S: Retinal venous changes in diabetes. Trans Ophthalmol Soc UK 1946;66:221–229.
49 Hughes S, Yang H, Chang-Ling T: Vascularization of the human fetal retina: roles of vasculogenesis and angiogenesis. Invest Ophthalmol Vis Sci 2000;41:1217–1228.

50 Martin A, Komada MR, Sane DC: Abnormal angiogenesis in diabetes mellitus. Med Res Rev 2003;23:117–145.
51 Taniguchi Y: Ultrastructure of newly formed blood vessels in diabetic retinopathy. Jap J Ophthalmol 1976;20:19–31.
52 Ballantyne AJ, Loewenstein A: Diseases of the retina. 1. The pathology of diabetic retinopathy. Trans Ophthalmol Soc UK 1943;63:95–115.
53 Bek T: Venous loops in diabetic retinopathy. Prevalence, distribution, and pattern of development. Acta Ophthalmol 1999;77:130–134.
54 Bandello F, Menchini F: Diabetic papillopathy as a risk factor for progression of diabetic retinopathy. Retina 2004;24:183–184.
55 Tagawa H, McMeel JW, Furukawas H, Quiroz H, Murakami K, Takahashi M, Trempe CL: Role of the vitreous in diabetic retinopathy. I. Vitreous changes in diabetic retinopathy and in physiologic aging. Ophthalmology 1986;93:596–601.
56 Shiraya T, Kato S, Fukushima H, Tanabe T: A case of diabetic retinopathy with both retinal neovascularization and complete posterior vitreous detachment. Eur J Ophthalmol 2006;16:644–646.
57 Hove M, Kristensen JK, Lauritzen T, Bek T: The relation between risk factors and the regional distribution of retinopathy lesions in type 2 diabetes. Acta Ophthalmol 2006;84:619–623.
58 Bek T, Helgesen A: The regional distribution of diabetic retinopathy lesions may predict risk factors for the progression of the disease. Acta Ophthalmol 2001;79:501–505.
59 Kohner EM, Patel V, Rassam SM: Role of blood flow and impaired autoregulation in the pathogenesis of diabetic retinopathy. Diabetes 1995;44:603–607.
60 Bek T, Hajari J, Jeppesen P: Interaction between flicker induced vasodilation and pressure autoregulation in diabetic retinopathy. Graefes Arch Clin Exp 2008;246:763–769.
61 Pahor D: Visual field loss after argon laser panretinal photocoagulation in diabetic retinopathy: full- versus mild-scatter coagulation. Int Ophthalmol 22:313–319.
62 Lovestam-Adrian M, Svendenius N, Agardh E: Contrast sensitivity and visual recovery time in diabetic patients treated with panretinal photocoagulation. Acta Ophthalmol 78:672–676.
63 Bek T: Localized retinal morphology and differential light sensitivity in diabetic retinopathy. Methodology and clinical results. Acta Ophtalmol 1992;70(suppl 207):1–36.

Prof. Toke Bek
Department of Ophthalmology
Århus University Hospital, Norrebrogade 44
DK–8000 Århus C (Denmark)
Tel. +45 8949 3223, Fax +45 8612 1653, E-Mail toke.bek@mail.tele.dk

Hammes H-P, Porta M (eds): Experimental Approaches to Diabetic Retinopathy.
Front Diabetes. Basel, Karger, 2010, vol 20, pp 20–41

Retinal Vascular Permeability in Health and Disease

Vassiliki Poulaki

Retina Research Laboratory, Massachusetts Eye and Ear Infirmary, Harvard Medical School, Boston, Mass., USA

Abstract

Homeostasis in the retina microenvironment is maintained by the proper function of the blood-retinal barrier (BRB), which regulates the movement of chemicals and cells between the intravascular compartment and the retina. The BRB consists of two major topographically distinct components: the endothelium of the retinal vessels (inner BRB) and the retinal pigment epithelium (outer BRB). The barrier function of the retinal vascular endothelium depends on its lack of fenestrations, whereas the ability of the retinal pigment epithelium to regulate solute transport depends on the apical tight junctions. The tight junctions are membrane fusion areas between adjacent cells that serve as a diffusion barrier for paracellular transport and as a 'molecular fence', restricting the free movement of transmembrane proteins, and thus maintaining cell polarity and the asymmetric distribution of transmembrane proteins. Among the most important proteins that are associated with tight junctions are occludin, zonula occludens and claudins. Pathologic increase in blood retinal permeability can be caused by endothelial or pericyte cell death, tight junction disassembly, or cytokines such as vascular endothelial growth factor. Several assays have been developed to allow detection, quantification and monitoring of BRB breakdown in experimental and clinical settings. Assays used in animal models include the injection of chromophores, such as Evans blue, horseradish peroxidase, and fluorescein; the imaging techniques include electron microscopy and MRI. In humans, fluorescein angiography, vitreous fluorophotometry and optical coherence tomography are most commonly used. The disruption of the BRB contributes to the pathophysiology of several retinal diseases such as diabetic retinopathy, age-related macula degeneration, retinopathy of prematurity, central serous chorioretinopathy, vascular occlusive and inflammatory diseases. Several medical and surgical treatments have been developed to restore normal BRB function. Traditional procedures such as laser photocoagulation and corticosteroids have been recently supplemented with vascular endothelial growth factor pathway inhibitors, anti-TNF-α agents, mammalian target of rapamycin inhibitors and PKCβ inhibitors. Early results from clinical trials offer hope for effective vision-preserving therapies.

Although the mammalian retina is constantly exposed to the rich choroidal circulation, it maintains a high level of electrolyte and metabolite balance that is crucial for the proper retinal function and ultimately vision. This homeostasis is maintained by the proper function of the blood-retinal barrier (BRB) that regulates the transport of cells and chemical substances from the circulation to the retina, therefore the retinal microenvironment. The molecular basis for the BRB are tight junctions (TJs) between endothelial cells in the inner retina, and between pigmented epithelial cells in the outer retina. The disruption of the BRB in the retinal vasculature or in neovessels underlies the pathophysiology of a variety of vision-threatening diseases of the retina. Restoration of the vascular stability and integrity improves visual outcomes and is currently a therapeutic goal for many ocular conditions.

Physiology of the Retinal Vascular Network

The retina is a highly specialized neural tissue that consists of seven layers: the nerve fiber layer, the ganglion cell layer, the inner plexiform layer, the inner nuclear layer, the outer plexiform layer, the outer nuclear layer and the photoreceptors (rods and cones). The majority of the retina blood supply (85%) is derived from the choroidal blood vessels, whereas the central retinal artery provides the remaining 15%. The central retinal artery gives out four main vessels as it runs through the optic nerve head and supplies three capillary networks: the radial peripapillary, the inner and the outer network. The most superficial capillary network is the radial peripapillary one, which runs in the inner part of the nerve fiber layer along the major arterial arcades. The inner capillary network runs in the ganglion cell layer, whereas the outer capillary network runs throughout the inner nuclear layer. The three networks form multiple anastomoses between them. The retinal area responsible for central vision is located in the center of the macula, called the fovea; it is avascular and the retinal vessels arc around it. The choroidal vasculature consists of fan-shaped lobules of capillaries derived from the long and short posterior ciliary arteries and from branches of the peripapillary arterial network.

Physiology of the Blood-Retinal Barrier

The BRB maintains a constant milieu by regulating the exchange of water, nutrients, metabolites, proteins and neurotransmitters, and the efflux of toxic byproducts of metabolism. Moreover, it shields the neural retina from the circulating blood by restricting the entry of toxins, inflammatory cytokines, antibodies and circulating immune cells. The concept of the existence of the blood-tissue barrier in neural tissues was first introduced in the literature in 1885 by Goodman who demonstrated that trypan blue injected intravenously in the rat stained all tissues except the brain [1, 2]. In 1965, Ashton and Cuhna-Vaz demonstrated that intravenously injected histamine increased the vascular permeability of various ocular tissues except the retina [3], leading to the concept of the BRB [2]. Subsequent morphological studies showed that the retinal endothelial cells demonstrate an epithelial-like structure with 'zonnulae occludentes' between them.

Maurice and Cunha-Vaz performed morphological studies and permeability measurements and proposed that the BRB consists of two major components: the endothelium of the retinal vessels (inner BRB) and the retinal pigment epithelium (RPE; outer BRB) [2]. These two components are topographically distinct (the former is responsible for BRB functions in the inner retina, whereas the latter for the outer retina) and mechanistically independent. Therefore, it should be emphasized that the two different yet parallel sources of perfusion in the retina (the choroidal blood vessels and the central retina artery) are dependent on different mechanisms of the BRB: the endothelial cells of the choroidal capillaries have fenestrations similar to those of endothelial cells elsewhere in the body and rely entirely on the adjacent RPEs for BRB functions. In contrast, the endothelial cells of the retinal network capillaries lack fenestrations and exhibit all the specialized barrier properties of the BRB, while their surrounding pericytes, which contribute to a second line of defense in the blood-brain barrier, are approximately four times as numerous in the retina as in the brain [4].

There are no diffusional barriers between the extracellular fluid of the retina and the adjacent vitreous, and the vitreous body does not hinder significantly the diffusion of solutes. It should be emphasized that not all aspects of the physiology of BRB have been well studied in a retina-related model. Several conclusions are derived from extrapolation based on observations in other natural barriers, such as the blood-brain barrier.

Molecular Biology of the Blood-Retinal Barrier

The main routes used by water, solutes and proteins to move across endothelial and epithelial cell layers can be classified as transcellular vs. paracellular flux. Transcellular (transfer across the cell) can be via passive diffusion, facilitated diffusion (channel-facilitated transport), active transport (receptor-mediated uptake), endocytosis/pinocytosis (membrane invaginations across the cell surface that pinch off to form vesicles that move to the cell interior and are released on the other side, allowing nonspecific transport of material), and finally via pores or fenestrations. It should be noted that RPE cells and endothelial cells in the BBB and BRB lack fenestrations [5] and have profoundly decreased pinocytosis activity, while the choriocapillaris is fenestrated [6]. It is possible that the choriocapillaris endothelial cell fenestrations are regulated by vascular endothelial growth factor (VEGF), as intravitreal injection of the anti-VEGF antibody bevacizumab in cynomolgus monkeys significantly reduced these fenestrations, an effect that may be of clinical relevance in the treatment of macular edema [7]. Because the choriocapillaris is fenestrated, it is the RPE cells that form the outer BRB and regulate the environment of the outer retina. Like all epithelia and endothelia, the ability of RPE to regulate transepithelial transport depends upon two properties: apical TJs to resist diffusion through the paracellular spaces of the monolayer, and an asymmetric distribution of proteins to regulate vectorial transport across the monolayer [8]. During development, these properties form gradually. Initially, the TJs are leaky, and the RPE exhibits only partial polarity. As the neural retina and choriocapillaris develop, there are progressive changes in the composition of the apical junctional complexes, the expression of cell adhesion proteins, and the distribution of membrane and cytoskeletal proteins [8]. Another aspect of RPE function is the active transport of water out of the retina into the choriocapillaris. This flow of water out of the retina helps maintain retinal attachment.

In addition to controlling the influx of solutes, the BRB also actively transports potentially noxious compounds out of the retina in order to maintain the ideal microenvironment for its function. Lactate is actively transported from the RPE cells to the choroid [9, 10]. The P-glycoprotein is present in the BRB and actively pumping lipophilic toxins and drugs out of the endothelial or RPE cell, back to the bloodstream [5, 11–13].

The paracellular flux (transfer between cells) is primarily regulated by the permeability of TJs. In pathologic situations, disassembly of the TJs and large gaps in the cellular continuum allow for breakdown of the barrier.

Tight Junctions

TJs are areas of apparent fusions between the closely apposed outer leaflets of plasma membranes of adjacent cells (endothelial and epithelial), where the intercellular space disappears forming continuous seals circling around the cell's circumference like a belt. TJs serve as a highly selective diffusion barrier and strictly control the paracellular flux of water and solutes [14], allowing the separation of fluids on either side that have a different chemical composition. They also function as a 'molecular fence' restricting the free movement of integral cell membrane proteins, thus maintaining a different protein composition between apical and basolateral membrane, which contributes to cell polarity. Over 40 proteins have been found to be associated with TJs, including transmembrane, scaffolding, and intracellular signaling proteins [14, 15], such as occludin, the zonula occludens (ZO) proteins, claudins, and others.

The link between BRB, TJ molecules and angiogenesis is a subject of intense investigation. In human placenta, junctional complexes regulate angiogenesis and vascular remodeling. According to Leach [16], there are two types of junctional adhesion phenotypes that are regulated by the differential expression of VEGF and angiopoietins 1 and 2. The 'activated' type has low immunoreactivity for TJ molecules such as occludin and claudin, and is found in highly angiogenic terminal capillaries, whereas the 'tight' type has high levels of these molecules and is found in quiescent capillaries [16].

Transmembrane Tight Junction Proteins

Occludin

Occludin, a 65-kDa protein, was the first transmembrane TJ protein discovered [17], and is present in TJs of both epithelial and endothelial cells. It has four transmembrane helices, a short intracellular loop, two extracellular loops, and 2 intracellular tails. The intracellular N-terminal cytoplasmic tail interacts with the E3 ubiquitin-protein ligase Itch, resulting in the ubiquitination of occludin, which promotes its degradation by the proteasome [18]. Cyclic AMP promotes disassembly of the TJs by promoting proteasome-mediated degradation of occludin [19]. This pathway provides a mechanism for cytokine-induced regulation of TJ function. The two extracellular loops can bind to the occludin molecule on the adjacent cell. The distal C-terminus forms a coiled-coil domain that participates in protein–protein interactions, binding directly to the intracellular protein ZO-1 [20]. VEGF promotes PKC-dependent serine/threonine phosphorylation of occludin [21, 22], which causes dissociation from ZO-1 [23], disruption of the TJ and increased permeability. This effect may explain the activity of PKC inhibitors against vascular leakage in diabetic retinopathy (DR) [21].

The occludin content at the TJ correlates with the tightness of the barrier, with higher levels in cells known to have a tight barrier, such as arterial endothelial cells and brain endothelium [14, 24, 25]. Occludin expression appears 1 week postnatally (in rat models), which correlates with maturation of the barrier [5, 24]. Suppression of occludin expression (using antisense technology or siRNA) results in decreased barrier capacity to solutes [25, 26]. In rats with streptozotocin-induced diabetes, decreased occludin content in the retina is noted and correlates with increased BRB permeability [14, 27, 28]. The localization of occludin also changes from continuous cell border to interrupted, punctate immunoreactivity in the arterioles [27]. This change in localization is associated with increased occludin phosphorylation at Ser490, which lies in the coiled-coil domain, and abolishes binding to ZO-1 [14]. In addition to VEGF [21], other stimuli that promote occludin phosphorylation and internalization are lysophosphatidic acid [29], histamine [29], oxidized phospholipids [30], and shear stress [31]. Conversely, hydrocortisone suppresses occludin phosphorylation, increases occludin expression and reduces BRB permeability [32], supporting the use of corticosteroids for the treatment of macular edema in DR [33].

Although occludin is an important component of TJs, it appears that it is not totally indispensable [34]. Occludin-deficient cells can still form functional TJs that recruit ZO-1, and occludin knock-out mice are viable, with TJs that appear morphologically normal and have normal transepithelial resistance (TER, a measure of permeability; although there is evidence of dysfunction of tissues that require barrier formation, such as testicular and gastric mucosa) [35]. Therefore, it appears that a high degree of redundancy in TJ composition exists, which can be explained by the fact that the carboxy tail of claudins can interact with ZO-1, -2, and -3 and recruit them to the TJ [36], thus substituting to a major degree for the role of occludin.

Claudins

The claudin family comprises at least 24 members that are differentially expressed in various tissues. Claudins are 20- to 27-kDa proteins with four transmembrane domains, two extracellular loops, and a short carboxy intercellular tail. Different cell types express different combinations of claudins [37]. The claudin expression pattern determines the barrier properties of individual TJ strands and is dynamically regulated during development, under normal conditions to respond to the selective permeability needs of the tissues, and during disease [37]. Claudins form both homopolymers and heteropolymers and bind across adjacent membranes, forming the TJ backbone [37–39]. Not all claudin combinations are compatible to form a functional TJ, and overexpression of an incompatible claudin type can result in a leaky TJ. For example, MDCK I cells normally express claudin-1 and claudin-4, and their TER values fall dramatically after overexpression of claudin-2, but not claudin-3 [40]. Several claudins participate in the formation of ion-selective channels, and genetic defects in these claudins are associated with disorders of ion transport and aberrant barrier function [37].

Claudin-5 is a critical component of TJs between endothelial cells, and its expression in the plasma membrane of retinal microvascular endothelial cells is significantly reduced under hypoxic conditions [41]. Inhibition of claudin-5 expression by RNAi resulted in a reduction of transendothelial electrical resistance, indicating a critical role of claudin-5 in the barrier property [41]. In claudin-5-deficient mice, the blood-brain barrier is selectively affected against small molecules (<800 Da), but not larger molecules [42]. In experimental autoimmune uveitis, expression of TJ proteins claudin-1, -3 and occludin-1 in the retina was found to be decreased [43].

Intracellular Tight Junction Proteins

Zonula Occludens Proteins

The 225-kDa ZO-1 was the first TJ protein to be characterized [44], and the related ZO-2 and ZO-3 were subsequently identified [45–47]. ZO-1, ZO-2 and ZO-3 are intracellular adaptor proteins that associate with the cytoplasmic surface of the TJ and are composed of three PDZ domains (PDZ1, PDZ2, PDZ3), one SH3 domain, and one guanylate kinase (GUK) domain that belong to the membrane-associated GUK protein family [14, 37, 46, 48]. ZO-1 is the central organizer of the TJ and forms a molecular scaffold that links the TJ to the cytoskeleton [5, 14]. Via its SH3-GUK region, it binds to occludin [49]. Via its PDZ-1 region, it binds to the COOH-terminal tail of the claudins [36], and via its PDZ-2 domain it binds to ZO-2 [50]. ZO-1 and ZO-2 bind directly to actin filaments, thus linking the TJ to the cytoskeleton [47, 51]. Removal of all three ZO proteins revealed that at least one of ZO-1 or ZO-2 is necessary for TJ formation and establishment of barrier properties [14, 52]. The cell membrane expression of ZO-1 in various cells correlates with the barrier properties of these tissues. In endothelial cells from various tissues with potent barriers, VEGF induces tyrosine phosphorylation and redistribution of ZO-1 from the cell border to the cell interior [22, 53].

Pathophysiology of the Blood-Retinal Barrier Breakdown

Two major pathways are responsible for hyperpermeability of retinal vessels in diseases of the retina, i.e. transcellular and paracellular transport [54]. Transcellular flux is very limited in BRB under normal conditions, due to the absence of fenestrations [5] and decreased pinocytosis.

However, this may change under pathologic conditions that lead to BRB breakdown. In a model of VEGF-induced retinopathy with microvascular leakage in monkeys, there was an increase in the number of pinocytotic vesicles at the endothelial luminal membrane, but no fenestrations or vesiculovacuolar organelles were found in the endothelial cells by electron microscopy [55]. The endothelium-specific antigen PAL-E, associated with transport vesicles in nonbarrier endothelium, which is almost absent from barrier capillaries in the normal brain and retina, is markedly and uniformly present in areas of vascular leakage in this model, as well as in human post-mortem eyes of individuals with DR [56–58].

Mechanisms of increased paracellular flux that lead to BRB breakdown are explained below.

Endothelial Cell Division or Cell Death

Large gaps in the capillary endothelial cell layer can be caused by endothelial cell division or cell death [5, 59], allowing leakage of fluid, protein and lipids. Endothelial cell death leads to the formation of acellular capillaries and pericyte ghosts. In a streptozotocin-induced model of diabetes, leukocyte adhesion to the diabetic retinal vasculature led to leukocyte-mediated, Fas-FasL-dependent apoptosis of endothelial cells [60]. Inhibition of FasL activity with a neutralizing antibody potently reduced retinal vascular endothelial cell injury, apoptosis, and BRB breakdown, but did not diminish leukocyte adhesion to the diabetic retinal vasculature [60]. Other causes of endothelial cell death could be oxidative stress [61–63], and advanced glycation endproducts (AGEs) [64]. BRB breakdown can also occur as a result of leukocyte extravasation during retinal inflammation [43].

Pericyte Loss

Pericytes are smooth muscle cells that form a sheath around the capillary endothelial cells. They help maintain vascular tone, provide structural support to the endothelium and release growth factors necessary for endothelial cell survival [65]. Pericyte loss is a hallmark of early DR [66]. Pericytes exposed to high glucose concentrations exhibit increased expression of Bax and TNF-α, and undergo apoptosis [67–69]. Other mechanisms of pericyte loss include oxidative stress, toxicity from polyols, AGEs and heavily oxidized-glycated LDL, saturated free fatty acids, upregulation of protein kinase C, and focal leukostasis [65, 66, 70–77].

Tight Junction Disassembly

Disassembly of the TJs is frequently observed and leads to barrier breakdown in various pathologic conditions. This can be attributed to changes in TJ protein content and/or cellular localization. Vascular segments at the early stage of vascular formation and regression have decreased occludin expression [78]. Moreover, it has been known for the past 20 years that phosphorylation of TJ proteins modulates its permeability [79, 80].

Histamine causes a reversible concentration-dependent reduction of ZO-1 protein content in cultured retinal vascular endothelial cells [81, 82]. In the same model, high glucose (20 mM) and low insulin (10^{-12} M) reduced ZO-1 protein content, while astrocyte-conditioned medium increased ZO-1 protein content [82].

VEGF also has potent effects on TJ protein expression and localization. In a rat model of streptozotocin-induced diabetes, BRB permeability was increased and retinal occludin content decreased, an effect that was reproduced in bovine retinal endothelial cells treated in culture with VEGF [83]. In brain microvessel endothelial cells (BMECs), VEGF increased sucrose permeability and caused a loss of occludin and ZO-1 from the endothelial cell junctions and changed the staining pattern of the cell boundary. Western blot analysis of BMEC lysates revealed that the level of occludin but not of ZO-1 was lowered by VEGF treatment [84]. Phosphorylation of occludin reduces its ability to bind ZO-1, ZO-2, and ZO-3 [85]. VEGF promotes PKC-dependent phosphorylation of occludin [21, 22], which causes dissociation from ZO-1 [23], disruption of the TJ and increased permeability. Moreover, phosphatidylinositol 3-kinase (PI3-kinase) may directly interact with occludin and phosphorylate it [86, 87].

Other stimuli that promote occludin phosphorylation and internalization are lysophosphatidic acid [29], histamine [29], oxidized phospholipids [30], and shear stress [31]. Hepatocyte growth factor also induces rapid phosphorylation of ZO-1 [88], occludin, and β-catenin in bovine RPE cells, leading to rapid TJ disassembly and protein redistribution from the membrane to the cytoplasm [89]. Conversely, hydrocortisone increases both occludin and ZO-1 presence at the cell membrane and reduces occludin phosphorylation [32].

Neovessels Are Immature and Leaky: The Role of VEGF

VEGF, the endothelial cell mitogen [90] that promotes the formation of new vessels, was actually originally identified as a permeability factor, and originally named vascular permeability factor [91, 92]. It exists in five different isoforms of 121, 145, 165, 189, and 206 amino acids, derived from alternatively spliced mRNAs, of which $VEGF_{165}$ is the predominant molecular species. It binds two high-affinity receptors, the 180-kDa fms-like tyrosine kinase (Flt-1, also known as VEGFR1) and the 200-kDa kinase insert domain-containing receptor (KDR), also known as fetal liver kinase (flk or VEGFR2), but KDR transduces the signals for endothelial proliferation and chemotaxis [93, 94]. VEGF participates in the pathogenesis and progression of a wide range of angiogenesis-dependent diseases, including cancer [95, 96], inflammation, and DR [97, 98]. VEGF gene transcription is stimulated by hypoxia (via HIF-1α binding to consensus and ancillary hypoxia-response elements in the VEGF promoter), hyperglycemia, reactive oxygen intermediates, AGEs, inflammatory mediators, hormones and growth factors (IGF-I and insulin), prostaglandins, and other proangiogenic stimuli. Also, hypoxia may increase the stability of VEGF mRNA [99, 100].

VEGF stimulates endothelial cell proliferation and neovascularization via a MAPK-dependent pathway [101], migration and vascular permeability [83]. A major reason why VEGF promotes vascular leakage and BRB breakdown is because the newly formed vessels are fragile and leak serous fluid and blood. Moreover, the formation of new vessels requires the degradation of the surrounding matrix and the activation of the existing vascular tree, with initial vasodilatation and increased vascular permeability [102]. The tissue edema and the increased hydrostatic pressure worsen hypoxia, further stimulating VEGF production. The neovessels may also cause vitreous traction and retinal detachment. Interestingly, neovessels, but not mature retinal or choroidal vessels, are sensitive to angiopoietin-2 that promotes their regression in the setting of a high angiopoietin-2/VEGF ratio, an observation that could have important therapeutic implications [103].

Macular Edema

The BRB breakdown and increased permeability leads to increased accumulation of fluid, as well as deposits of proteinaceous and lipid material in the extracellular space of the retina. The resulting edema raises the hydrostatic pressure and inhibits the flow of oxygen and nutrients. Edema in the area of the macula leads to central vision loss and is an indication for treatment.

Assays for Studying the Permeability of the Blood-Retinal Barrier

Our ability to detect, quantify and monitor BRB breakdown depends on the availability of appropriate imaging techniques. Accurate quantification of macular edema is important for making the decision to start treatment, assessing response to therapy, and also for appropriate enrollment in clinical trials.

Assays Used in Animal Models

Evans Blue

The Evans blue (EB) method is used to visualize and quantify the BRB breakdown ex vivo in retinal flat mount preparations [104]. With this method, EB is injected in the animal intravenously and binds irreversibly to serum albumin. Therefore, its distribution reflects the albumin exchange between the intravascular and extravascular tissue components [105]. The amount of EB measured in retinal extracts represents retained and, therefore, extravasated EB, which gives an estimate of the BRB permeability.

Fluorescein-Labeled Lectins

Similar to the EB method, the FITC-dextran method is used to quantify the BRB breakdown ex vivo. Fluorescein-labeled dextrans are complex polysaccharides that can be manufactured to have a molecular weight and a size suitable to prevent extravasation when the barrier is intact. Therefore, as with EB, the amount of FITC-dextran retained and measured in retinal extracts reflects extravasation, and is an estimate of the extent of BRB breakdown.

Horseradish Peroxidase Tracer Method

Horseradish peroxidase (HRP) is an enzyme that is similar in size to albumin and can be used to histochemically identify areas of BRB breakdown. HRP is injected in vivo and extravasates in areas with abnormal permeability. The enzymatic activity of HRP is preserved in paraffin-embedded tissues and can be detected upon exposure to an appropriate enzymatic substrate [104].

Electron Microscope Studies

In this technique, lanthanum nitrate is injected into the vasculature, and subsequently the retina is removed. Retinal microvessels are isolated with the freeze-fracture method. The distribution of lanthanum in electron microscopy slides determines the degree and site of BRB breakdown and permeability. Electron microscopy can be used to demonstrate pinocytic vesicles, as well as alterations in the morphology of the basement membrane and the integrity of endothelial cell TJ. Electron microscopy immunocytochemistry can provide a more detailed picture of a limited area of interest, giving insight into the mechanisms of extravasation at the ultrastructural level [106].

Magnetic Resonance Imaging

Dynamic contrast-enhanced magnetic resonance imaging provides a sensitive, noninvasive, and linear assay that accurately measures passive BRB permeability surface area product (BRB PS) in retinopathy models in vivo [107]. Gadolinium diethylenetriamine-pentaacetic acid (Gd-DTPA) is injected intravenously and normally does not penetrate nonfenestrated vessels or barriers. In areas where the BRB is compromised, Gd-DTPA extravasates in the vitreous and can be measured as a T_1-weighted image [108].

Assays Used Clinically in Humans

Visual acuity examination and fundus photography, although not sensitive, can confirm the presence of macular edema, which is an important clinical manifestation of BRB. The gold standard for assessing BRB breakdown in humans is fluorescein angiography. The method uses the fluorescein dye that extravasates in areas of leakage, and allows the localization of the BRB breakdown, but is not easily quantifiable. Another method that allows for quantification of the BRB is vitreous fluorophotometry that measures the fluorescein concentration in the vitreous in vivo [2].

The method that revolutionalized the way we detect and quantify macular edema is the optical coherence tomography (OCT). OCT uses infrared light that is reflected off the internal microstructures of the retina. The reflected light is collected in multiple sensors and is used to reconstitute a high resolution picture of the ocular microanatomic structures and provide information for the retinal thickness and the existence of fluid. When combined with fluorescein angiography in latest models, it can also localize the areas of abnormal vascular permeability [109].

Retinal Diseases Where the Blood-Retinal Barrier Is Impaired

Diabetic Retinopathy

BRB breakdown is one of the hallmarks of DR. DR is classified into two main groups: nonproliferative (mild, moderate, moderately severe and severe) and proliferative (mild, moderate and high risk) DR. Nonproliferative DR is characterized by increased vascular permeability, dilation and tortuosity of the retinal veins, abnormal vascular communications between arterioles and venules, microaneurysms, intraretinal hemorrhages. 'Cotton-wool' spots and soft exudates represent ischemic areas of the nerve-fiber retina layer. Microvascular angiopathy results in exudation of plasma from breakdown of the BRB. The reabsorption of the exuded fluid results in the deposition of protein and lipid exudates ('hard exudates'). Proliferative DR (PDR) is marked by the formation of neovessels in the area of the optic disk or elsewhere. Chronic hyperglycemia results in the formation of vascular microaneurysms, venular dilatation, thickening of the retinal basement membrane, microvascular contractile cell (pericyte) death, leading to acellular capillaries, which tend to undergo occlusion, causing retinal ischemia. Platelet microthrombi can form, leading to capillary occlusion [110]. Hemorrhages and/or extravasation of fluid and retinal edema promote more hypoxia. Growth of new blood vessels in the retina in response to retinal hypoxia is the hallmark of PDR.

Retinal VEGF expression temporally and spatially correlates with neovascularization in PDR [111]. Within 1 week of experimental diabetes in relevant animal models, retinal VEGF levels increase [112] and serve to stimulate intercellular adhesion molecule-1 expression in the retinal vasculature, which promotes leukocyte binding to the diabetic retinal vasculature (leukostasis) [113]. Leukocytes then trigger a Fas/FasL-mediated endothelial cell death, and breakdown of the BRB [60]. Diabetic retinal leukostasis is temporally and spatially associated with retinal endothelial cell injury and death. Hypoxic retinal pericytes and retinal pigment epithelial cells stimulate retinal endothelial cell growth in a VEGF-dependent manner [114]. As mentioned already, data from experimental animal models of DR suggest that VEGF leads to decreases in retinal occludin content [83], possibly due to PKC-dependent phosphorylation of occludin [21, 22], which causes dissociation from ZO-1 [23], disruption of the TJ and increased permeability.

Macular Degeneration

Age-related macula degeneration (AMD) is the leading cause of vision loss among the elderly in the developed world. AMD consists of a collection of inherited multifactorial diseases that share a positive family history, advanced age predilection, a characteristic macular appearance with yellowish deposits and RPE changes. In the majority of AMD patients, there are mutations in one the three following genes: CFH (complement factor H), BF (complement factor B) and LOC [115]. CFH is a member of the complement that, when mutated, is less effective in limiting the immune response and inflammation in the subretinal space. Dry AMD is characterized by the appearance of drusen in the macular area, i.e. collections of apolipoproteins, lipids, amyloid and inflammatory mediators. While the traditional notion was that drusen represents waste material, it was recently shown that it is derived from the inflammation in the subretinal space [116]. As the drusen enlarge and coalesce, they cause death of the RPE and overlying photoreceptors, resulting in geographic atrophy, or they facilitate the invasion of abnormal blood vessels from the choroid to the subretinal space, that characterizes the wet form of AMD.

One of the key pathophysiological features of wet AMD is the breakdown of the BRB and the endothelial cell proliferation with subsequent neuroretinal damage. Recently, in vitro experiments involving cocultures of endothelial cells and RPE cells on amniotic membranes elucidated the role of the outer BRB in macula degeneration [117]. In this model, endothelial cells assume a fenestrated phenotype similar to those of the choriocapillaris, with paracellular clefts and well-defined tight junctional complexes consisting of ZO-1, occludin and V-cadherin. Interestingly, the cocultures had barrier capabilities when a barrier membrane like amnion (that corresponds to Bruch's membrane in vivo) separated the two cellular populations. However, when the two cell categories (RPE and endothelial cells) were cocultured without a barrier membrane, they developed no barrier capabilities, and mimicked Bruch's disruption in wet AMD, with endothelial cell proliferation and migration. It has been proposed that pigment epithelium-derived factor secreted from the RPE plays a role in inhibiting this response [118]. The BRB is also influenced by age-related changes in Bruch's membrane that result in significant decline in its hydraulic conductivity, with decreased capacity of exchange of fluids and electrolytes between the choriocapillaris and retinal epithelium and subsequent entrapment of fluid and lipids beneath the epithelium [119].

The Fas/FasL system is also implicated in the BRB breakdown in macular degeneration. FasL expressed in the RPE acts as a 'barrier' for the invasion of Fas-bearing endothelial cells in the subretinal space. When the RPE cells do not function normally or die in macula degeneration, Fas-positive endothelial cells can invade the subretinal space and proliferate. Macrophages infiltrate the retina, especially in areas of choroidal neovascularization (CNV), and play a key role in the disruption of the BRB [120]. The neovascular complex secretes cytokines such as VEGF, TNF-α, MCP-1 and interleukins that upregulate adhesion molecules in the endothelial cells and recruit macrophages [121]. These in turn secrete more VEGF, which further enhances the CNV formation and induces more endothelial cell damage through multiple mechanisms that include oxidative stress and the Fas/FasL pathway [60]. Recently, the role of the renin/angiotensin system was established in the macrophage infiltration in AMD [122]. The vascular endothelium expresses angiotensin receptors, and angiotensin II type 1 receptor blockade inhibits macrophage infiltration, growth factor upregulation and CNV formation [122]. The activation of endothelial cells and retinal infiltration with monocytes closely correlates with angiogenesis, as inhibition of this adhesion or infiltration results in decreased neovascular membrane formation [120]. Adhesion molecules expressed in the endothelium and monocytes, such as intercellular adhesion molecule-1 and CD18, play a role in this process [120]. Activation of Müller cells by monocytes might reduce the production of neurotrophic factors, such as fibroblast growth factor, which are essential to photoreceptor survival [123]. Interactions between macrophages and glial cells have been shown to participate in cellular pathways that lead to neuronal damage in retinal degeneration [124].

Retinopathy of Prematurity

Retinopathy of prematurity (ROP) is a vascular disorder that affects the eyes of premature infants and is a major cause of blindness in children in the developed and the developing world. The disease was originally thought to be caused by excessive oxygen supplementation after delivery, but it was later found that low birth weight and gestation age at birth are stronger risk factors. ROP has two phases; in the first phase, an insult (relative hyperoxia in the extrauterine environment, low IGF/GH levels) decrease the effective levels of VEGF and results in reduction or arrest of the vessel growth. In the second phase of ROP, the production of large amounts of vasoproliferative growth factors, such as VEGF, from the hypoxic retina results in neovessel formation. These new vessels are immature, leak blood and fluid, and can cause retinal edema, hemorrhage, fibrovascular proliferation with subsequent traction retinal detachment that has detrimental effects on visual function. It is known that astrocytes and Müller cells form the glia limitans of the vessels in the outer and inner nuclear layer and they induce barrier capabilities in the endothelial cells they contact. During the hypoxia phase of ROP, the neurons survive whereas the astrocytes degenerate, and this could facilitate the abnormal BRB permeability. The neovessels that are formed during the hypoxia phase show abnormal permeability at the neovascular 'front', where they lack contact with the Müller cells and astroglia. The proliferative vasculature regains its barrier capabilities when astrocytes recolonize the retina as they recover from hypoxia.

The above are corroborated by Ritter et al. [125], who found that bone marrow-derived progenitor cells accelerated retinal repair and increase the physiological retinal vascularization in a HIF-1α-dependent manner, while at the same time decreasing the pathological preretinal neovascularization, without causing any long-term toxicity. According to this study, these cells differentiate into microglia that restore the appropriate angiogenic 'gradients' and normalize angiogenesis. In addition, endothelial cell damage from the oxidative stress during the hyperoxic phase (peroxynitrite and nitric oxide, free radical formation) contributes to the blood barrier breakdown. The increase in permeability factors, such as angiopoietin-2, PDGF, endothelin-1, PAF and VEGF, and the decrease in vessel stabilizing factors, such as angiopoietin-1, make the vasculature more 'unstable' and contribute to the increased vascular leakage. Angiopoietin-2, Tie-2 and VEGF colocalize in the fibrovascular membranes from patients with ROP [126].

Vascular Occlusive Diseases

Retinal vein occlusion is a frequent vascular condition of the retina. Although we know that thrombosis plays a central role in its pathogenesis, it is uncertain whether this is the real primary cause of this condition. The pathogenesis of the vascular occlusive retinal diseases also involves venous outflow obstruction, reduced blood flow, increased pressure in the retinal venous circulation that damages the vessels, and exudation of fluid and proteins into the interstitial space. The marked extracellular exudation results in capillary nonperfusion and retinal ischemia. In some patients, the retinal ischemia increases over time, and neovascularization occurs with the known detrimental sequelae for vision. Detailed histopathological studies in monkeys with experimental vein occlusion demonstrated that retinal leakage resulting in retinal edema can occur as early as 1–6 h after the occlusion. The early leakage in vascular occlusion is likely due to the formation of intracellular gaps by the breakdown of endothelial TJs [127]. Although no gross endothelial capillary destruction was seen by 6 h, there is still a possibility of focal rhexis that was quickly repaired and cannot be detected. At 7 h to 1 week, degenerative changes in the endothelium could be seen, with hemorrhage and exudation that caused secondary capillary nonperfusion that initially was reversible. The endothelial destruction with subsequent exposure of the basement membrane contributes to the formation of platelet thrombi and adds more insult to the hypoxic retina. Within 1–5 weeks, there is permanent capillary closure and the effects of ischemia are more pronounced. Earlier animal models have shown that destruction of the RPE layer facilitates the absorption of the accumulated fluid, as the oncotic pressure of the choroid drives the passage of the subretinal fluid over the damaged RPE [128].

In addition to hemodynamic factors, chemical mediators also play a role in the disruption of the BRB in retinal vascular occlusions. Since retinal ischemia is a key characteristic even in the cases of nonischemic vein occlusions at different degrees, VEGF, which is a hypoxia-responsive factor, increases early in the course of this condition and contributes to the BRB breakdown. VEGF levels increase in the aqueous of patients with vascular occlusions and correlate inversely with the visual acuity [129]. IL-6, IL-2 and TNF-α share many characteristics with VEGF, are also controlled by hypoxia, and were found at increased levels in aqueous humor of patients with vein occlusions both early and late during the course of the disease [130, 131].

Inflammatory Retinal Disorders
Uveitis is one of the leading causes of blindness in the world. It is characterized by intraocular inflammation that can lead to edema, high intraocular pressure, and, ultimately, destruction of the intraocular tissues and blindness. Uveitis is associated with a number of inflammatory diseases, including Behçet's, ankylosing spondylitis, juvenile rheumatoid arthritis, Reiter's syndrome, and inflammatory bowel disease. BRB breakdown that results in exudation of fluid, protein and blood, occurs early in uveitis and characterizes the disease. Mechanisms similar to those described above for other vascular retinopathies also play a role in uveitis-induced macular edema, including dysfunction of the TJs of the RPE and the endothelium, with subsequent leakage of micro- and macromolecules through them, upregulation of vesicular transport, and permeation of the surface membranes of the RPE and endothelium [132]. A number of candidate molecules have been shown to contribute to the BRB breakdown: adenosine, TNF-α, VEGF, IL-1β, and prostaglandins [133–135]. Upon intravitreal administration of each of the above factors, a functional opening of the TJs of the retinal endothelium was noted, with an increase in the vesicular-mediated transport [135, 136]. VEGF and TNF-α may also function as mediators of the immune response by upregulating adhesion molecules, and therefore activating leukocytes and vascular endothelium, and promoting leukocyte adhesion to the activated vascular endothelium [137, 138]. The role of TJ adhesion proteins was studied in animal models of uveitis. VEGF and TNF-α increase the activation of NF-κB, HIF-1α, p38, PI-3K and MAPK, and result in the phosphorylation of ZO-1 and occludin. The phosphorylated adhesion proteins dissociate from the TJ complex, resulting in the breakdown of the BRB [139].

Post-Intraocular Surgery
Subclinical macular edema, which is only detectable by fluorescein angiography, can complicate 20% of cases after cataract extraction, and can be sufficient to cause significant decrease in visual acuity in 2% of cases. Among the molecules that have been implicated in the pathophysiology of this phenomenon, prostaglandins have a prominent role [140]. Risk factors for postsurgical macular edema include vitreous loss during the surgery, vitreous adhesion to the cataract wound, retained lens material, and pre-existing conditions such as DR and uveitis.

Laser Surgery
It is known that laser photocoagulation can aggravate macular edema in diabetic patients. The mechanism of this phenomenon is not clearly understood, but it is believed that inflammatory mediators from the increased macular flow induced by the laser photocoagulation contribute to the exudation of fluid in the macula.

Central Serous Choroidoretinopathy
Central serous choroidoretinopathy is characterized by a detachment of the neurosensory retina over an area of leakage from the choriocapillaris through the RPE. Multiple hypotheses have been proposed to explain the accumulation of fluid in the neurosensory retina, and dysfunction in

either the choroid or the RPE is central in the majority of them. Primary dysfunction of the RPE can result in abnormal ion transport, decreased pumping of the subretinal fluid to the choroid and neurosensory detachment. Alternatively, focal choroidal ischemia can lead to secondary RPE dysfunction that leads to the same end result. Both theories are supported by ICG studies that showed multifocal choroidal hyperpermeability and choroidal hypofluorescence that suggest choroidal ischemia, and ERG studies are suggestive of bilateral diffuse retinal dysfunction. The observation that hypertension and type A personalities are predisposing factors for central serous choroidoretinopathy led to the speculation that elevated adrenal hormones such as cortisol and epinephrine can be responsible for the deregulation of the choroidal circulation [141].

Blood-Retinal Barrier Breakdown and Drug Delivery

In addition to contributing to the pathophysiology of retinopathies, dysfunctional retinal vessels can be a significant barrier to effective penetration of therapeutic agents, because it results in irregular blood flow and high interstitial fluid pressure [142]. Conversely, VEGF inhibition can effect transient 'normalization' of the vasculature, thereby improving perfusion and, consequently, delivery of systemic therapy.

Similar approaches are under investigation in cancer therapy, where anti-angiogenic therapy can lead to maturation of intratumoral vasculature and improved delivery of cytotoxic chemotherapy [143]. Also, improved delivery of oxygen and nutrients may stimulate the tumor cells to become more metabolically active and therefore sensitive to cytotoxic chemotherapy [144]. Drugs that induce vascular normalization can alleviate hypoxia and increase the efficacy of conventional therapies if both are carefully scheduled. Various studies have examined the feasibility of combining anti-VEGF therapy with cytotoxic or biological agents. Combining bevacizumab with doxorubicin, topotecan, paclitaxel, docetaxel, or radiotherapy resulted in improved intratumoral blood flow; reduction in interstitial fluid pressure; increase in intratumoral penetration of systemically administered chemotherapy; additive or synergistic tumor growth inhibition [145]; increased smooth muscle cell coverage of tumor vessels, and decreased vessel permeability and intratumoral hypoxia [146, 147]. Such findings raise the hypothesis that similar principles may apply in the retina as well. It is possible that the normalization of the BRB by antiangiogenic agents may improve drug delivery of systemic therapy.

Medical and Surgical Treatments for Blood-Retinal Barrier Breakdown

Laser Photocoagulation

The increased vascular permeability that results in macular edema responds to laser photocoagulation with either argon green or diode laser. The Early Treatment Diabetic Retinopathy Study investigated the role of laser photocoagulation in the treatment of diabetic macular edema (DME), and demonstrated that laser treatment reduces the risk of moderate visual loss (defined as loss of 15 letters or 3 lines) in 3 years by half [148]. However, in that study, only about 10% of subjects improved [149]. A prospective randomized trial conducted by the Diabetic Retinopathy Clinical Research Network compared focal/grid photocoagulation vs. 1 mg intravitreal triamcinolone vs. 4 mg intravitreal triamcinolone [150]. At 4 months, mean visual acuity was better in the 4 mg triamcinolone group than in the laser group or the 1 mg triamcinolone group. By 1 year, there were no significant differences between groups in mean visual acuity. At the 16-month visit and extending through the primary outcome visit at 2 years, mean visual acuity was better in the laser group than in the 2 triamcinolone groups [149,

150]. Optical coherence tomography results generally paralleled the visual acuity results. These findings have re-enforced the interest in laser photocoagulation therapies for DME [149].

Laser photocoagulation is also effective in the treatment of macular edema caused by branch retinal vein occlusion when the vision is less than 20/40 [151], whereas it is ineffective in the treatment of macula edema caused by central retinal occlusion [152].

Focal laser may decrease retinal edema in part due to closure of leaky microaneurysms, but the detailed mechanisms with which it works are not fully known. Clinical studies in normal volunteers and histopathological studies have established the alterations in retinal and choroidal vasculature after laser photocoagulation [153]. It was also proposed that the laser-induced destruction of the retinal tissue results in vasoconstriction due to an autoregulatory mechanism that in turn contributes to the reduced plasma exudation and therefore reduced edema [154]. Various cytokines that decrease vascular permeability, such as pigment epithelium-derived factor, angiostatin and TGF-β, are upregulated with laser photocoagulation, whereas cytokines that increase vascular permeability, such as VEGF and IL-8, are decreased [155].

Corticosteroids

Corticosteroids have been increasingly used for the treatment of macular edema and abnormal vascular permeability. They have anti-inflammatory properties and help restore the integrity of the BRB. Steroids also increase occludin expression in primary retinal endothelial cells and strengthen the TJs [156]. Treatment of bovine retinal endothelial cell monolayers with hydrocortisone for 2 days significantly decreased water and solute transport across cell monolayers, and induced an increase in occludin mRNA and protein cell content [32]. Both occludin and ZO-1 presence at the cell membrane increased significantly [32]. Additionally, 4 h of hydrocortisone treatment significantly reduced occludin phosphorylation [32]. Intravitreal injection of corticosteroids inhibits leukocyte recruitment in the diabetic retina in animal models [157].

Corticosteroids have been used in multiple formulations for the treatment of BRB breakdown and DME [33]. Improvement in visual acuity in eyes with clinically significant DME has been reported after intravitreal injection of 1–4 mg of triamcinolone acetonide (TA) [33]. However, as mentioned above, the prospective Diabetic Retinopathy Clinical Research Network study recently compared focal/grid photocoagulation vs. 1 mg intravitreal triamcinolone vs. 4 mg intravitreal triamcinolone [150] and found that, while at 4 months mean visual acuity was better in the 4 mg triamcinolone group than in the laser group, by the 16-month visit and extending through the primary outcome visit at 2 years, mean visual acuity was better in the laser group than in the two triamcinolone groups [149, 150]. These findings have emphasized the need for longer follow-up studies [149]. A phase I randomized prospective study that compares intravitreal TA with intravitreal bevacizumab (IBEME) in refractory DME is currently ongoing.

Nova63035 (Novagali) is a sustained release, injectable emulsion that contains a tissue-activated corticosteroid prodrug, intended to be activated in the retina and choroid. A phase I study is currently underway to assess the safety and tolerability of this medication in patients with DME. TA has also been used intravitreally and there is growing evidence that it effectively reduces macular thickness and improves vision in DME.

Corticosteroids have also been used intravitreally in the form of drug-delivery implants that overcome the problem of frequent intravitreal injections and systemic side effects. Posurdex (Allergan), a sustained-release dexamethasone formulation, Retisert (Bausch and Lomb), a fluocinolone acetonide sustained delivery formulation, Medidur (Alimera), a fluocinolone-based implant, and Ivation (SurModics), a sustained triamcinolone release formulation, are all currently used in clinical trials for DME. The implants have shown promising results, decreasing macular thickness and restoring vision in patients with DME, but they have significant side effects such as cataract and glaucoma.

VEGF Inhibitors

VEGF plays a crucial role in the pathogenesis of macular edema by promoting the phosphorylation of TJ proteins such as occludin and claudins and increasing permeability. VEGF inhibitors restore vision and decrease macular thickness in patients with macular edema [158–164]. Ranibizumab (Lucentis, Genentech) [165, 166] and bevacizumab (Avastin, Genentech) [166] are antibodies against all forms of VEGF-A. They are currently in phase II and III trials where they are being compared with focal photocoagulation in multiple treatment schedules and dosages to assess their effectiveness in DME.

Other VEGF inhibitors that are currently being tested in DME are pegaptanib sodium (Macugen) [167], an anti-VEGF aptamer that binds and blocks $VEGF_{165}$; bevasiranib (OPKO), a siRNA against VEGF, and VEGF trap (Regeneron) [168], a soluble VEGF receptor fusion protein that binds VEGF-A and placental growth factor.

Nonsteroidal Anti-Inflammatory Drugs

Nonsteroidal anti-inflammatory drugs inhibit COX-2-mediated prostaglandin synthesis, and decrease retinal vascular hyperpermeability in preclinical models [169, 170]. Nepafenac [171] and bromfenac [172] are administered as ophthalmic drops, with a good pharmacokinetic profile and penetration in the posterior segment. Bromfenac is currently being studied in a nonrandomized open-label phase I trial to assess activity and safety in patients with refractory DME. Nepafenac is Food and Drug Association (FDA) approved for postoperative pain and inflammation in patients after cataract surgery and is currently used for the treatment of postsurgical macular edema.

Anti-TNF-α

TNF-α is an inflammatory cytokine that stimulates the acute phase reaction and plays a key role in the disruption of BRB breakdown in a variety of ocular conditions. Infliximab is a genetically engineered monoclonal anti-TNF-α antibody. Used systemically, it has shown preliminary evidence of activity in case series of patients with chronic cystoid macular edema associated with uveitis [173], DME [174] or AMD [175]. However, infliximab is a potent immunosuppressive agent and its systemic use carries significant risks [176]. There is currently an ongoing open-label phase I study designed to evaluate the safety and efficacy of intravitreally administered infliximab in patients with refractory DME or CNV secondary to AMD.

Mammalian Target of Rapamycin Inhibitors

Sirolimus (rapamycin, Macusight) is an inhibitor of the mammalian target of rapamycin and has been approved by the FDA for prevention of rejection of renal transplants. Sirolimus has demonstrated antiangiogenic and antipermeability properties, and promise in a phase I study in the treatment of patients with refractory clinically significant macular edema. The drug was well tolerated and safe when delivered subconjunctivally or intravitreally and has a prolonged action. Improvements in visual acuity and reductions in foveal thickness were noted up to 3 months after a single administration [177]. Currently, a phase II randomized, double-blind, placebo-controlled, dose-ranging study is underway to assess the safety and efficacy of sirolimus injected subconjunctivally in patients with DME. In parallel, Quark Pharmaceuticals and Pfizer have developed a siRNA drug candidate (PF-4523655) that targets RTP801, a regulator of the mammalian target of rapamycin pathway, and currently is in a phase II trial in patients with wet AMD. A phase I/II trial has already been completed and showed that PF-4523655 is safe and well tolerated in patients with wet AMD who failed to respond to currently approved therapies.

PKCβ Inhibitors

Protein kinase Cβ plays a central role in the pathophysiology of DR [178]. Ruboxistaurin is a PKCβ inhibitor that can be administered orally and has shown efficacy in decreasing macular edema in two separate phase III trials [179]. Ruboxistaurin reduces retinal vascular leakage, as measured by vitreous fluorometry [180]. However, in a recent 30-month study, ruboxistaurin did not delay disease progression or need for photocoagulation [181]. The drug is currently FDA approved for macular edema, although the FDA has requested additional data from a 3-year phase III trial.

Conclusions

The BRB plays a crucial role in the proper function of the retina. Disruption of the BRB is present in many retinopathies and contributes to vision loss. The elucidation of the mechanisms of pathologic angiogenesis and increased vascular permeability in the diseased retina provides several molecular targets for therapeutic intervention. Early clinical results offer significant hope for effective, vision-preserving therapies.

References

1 Goldmann EE: Vitalbarfung am Zentralnervensystem. Abhandl Konigl Preuss Akad Wiss 1913;1:1–60.

2 Cunha-Vaz JG: The blood-retinal barriers system. Basic concepts and clinical evaluation. Exp Eye Res 2004;78:715–721.

3 Ashton N, Cunha-Vaz JG: Effect of histamine on the permeability of the ocular vessels. Arch Ophthalmol 1965;73:211–223.

4 Stewart PA, Tuor UI: Blood-eye barriers in the rat: correlation of ultrastructure with function. J Comp Neurol 1994;340:566–576.

5 Phillips BE, Antonetti DA: Blood-retinal barrier, retinal vascular leakage and macular edema; in Joussen A, et al (eds): Retinal Vascular Disease. Berlin, Springer, 2007.

6 Burns MS, Hartz MJ: The retinal pigment epithelium induces fenestration of endothelial cells in vivo. Curr Eye Res 1992;11:863–873.

7 Peters S, Heiduschka P, Julien S, Ziemssen F, Fietz H, Bartz-Schmidt KU, Schraermeyer U: Ultrastructural findings in the primate eye after intravitreal injection of bevacizumab. Am J Ophthalmol 2007;143:995–1002.

8 Rizzolo LJ: Polarity and the development of the outer blood-retinal barrier. Histol Histopathol 1997;12:1057–1067.

9 Philp NJ, Yoon H, Grollman EF: Monocarboxylate transporter MCT1 is located in the apical membrane and MCT3 in the basal membrane of rat RPE. Am J Physiol 1998;274:R1824–R1828.

10 Philp NJ, Wang D, Yoon H, Hjelmeland LM: Polarized expression of monocarboxylate transporters in human retinal pigment epithelium and ARPE-19 cells. Invest Ophthalmol Vis Sci 2003;44:1716–1721.

11 Greenwood J: Characterization of a rat retinal endothelial cell culture and the expression of P-glycoprotein in brain and retinal endothelium in vitro. J Neuroimmunol 1992;39:123–132.

12 Kennedy BG, Mangini NJ: P-glycoprotein expression in human retinal pigment epithelium. Mol Vis 2002;8:422–430.

13 Maines LW, Antonetti DA, Wolpert EB, Smith CD: Evaluation of the role of P-glycoprotein in the uptake of paroxetine, clozapine, phenytoin and carbamazapine by bovine retinal endothelial cells. Neuropharmacology 2005;49:610–617.

14 Erickson KK, Sundstrom JM, Antonetti DA: Vascular permeability in ocular disease and the role of tight junctions. Angiogenesis 2007;10:103–117.

15 Gonzalez-Mariscal L, Betanzos A, Nava P, Jaramillo BE: Tight junction proteins. Prog Biophys Mol Biol 2003;81:1–44.

16 Leach L: The phenotype of the human materno-fetal endothelial barrier: molecular occupancy of paracellular junctions dictate permeability and angiogenic plasticity. J Anat 2002;200:599–606.

17 Furuse M, Hirase T, Itoh M, Nagafuchi A, Yonemura S, Tsukita S, Tsukita S: Occludin: a novel integral membrane protein localizing at tight junctions. J Cell Biol 1993;123:1777–1788.

18 Traweger A, Fang D, Liu YC, Stelzhammer W, Krizbai IA, Fresser F, Bauer HC, Bauer H: The tight junction-specific protein occludin is a functional target of the E3 ubiquitin-protein ligase itch. J Biol Chem 2002;277:10201–10208.

19 Lui WY, Lee WM: cAMP perturbs inter-Sertoli tight junction permeability barrier in vitro via its effect on proteasome-sensitive ubiquitination of occludin. J Cell Physiol 2005;203:564–572.

20 Furuse M, Itoh M, Hirase T, Nagafuchi A, Yonemura S, Tsukita S, Tsukita S: Direct association of occludin with ZO-1 and its possible involvement in the localization of occludin at tight junctions. J Cell Biol 1994;127:1617–1626.

21 Harhaj NS, Felinski EA, Wolpert EB, Sundstrom JM, Gardner TW, Antonetti DA: VEGF activation of protein kinase C stimulates occludin phosphorylation and contributes to endothelial permeability. Invest Ophthalmol Vis Sci 2006;47:5106–5115.
22 Antonetti DA, Barber AJ, Hollinger LA, Wolpert EB, Gardner TW: Vascular endothelial growth factor induces rapid phosphorylation of tight junction proteins occludin and zonula occluden 1. A potential mechanism for vascular permeability in diabetic retinopathy and tumors. J Biol Chem 1999;274:23463–23467.
23 Rao RK, Basuroy S, Rao VU, Karnaky Jr KJ, Gupta A: Tyrosine phosphorylation and dissociation of occludin-ZO-1 and E-cadherin-beta-catenin complexes from the cytoskeleton by oxidative stress. Biochem J 2002;368:471–481.
24 Hirase T, Staddon JM, Saitou M, Ando-Akatsuka Y, Itoh M, Furuse M, Fujimoto K, Tsukita S, Rubin LL: Occludin as a possible determinant of tight junction permeability in endothelial cells. J Cell Sci 1997;110(Pt 14):1603–1613.
25 Kevil CG, Okayama N, Trocha SD, Kalogeris TJ, Coe LL, Specian RD, Davis CP, Alexander JS: Expression of zonula occludens and adherens junctional proteins in human venous and arterial endothelial cells: role of occludin in endothelial solute barriers. Microcirculation 1998;5:197–210.
26 Yu AS, McCarthy KM, Francis SA, McCormack JM, Lai J, Rogers RA, Lynch RD, Schneeberger EE: Knockdown of occludin expression leads to diverse phenotypic alterations in epithelial cells. Am J Physiol Cell Physiol 2005;288:C1231–C1241.
27 Barber AJ, Antonetti DA, Gardner TW: Altered expression of retinal occludin and glial fibrillary acidic protein in experimental diabetes. The Penn State Retina Research Group. Invest Ophthalmol Vis Sci 2000;41:3561–3568.
28 Barber AJ, Antonetti DA: Mapping the blood vessels with paracellular permeability in the retinas of diabetic rats. Invest Ophthalmol Vis Sci 2003;44:5410–5416.
29 Hirase T, Kawashima S, Wong EY, Ueyama T, Rikitake Y, Tsukita S, Yokoyama M, Staddon JM: Regulation of tight junction permeability and occludin phosphorylation by Rhoa-p160ROCK-dependent and -independent mechanisms. J Biol Chem 2001;276:10423–10431.
30 DeMaio L, Rouhanizadeh M, Reddy S, Sevanian A, Hwang J, Hsiai TK: Oxidized phospholipids mediate occludin expression and phosphorylation in vascular endothelial cells. Am J Physiol Heart Circ Physiol 2006;290:H674–H683.
31 DeMaio L, Chang YS, Gardner TW, Tarbell JM, Antonetti DA: Shear stress regulates occludin content and phosphorylation. Am J Physiol Heart Circ Physiol 2001;281:H105–H113.
32 Antonetti DA, Wolpert EB, DeMaio L, Harhaj NS, Scaduto RC Jr: Hydrocortisone decreases retinal endothelial cell water and solute flux coincident with increased content and decreased phosphorylation of occludin. J Neurochem 2002;80:667–677.
33 Chieh JJ, Roth DB, Liu M, Belmont J, Nelson M, Regillo C, Martidis A: Intravitreal triamcinolone acetonide for diabetic macular edema. Retina 2005;25:828–834.
34 Schulzke JD, Gitter AH, Mankertz J, Spiegel S, Seidler U, Amasheh S, Saitou M, Tsukita S, Fromm M: Epithelial transport and barrier function in occludin-deficient mice. Biochim Biophys Acta 2005;1669:34–42.
35 Saitou M, Fujimoto K, Doi Y, Itoh M, Fujimoto T, Furuse M, Takano H, Noda T, Tsukita S: Occludin-deficient embryonic stem cells can differentiate into polarized epithelial cells bearing tight junctions. J Cell Biol 1998;141:397–408.
36 Itoh M, Furuse M, Morita K, Kubota K, Saitou M, Tsukita S: Direct binding of three tight junction-associated MAGUKs, ZO-1, ZO-2, and ZO-3, with the COOH termini of claudins. J Cell Biol 1999;147:1351–1363.
37 Turksen K, Troy TC: Barriers built on claudins. J Cell Sci 2004;117:2435–2447.
38 Furuse M, Sasaki H, Fujimoto K, Tsukita S: A single gene product, claudin-1 or -2, reconstitutes tight junction strands and recruits occludin in fibroblasts. J Cell Biol 1998;143:391–401.
39 Furuse M, Fujita K, Hiiragi T, Fujimoto K, Tsukita S: Claudin-1 and -2:novel integral membrane proteins localizing at tight junctions with no sequence similarity to occludin. J Cell Biol 1998;141:1539–1550.
40 Furuse M, Furuse K, Sasaki H, Tsukita S: Conversion of zonulae occludentes from tight to leaky strand type by introducing claudin-2 into Madin-Darby canine kidney I cells. J Cell Biol 2001;153:263–272.
41 Koto T, Takubo K, Ishida S, Shinoda H, Inoue M, Tsubota K, Okada Y, Ikeda E: Hypoxia disrupts the barrier function of neural blood vessels through changes in the expression of claudin-5 in endothelial cells. Am J Pathol 2007;170:1389–1397.
42 Nitta T, Hata M, Gotoh S, Seo Y, Sasaki H, Hashimoto N, Furuse M, Tsukita S: Size-selective loosening of the blood-brain barrier in claudin-5-deficient mice. J Cell Biol 2003;161:653–660.
43 Xu H, Dawson R, Crane IJ, Liversidge J: Leukocyte diapedesis in vivo induces transient loss of tight junction protein at the blood-retina barrier. Invest Ophthalmol Vis Sci 2005;46:2487–2494.
44 Stevenson BR, Siliciano JD, Mooseker MS, Goodenough DA: Identification of ZO-1: a high molecular weight polypeptide associated with the tight junction (zonula occludens) in a variety of epithelia. J Cell Biol 1986;103:755–766.
45 Jesaitis LA, Goodenough DA: Molecular characterization and tissue distribution of ZO-2, a tight junction protein homologous to ZO-1 and the Drosophila discs-large tumor suppressor protein. J Cell Biol 1994;124:949–961.
46 Haskins J, Gu L, Wittchen ES, Hibbard J, Stevenson BR: ZO-3, a novel member of the MAGUK protein family found at the tight junction, interacts with ZO-1 and occludin. J Cell Biol 1998;141:199–208.
47 Itoh M, Morita K, Tsukita S: Characterization of ZO-2 as a MAGUK family member associated with tight as well as adherens junctions with a binding affinity to occludin and alpha catenin. J Biol Chem 1999;274:5981–5986.
48 Gonzalez-Mariscal L, Betanzos A, Avila-Flores A: MAGUK proteins: structure and role in the tight junction. Semin Cell Dev Biol 2000;11:315–324.

49 Schmidt A, Utepbergenov DI, Mueller SL, Beyermann M, Schneider-Mergener J, Krause G, Blasig IE: Occludin binds to the SH3-hinge-GuK unit of zonula occludens protein 1:potential mechanism of tight junction regulation. Cell Mol Life Sci 2004;61:1354–1365.
50 Utepbergenov DI, Fanning AS, Anderson JM: Dimerization of the scaffolding protein ZO-1 through the second PDZ domain. J Biol Chem 2006;281:24671–24677.
51 Itoh M, Nagafuchi A, Moroi S, Tsukita S: Involvement of ZO-1 in cadherin-based cell adhesion through its direct binding to alpha catenin and actin filaments. J Cell Biol 1997;138:181–192.
52 Umeda K, Matsui T, Nakayama M, Furuse K, Sasaki H, Furuse M, Tsukita S: Establishment and characterization of cultured epithelial cells lacking expression of ZO-1. J Biol Chem 2004;279:44785–44794.
53 Fischer S, Wobben M, Marti HH, Renz D, Schaper W: Hypoxia-induced hyperpermeability in brain microvessel endothelial cells involves VEGF-mediated changes in the expression of zonula occludens-1. Microvasc Res 2002;63:70–80.
54 Joussen AM, Smyth N, Niessen C: Pathophysiology of diabetic macular edema. Dev Ophthalmol 2007;39:1–12.
55 Hofman P, Blaauwgeers HG, Tolentino MJ, Adamis AP, Nunes Cardozo BJ, Vrensen GF, Schlingemann RO: VEGF-A induced hyperpermeability of blood-retinal barrier endothelium in vivo is predominantly associated with pinocytotic vesicular transport and not with formation of fenestrations. Vascular endothelial growth factor-A. Curr Eye Res 2000;21:637–645.
56 Schlingemann RO, Hofman P, Vrensen GF, Blaauwgeers HG: Increased expression of endothelial antigen PAL-E in human diabetic retinopathy correlates with microvascular leakage. Diabetologia 1999;42:596–602.
57 Hofman P, Blaauwgeers HG, Vrensen GF, Schlingemann RO: Role of VEGF-A in endothelial phenotypic shift in human diabetic retinopathy and VEGF-A-induced retinopathy in monkeys. Ophthalmic Res 2001;33:156–162.
58 Witmer AN, Blaauwgeers HG, Weich HA, Alitalo K, Vrensen GF, Schlingemann RO: Altered expression patterns of VEGF receptors in human diabetic retina and in experimental VEGF-induced retinopathy in monkey. Invest Ophthalmol Vis Sci 2002;43:849–857.
59 Guo P, Weinstein AM, Weinbaum S: A dual-pathway ultrastructural model for the tight junction of rat proximal tubule epithelium. Am J Physiol Renal Physiol 2003;285:F241–F257.
60 Joussen AM, Poulaki V, Mitsiades N, Cai WY, Suzuma I, Pak J, Ju ST, Rook SL, Esser P, Mitsiades CS, Kirchhof B, Adamis AP, Aiello LP: Suppression of Fas-FasL-induced endothelial cell apoptosis prevents diabetic blood-retinal barrier breakdown in a model of streptozotocin-induced diabetes. FASEB J 2003;17:76–78.
61 el-Remessy AB, Bartoli M, Platt DH, Fulton D, Caldwell RB: Oxidative stress inactivates VEGF survival signaling in retinal endothelial cells via PI 3-kinase tyrosine nitration. J Cell Sci 2005;118:243–252.
62 Kowluru RA: Diabetic retinopathy: mitochondrial dysfunction and retinal capillary cell death. Antioxid Redox Signal 2005;7:1581–1587.
63 Kowluru RA, Atasi L, Ho YS: Role of mitochondrial superoxide dismutase in the development of diabetic retinopathy. Invest Ophthalmol Vis Sci 2006;47:1594–1599.
64 Kowluru RA: Effect of advanced glycation end products on accelerated apoptosis of retinal capillary cells under in vitro conditions. Life Sci 2005;76:1051–1060.
65 Ejaz S, Chekarova I, Ejaz A, Sohail A, Lim CW: Importance of pericytes and mechanisms of pericyte loss during diabetes retinopathy. Diabetes Obes Metab 2008;10:53–63.
66 Joussen AM, Poulaki V, Le ML, Koizumi K, Esser C, Janicki H, Schraermeyer U, Kociok N, Fauser S, Kirchhof B, Kern TS, Adamis AP: A central role for inflammation in the pathogenesis of diabetic retinopathy. FASEB J 2004;18:1450–1452.
67 Li W, Liu X, Yanoff M, Cohen S, Ye X: Cultured retinal capillary pericytes die by apoptosis after an abrupt fluctuation from high to low glucose levels: a comparative study with retinal capillary endothelial cells. Diabetologia 1996;39:537–547.
68 Podesta F, Romeo G, Liu WH, Krajewski S, Reed JC, Gerhardinger C, Lorenzi M: Bax is increased in the retina of diabetic subjects and is associated with pericyte apoptosis in vivo and in vitro. Am J Pathol 2000;156:1025–1032.
69 Romeo G, Liu WH, Asnaghi V, Kern TS, Lorenzi M: Activation of nuclear factor-kappaB induced by diabetes and high glucose regulates a proapoptotic program in retinal pericytes. Diabetes 2002;51:2241–2248.
70 Naruse K, Nakamura J, Hamada Y, Nakayama M, Chaya S, Komori T, Kato K, Kasuya Y, Miwa K, Hotta N: Aldose reductase inhibition prevents glucose-induced apoptosis in cultured bovine retinal microvascular pericytes. Exp Eye Res 2000;71:309–315.
71 Stitt AW, Hughes SJ, Canning P, Lynch O, Cox O, Frizzell N, Thorpe SR, Cotter TG, Curtis TM, Gardiner TA: Substrates modified by advanced glycation end-products cause dysfunction and death in retinal pericytes by reducing survival signals mediated by platelet-derived growth factor. Diabetologia 2004;47:1735–1746.
72 Murata M, Ohta N, Fujisawa S, Tsai JY, Sato S, Akagi Y, Takahashi Y, Neuenschwander H, Kador PF: Selective pericyte degeneration in the retinal capillaries of galactose-fed dogs results from apoptosis linked to aldose reductase-catalyzed galactitol accumulation. J Diabetes Complications 2002;16:363–370.
73 Song W, Barth JL, Lu K, Yu Y, Huang Y, Gittinger CK, Argraves WS, Lyons TJ: Effects of modified low-density lipoproteins on human retinal pericyte survival. Ann N Y Acad Sci 2005;1043:390–395.
74 Miwa K, Nakamura J, Hamada Y, Naruse K, Nakashima E, Kato K, Kasuya Y, Yasuda Y, Kamiya H, Hotta N: The role of polyol pathway in glucose-induced apoptosis of cultured retinal pericytes. Diabetes Res Clin Pract 2003;60:1–9.
75 Yamagishi S, Amano S, Inagaki Y, Okamoto T, Koga K, Sasaki N, Yamamoto H, Takeuchi M, Makita Z: Advanced glycation end products-induced apoptosis and overexpression of vascular endothelial growth factor in bovine retinal pericytes. Biochem Biophys Res Commun 2002;290:973–978.

76 Pomero F, Allione A, Beltramo E, Buttiglieri S, D'Alu F, Ponte E, Lacaria A, Porta M: Effects of protein kinase C inhibition and activation on proliferation and apoptosis of bovine retinal pericytes. Diabetologia 2003;46:416–419.
77 Cacicedo JM, Benjachareowong S, Chou E, Ruderman NB, Ido Y: Palmitate-induced apoptosis in cultured bovine retinal pericytes: roles of NAD(P)H oxidase, oxidant stress, and ceramide. Diabetes 2005;54:1838–1845.
78 Morcos Y, Hosie MJ, Bauer HC, Chan-Ling T: Immunolocalization of occludin and claudin-1 to tight junctions in intact CNS vessels of mammalian retina. J Neurocytol 2001;30:107–123.
79 Staddon JM, Herrenknecht K, Smales C, Rubin LL: Evidence that tyrosine phosphorylation may increase tight junction permeability. J Cell Sci 1995;108(Pt 2):609–619.
80 Stevenson BR, Anderson JM, Braun ID, Mooseker MS: Phosphorylation of the tight-junction protein ZO-1 in two strains of Madin-Darby canine kidney cells which differ in transepithelial resistance. Biochem J 1989;263:597–599.
81 Gardner TW, Lesher T, Khin S, Vu C, Barber AJ, Brennan WA Jr: Histamine reduces ZO-1 tight-junction protein expression in cultured retinal microvascular endothelial cells. Biochem J 1996;320(Pt 3):717–721.
82 Gardner TW: Histamine, ZO-1 and increased blood-retinal barrier permeability in diabetic retinopathy. Trans Am Ophthalmol Soc 1995;93:583–621.
83 Antonetti DA, Barber AJ, Khin S, Lieth E, Tarbell JM, Gardner TW: Vascular permeability in experimental diabetes is associated with reduced endothelial occludin content: vascular endothelial growth factor decreases occludin in retinal endothelial cells. Penn State Retina Research Group. Diabetes 1998;47:1953–1959.
84 Wang W, Dentler WL, Borchardt RT: VEGF increases BMEC monolayer permeability by affecting occludin expression and tight junction assembly. Am J Physiol Heart Circ Physiol 2001;280:H434–H440.
85 Kale G, Naren AP, Sheth P, Rao RK: Tyrosine phosphorylation of occludin attenuates its interactions with ZO-1, ZO-2, and ZO-3. Biochem Biophys Res Commun 2003;302:324–329.
86 Nusrat A, Chen JA, Foley CS, Liang TW, Tom J, Cromwell M, Quan C, Mrsny RJ: The coiled-coil domain of occludin can act to organize structural and functional elements of the epithelial tight junction. J Biol Chem 2000;275:29816–29822.
87 Sheth P, Basuroy S, Li C, Naren AP, Rao RK: Role of phosphatidylinositol 3-kinase in oxidative stress-induced disruption of tight junctions. J Biol Chem 2003;278:49239–49245.
88 Grisendi S, Arpin M, Crepaldi T: Effect of hepatocyte growth factor on assembly of zonula occludens-1 protein at the plasma membrane. J Cell Physiol 1998;176:465–471.
89 Jin M, Barron E, He S, Ryan SJ, Hinton DR: Regulation of RPE intercellular junction integrity and function by hepatocyte growth factor. Invest Ophthalmol Vis Sci 2002;43:2782–2790.
90 Folkman J: Tumor angiogenesis; in Bast RC, Kufe DW, Pollock RE, Weichselbaum RR, Holland JF, Frei E, Gansler TS (eds): Cancer Medicine. Hamilton, Decker, 2000, pp 132–152.
91 Senger DR, Galli SJ, Dvorak AM, Perruzzi CA, Harvey VS, Dvorak HF: Tumor cells secrete a vascular permeability factor that promotes accumulation of ascites fluid. Science 1983;219:983–985.
92 Senger DR, Perruzzi CA, Feder J, Dvorak HF: A highly conserved vascular permeability factor secreted by a variety of human and rodent tumor cell lines. Cancer Res 1986;46:5629–5632.
93 Leung DW, Cachianes G, Kuang WJ, Goeddel DV, Ferrara N: Vascular endothelial growth factor is a secreted angiogenic mitogen. Science 1989;246:1306–1309.
94 Ferrara N, Houck K, Jakeman L, Leung DW: Molecular and biological properties of the vascular endothelial growth factor family of proteins. Endocr Rev 1992;13:18–32.
95 Folkman J: Angiogenesis in cancer, vascular, rheumatoid and other disease. Nat Med 1995;1:27–31.
96 Folkman J: Seminars in Medicine of the Beth Israel Hospital, Boston. Clinical applications of research on angiogenesis. N Engl J Med 1995;333:1757–1763.
97 Joussen AM, Poulaki V, Qin W, Kirchhof B, Mitsiades N, Wiegand SJ, Rudge J, Yancopoulos GD, Adamis AP: Retinal vascular endothelial growth factor induces intercellular adhesion molecule-1 and endothelial nitric oxide synthase expression and initiates early diabetic retinal leukocyte adhesion in vivo. Am J Pathol 2002;160:501–509.
98 Poulaki V, Joussen AM, Mitsiades N, Mitsiades CS, Iliaki EF, Adamis AP: Insulin-like growth factor-I plays a pathogenetic role in diabetic retinopathy. Am J Pathol 2004;165:457–469.
99 Levy AP, Levy NS, Goldberg MA: Post-transcriptional regulation of vascular endothelial growth factor by hypoxia. J Biol Chem 1996;271:2746–2753.
100 Levy AP, Levy NS, Goldberg MA: Hypoxia-inducible protein binding to vascular endothelial growth factor mRNA and its modulation by the von Hippel-Lindau protein. J Biol Chem 1996;271:25492–25497.
101 Murata M, Kador PF, Sato S: Vascular endothelial growth factor (VEGF) enhances the expression of receptors and activates mitogen-activated protein (MAP) kinase of dog retinal capillary endothelial cells. J Ocul Pharmacol Ther 2000;16:383–391.
102 Conway EM, Collen D, Carmeliet P: Molecular mechanisms of blood vessel growth. Cardiovasc Res 2001;49:507–521.
103 Oshima Y, Oshima S, Nambu H, Kachi S, Takahashi K, Umeda N, Shen J, Dong A, Apte RS, Duh E, Hackett SF, Okoye G, Ishibashi K, Handa J, Melia M, Wiegand S, Yancopoulos G, Zack DJ, Campochiaro PA: Different effects of angiopoietin-2 in different vascular beds: new vessels are most sensitive. FASEB J 2005;19:963–965.
104 Vinores SA: Assessment of blood-retinal barrier integrity. Histol Histopathol 1995;10:141–154.
105 Radius RL, Anderson DR: Distribution of albumin in the normal monkey eye as revealed by Evans blue fluorescence microscopy. Invest Ophthalmol Vis Sci 1980;19:238–243.
106 Vinores SA, Derevjanik NL, Mahlow J, Berkowitz BA, Wilson CA: Electron microscopic evidence for the mechanism of blood-retinal barrier breakdown in diabetic rabbits: comparison with magnetic resonance imaging. Pathol Res Pract 1998;194:497–505.

107 Berkowitz BA, Roberts R, Luan H, Peysakhov J, Mao X, Thomas KA: Dynamic contrast-enhanced MRI measurements of passive permeability through blood retinal barrier in diabetic rats. Invest Ophthalmol Vis Sci 2004;45:2391–2398.
108 Trick GL, Liggett J, Levy J, Adamsons I, Edwards P, Desai U, Tofts PS, Berkowitz BA: Dynamic contrast enhanced MRI in patients with diabetic macular edema: initial results. Exp Eye Res 2005;81:97–102.
109 Massin P, Girach A, Erginay A, Gaudric A: Optical coherence tomography: a key to the future management of patients with diabetic macular oedema. Acta Ophthalmol Scand 2006;84:466–474.
110 Ishibashi T, Tanaka K, Taniguchi Y: Platelet aggregation and coagulation in the pathogenesis of diabetic retinopathy in rats. Diabetes 1981;30:601–606.
111 Pe'er J, Shweiki D, Itin A, Hemo I, Gnessin H, Keshet E: Hypoxia-induced expression of vascular endothelial growth factor by retinal cells is a common factor in neovascularizing ocular diseases. Lab Invest 1995;72:638–645.
112 Miller JW, Adamis AP, Shima DT, D'Amore PA, Moulton RS, O'Reilly MS, Folkman J, Dvorak HF, Brown LF, Berse B, et al: Vascular endothelial growth factor/vascular permeability factor is temporally and spatially correlated with ocular angiogenesis in a primate model. Am J Pathol 1994;145:574–584.
113 Miyamoto K, Khosrof S, Bursell SE, Moromizato Y, Aiello LP, Ogura Y, Adamis AP: Vascular endothelial growth factor (VEGF)-induced retinal vascular permeability is mediated by intercellular adhesion molecule-1 (ICAM-1). Am J Pathol 2000;156:1733–1739.
114 Aiello LP, Northrup JM, Keyt BA, Takagi H, Iwamoto MA: Hypoxic regulation of vascular endothelial growth factor in retinal cells. Arch Ophthalmol 1995;113:1538–1544.
115 Klein RJ, Zeiss C, Chew EY, Tsai JY, Sackler RS, Haynes C, Henning AK, SanGiovanni JP, Mane SM, Mayne ST, Bracken MB, Ferris FL, Ott J, Barnstable C, Hoh J: Complement factor H polymorphism in age-related macular degeneration. Science 2005;308:385–389.
116 Johnson PT, Betts KE, Radeke MJ, Hageman GS, Anderson DH, Johnson LV: Individuals homozygous for the age-related macular degeneration risk-conferring variant of complement factor H have elevated levels of CRP in the choroid. Proc Natl Acad Sci USA 2006;103:17456–17461.
117 Hamilton RD, Foss AJ, Leach L: Establishment of a human in vitro model of the outer blood-retinal barrier. J Anat 2007;211:707–716.
118 Steele FR, Chader GJ, Johnson LV, Tombran-Tink J: Pigment epithelium-derived factor: neurotrophic activity and identification as a member of the serine protease inhibitor gene family. Proc Natl Acad Sci USA 1993;90:1526–1530.
119 Moore DJ, Hussain AA, Marshall J: Age-related variation in the hydraulic conductivity of Bruch's membrane. Invest Ophthalmol Vis Sci 1995;36:1290–1297.
120 Sakurai E, Taguchi H, Anand A, Ambati BK, Gragoudas ES, Miller JW, Adamis AP, Ambati J: Targeted disruption of the CD18 or ICAM-1 gene inhibits choroidal neovascularization. Invest Ophthalmol Vis Sci 2003;44:2743–2749.
121 Tsutsumi C, Sonoda KH, Egashira K, Qiao H, Hisatomi T, Nakao S, Ishibashi M, Charo IF, Sakamoto T, Murata T, Ishibashi T: The critical role of ocular-infiltrating macrophages in the development of choroidal neovascularization. J Leukoc Biol 2003;74:25–32.
122 Nagai N, Oike Y, Izumi-Nagai K, Urano T, Kubota Y, Noda K, Ozawa Y, Inoue M, Tsubota K, Suda T, Ishida S: Angiotensin II type 1 receptor-mediated inflammation is required for choroidal neovascularization. Arterioscler Thromb Vasc Biol 2006;26:2252–2259.
123 Campochiaro PA, Chang M, Ohsato M, Vinores SA, Nie Z, Hjelmeland L, Mansukhani A, Basilico C, Zack DJ: Retinal degeneration in transgenic mice with photoreceptor-specific expression of a dominant-negative fibroblast growth factor receptor. J Neurosci 1996;16:1679–1688.
124 Harada T, Harada C, Kohsaka S, Wada E, Yoshida K, Ohno S, Mamada H, Tanaka K, Parada LF, Wada K: Microglia-Muller glia cell interactions control neurotrophic factor production during light-induced retinal degeneration. J Neurosci 2002;22:9228–9236.
125 Ritter MR, Banin E, Moreno SK, Aguilar E, Dorrell MI, Friedlander M: Myeloid progenitors differentiate into microglia and promote vascular repair in a model of ischemic retinopathy. J Clin Invest 2006;116:3266–3276.
126 Umeda N, Ozaki H, Hayashi H, Miyajima-Uchida H, Oshima K: Colocalization of Tie2, angiopoietin 2 and vascular endothelial growth factor in fibrovascular membrane from patients with retinopathy of prematurity. Ophthalmic Res 2003;35:217–223.
127 Ryan GB, Majno G: Acute inflammation. A review. Am J Pathol 1977;86:183–276.
128 Ieki Y, Nishiwaki H, Miura S, Hirata Y, Sakata I, Nonaka A, Kiryu J, Honda Y: Quantitative evaluation for blood-retinal barrier breakdown in experimental retinal vein occlusion produced by photodynamic thrombosis using a new photosensitizer. Curr Eye Res 2002;25:317–323.
129 Campochiaro PA, Hafiz G, Shah SM, Nguyen QD, Ying H, Do DV, Quinlan E, Zimmer-Galler I, Haller JA, Solomon SD, Sung JU, Hadi Y, Janjua KA, Jawed N, Choy DF, Arron JR: Ranibizumab for macular edema due to retinal vein occlusions: implication of VEGF as a critical stimulator. Mol Ther 2008;16:791–799.
130 Chen KH, Wu CC, Roy S, Lee SM, Liu JH: Increased interleukin-6 in aqueous humor of neovascular glaucoma. Invest Ophthalmol Vis Sci 1999;40:2627–2632.
131 Ki IY, Arimura N, Noda Y, Yamakiri K, Doi N, Hashiguchi T, Maruyama I, Shimura M, Sakamoto T: Stromal-derived factor-1 and inflammatory cytokines in retinal vein occlusion. Curr Eye Res 2007;32:1065–1072.
132 Guex-Crosier Y: The pathogenesis and clinical presentation of macular edema in inflammatory diseases. Doc Ophthalmol 1999;97:297–309.
133 Campochiaro PA, Sen HA: Adenosine and its agonists cause retinal vasodilation and hemorrhages. Implications for ischemic retinopathies. Arch Ophthalmol 1989;107:412–416.
134 Hangai M, Yoshimura N, Honda Y: Increased cytokine gene expression in rat retina following transient ischemia. Ophthalmic Res 1996;28:248–254.

135 Vinores SA, Sen H, Campochiaro PA: An adenosine agonist and prostaglandin E1 cause breakdown of the blood-retinal barrier by opening tight junctions between vascular endothelial cells. Invest Ophthalmol Vis Sci 1992;33:1870–1878.

136 Luna JD, Chan CC, Derevjanik NL, Mahlow J, Chiu C, Peng B, Tobe T, Campochiaro PA, Vinores SA: Blood-retinal barrier (BRB) breakdown in experimental autoimmune uveoretinitis: comparison with vascular endothelial growth factor, tumor necrosis factor alpha, and interleukin-1beta-mediated breakdown. J Neurosci Res 1997;49:268–280.

137 Melder RJ, Koenig GC, Witwer BP, Safabakhsh N, Munn LL, Jain RK: During angiogenesis, vascular endothelial growth factor and basic fibroblast growth factor regulate natural killer cell adhesion to tumor endothelium. Nat Med 1996;2:992–997.

138 Melder RJ, Koenig GC, Munn LL, Jain RK: Adhesion of activated natural killer cells to tumor necrosis factor-alpha-treated endothelium under physiological flow conditions. Nat Immun 1996;15:154–163.

139 Poulaki V, Iliaki E, Mitsiades N, Mitsiades CS, Paulus YN, Bula DV, Gragoudas ES, Miller JW: Inhibition of Hsp90 attenuates inflammation in endotoxin-induced uveitis. FASEB J 2007;21:2113–2123.

140 Flach AJ, Jampol LM, Weinberg D, Kraff MC, Yannuzzi LA, Campo RV, Neumann AC, Cupples HP, Lefler WH, Pulido JS, et al: Improvement in visual acuity in chronic aphakic and pseudophakic cystoid macular edema after treatment with topical 0.5% ketorolac tromethamine. Am J Ophthalmol 1991;112:514–519.

141 Tewari HK, Gadia R, Kumar D, Venkatesh P, Garg SP: Sympathetic-parasympathetic activity and reactivity in central serous chorioretinopathy: a case-control study. Invest Ophthalmol Vis Sci 2006;47:3474–3478.

142 Dickson PV, Hamner JB, Sims TL, Fraga CH, Ng CY, Rajasekeran S, Hagedorn NL, McCarville MB, Stewart CF, Davidoff AM: Bevacizumab-induced transient remodeling of the vasculature in neuroblastoma xenografts results in improved delivery and efficacy of systemically administered chemotherapy. Clin Cancer Res 2007;13:3942–3950.

143 Jain RK: Normalization of tumor vasculature: an emerging concept in antiangiogenic therapy. Science 2005;307:58–62.

144 Jain RK: Antiangiogenic therapy for cancer: current and emerging concepts. Oncology (Williston Park) 2005;19:7–16.

145 Gerber HP, Ferrara N: Pharmacology and pharmacodynamics of bevacizumab as monotherapy or in combination with cytotoxic therapy in preclinical studies. Cancer Res 2005;65:671–680.

146 Dickson PV, Hagedorn NL, Hamner JB, Fraga CH, Ng CY, Stewart CF, Davidoff AM: Interferon beta-mediated vessel stabilization improves delivery and efficacy of systemically administered topotecan in a murine neuroblastoma model. J Pediatr Surg 2007;42:160–165; discussion 165.

147 Dickson PV, Hamner JB, Streck CJ, Ng CY, McCarville MB, Calabrese C, Gilbertson RJ, Stewart CF, Wilson CM, Gaber MW, Pfeffer LM, Skapek SX, Nathwani AC, Davidoff AM: Continuous delivery of IFN-beta promotes sustained maturation of intratumoral vasculature. Mol Cancer Res 2007;5:531–542.

148 Photocoagulation for diabetic macular edema. Early Treatment Diabetic Retinopathy Study report number 1. Early Treatment Diabetic Retinopathy Study research group. Arch Ophthalmol 1985;103:1796–1806.

149 Schachat AP: A new look at an old treatment for diabetic macular edema. Ophthalmology 2008;115:1445–1446.

150 A randomized trial comparing intravitreal triamcinolone acetonide and focal/grid photocoagulation for diabetic macular edema. Ophthalmology 2008;115:1447–1449, 1449.e1441–1410.

151 Rehak J, Rehak M: Branch retinal vein occlusion: pathogenesis, visual prognosis, and treatment modalities. Curr Eye Res 2008;33:111–131.

152 Mohamed Q, McIntosh RL, Saw SM, Wong TY: Interventions for central retinal vein occlusion: an evidence-based systematic review. Ophthalmology 2007;114:507–519, 524.

153 Apple DJ, Goldberg MF, Wyhinny G: Histopathology and ultrastructure of the argon laser lesion in human retinal and choroidal vasculatures. Am J Ophthalmol 1973;75:595–609.

154 Arnarsson A, Stefansson E: Laser treatment and the mechanism of edema reduction in branch retinal vein occlusion. Invest Ophthalmol Vis Sci 2000;41:877–879.

155 Fong DS, Strauber SF, Aiello LP, Beck RW, Callanan DG, Danis RP, Davis MD, Feman SS, Ferris F, Friedman SM, Garcia CA, Glassman AR, Han DP, Le D, Kollman C, Lauer AK, Recchia FM, Solomon SD: Comparison of the modified Early Treatment Diabetic Retinopathy Study and mild macular grid laser photocoagulation strategies for diabetic macular edema. Arch Ophthalmol 2007;125:469–480.

156 Felinski EA, Antonetti DA: Glucocorticoid regulation of endothelial cell tight junction gene expression: novel treatments for diabetic retinopathy. Curr Eye Res 2005;30:949–957.

157 Tamura H, Miyamoto K, Kiryu J, Miyahara S, Katsuta H, Hirose F, Musashi K, Yoshimura N: Intravitreal injection of corticosteroid attenuates leukostasis and vascular leakage in experimental diabetic retina. Invest Ophthalmol Vis Sci 2005;46:1440–1444.

158 Rosenfeld PJ, Brown DM, Heier JS, Boyer DS, Kaiser PK, Chung CY, Kim RY: Ranibizumab for neovascular age-related macular degeneration. N Engl J Med 2006;355:1419–1431.

159 Chun DW, Heier JS, Topping TM, Duker JS, Bankert JM: A pilot study of multiple intravitreal injections of ranibizumab in patients with center-involving clinically significant diabetic macular edema. Ophthalmology 2006;113:1706–1712.

160 Lantry LE: Ranibizumab, a mAb against VEGF-A for the potential treatment of age-related macular degeneration and other ocular complications. Curr Opin Mol Ther 2007;9:592–602.

161 Pieramici DJ, Rabena M, Castellarin AA, Nasir M, See R, Norton T, Sanchez A, Risard S, Avery RL: Ranibizumab for the treatment of macular edema associated with perfused central retinal vein occlusions. Ophthalmology 2008;115:e47–e54.

162 Spaide RF, Chang LK, Klancnik JM, Yannuzzi LA, Sorenson J, Slakter JS, Freund KB, Klein R: Prospective study of intravitreal ranibizumab as a treatment for decreased visual acuity secondary to central retinal vein occlusion. Am J Ophthalmol 2009;147:298–306.

163 Ng EW, Adamis AP: Anti-VEGF aptamer (pegaptanib) therapy for ocular vascular diseases. Ann N Y Acad Sci 2006;1082:151–171.
164 Ng EW, Shima DT, Calias P, Cunningham ET Jr, Guyer DR, Adamis AP: Pegaptanib, a targeted anti-VEGF aptamer for ocular vascular disease. Nat Rev Drug Discov 2006;5:123–132.
165 Campochiaro PA: Targeted pharmacotherapy of retinal diseases with ranibizumab. Drugs Today (Barc) 2007;43:529–537.
166 Jager RD, Mieler WF, Miller JW: Age-related macular degeneration. N Engl J Med 2008;358:2606–2617.
167 Fine SL, Martin DF, Kirkpatrick P: Pegaptanib sodium. Nat Rev Drug Discov 2005;4:187–188.
168 Holash J, Davis S, Papadopoulos N, Croll SD, Ho L, Russell M, Boland P, Leidich R, Hylton D, Burova E, Ioffe E, Huang T, Radziejewski C, Bailey K, Fandl JP, Daly T, Wiegand SJ, Yancopoulos GD, Rudge JS: VEGF-Trap: a VEGF blocker with potent antitumor effects. Proc Natl Acad Sci USA 2002;99:11393–11398.
169 Joussen AM, Poulaki V, Mitsiades N, Kirchhof B, Koizumi K, Dohmen S, Adamis AP: Nonsteroidal anti-inflammatory drugs prevent early diabetic retinopathy via TNF-alpha suppression. FASEB J 2002;16:438–440.
170 Castro MR, Lutz D, Edelman JL: Effect of COX inhibitors on VEGF-induced retinal vascular leakage and experimental corneal and choroidal neovascularization. Exp Eye Res 2004;79:275–285.
171 Ke TL, Graff G, Spellman JM, Yanni JM: Nepafenac, a unique nonsteroidal prodrug with potential utility in the treatment of trauma-induced ocular inflammation: II. In vitro bioactivation and permeation of external ocular barriers. Inflammation 2000;24:371–384.
172 Baklayan GA, Patterson HM, Song CK, Gow JA, McNamara TR: 24-hour evaluation of the ocular distribution of (14) c-labeled bromfenac following topical instillation into the eyes of New Zealand white rabbits. J Ocul Pharmacol Ther 2008;24:392–398.
173 Markomichelakis NN, Theodossiadis PG, Pantelia E, Papaefthimiou S, Theodossiadis GP, Sfikakis PP: Infliximab for chronic cystoid macular edema associated with uveitis. Am J Ophthalmol 2004;138:648–650.
174 Sfikakis PP, Markomichelakis N, Theodossiadis GP, Grigoropoulos V, Katsilambros N, Theodossiadis PG: Regression of sight-threatening macular edema in type 2 diabetes following treatment with the anti-tumor necrosis factor monoclonal antibody infliximab. Diabetes Care 2005;28:445–447.
175 Markomichelakis NN, Theodossiadis PG, Sfikakis PP: Regression of neovascular age-related macular degeneration following infliximab therapy. Am J Ophthalmol 2005;139:537–540.
176 Lin J, Ziring D, Desai S, Kim S, Wong M, Korin Y, Braun J, Reed E, Gjertson D, Singh RR: TNFalpha blockade in human diseases: an overview of efficacy and safety. Clin Immunol 2008;126:13–30.
177 Blumenkranz MS, Dugel PU, Solley WA, et al: Rapamycin (sirolimus) for the treatment of diabetic macular edema: preliminary results of a prospective phase I safety trial. Annu Meet Retina Soc, Boston, 2007.
178 Aiello LP, Clermont A, Arora V, Davis MD, Sheetz MJ, Bursell SE: Inhibition of PKC beta by oral administration of ruboxistaurin is well tolerated and ameliorates diabetes-induced retinal hemodynamic abnormalities in patients. Invest Ophthalmol Vis Sci 2006;47:86–92.
179 The effect of ruboxistaurin on visual loss in patients with moderately severe to very severe nonproliferative diabetic retinopathy: initial results of the Protein Kinase C beta Inhibitor Diabetic Retinopathy Study (PKC-DRS) multicenter randomized clinical trial. Diabetes 2005;54:2188–2197.
180 Strom C, Sander B, Klemp K, Aiello LP, Lund-Andersen H, Larsen M: Effect of ruboxistaurin on blood-retinal barrier permeability in relation to severity of leakage in diabetic macular edema. Invest Ophthalmol Vis Sci 2005;46:3855–3858.
181 Effect of ruboxistaurin in patients with diabetic macular edema: thirty-month results of the randomized PKC-DMES clinical trial. Arch Ophthalmol 2007;125:318–324.

Vassiliki Poulaki, MD, PhD
Retina Research Laboratory, Massachusetts Eye and Ear Infirmary
Harvard Medical School
325 Cambridge Street, Boston, MA 02114 (USA)
Tel. +1 617 573 3078, Fax +1 617 812 7701, E-Mail poulakiv@hotmail.com

Hammes H-P, Porta M (eds): Experimental Approaches to Diabetic Retinopathy.
Front Diabetes. Basel, Karger, 2010, vol 20, pp 42–60

In vivo Models of Diabetic Retinopathy

Ling Zheng[a] · Timothy S. Kern[b–d]

[a]College of Life Sciences, Wuhan University, Wuhan, China, Departments of [b]Medicine, and [c]Ophthalmology, Case Western Reserve University, and [d]Louis Stokes Cleveland Department of Veterans Affairs Medical Center, Cleveland, Ohio, USA

Abstract

Diabetic animal models studied to date have developed some lesions characteristic of the early stages of diabetic retinopathy. This spectrum of lesions includes degenerate and nonperfused (acellular) capillaries, loss of capillary cells, thickening of basement membranes, and in longer-lived species, microaneurysms and intra-retinal microvascular abnormalities. To date, none of these diabetic animal models has been found to reliably develop preretinal neovascularization (an advanced stage of the retinopathy), likely due in part to less vaso-obliteration occurring during the short duration of diabetes that these models have been studied compared to diabetic patients. Although not diabetic, some animal models develop a diabetic-like preretinal neovascularization, and these models have been used to study ways to inhibit the neovascularization. Animal models are being used to provide valuable insight into the roles of specific biochemical pathways or physiological abnormalities in the development of diabetic retinopathy. Distinct advantages and disadvantages of each of these models are outlined in this review, thus providing information that should be valuable for planning experimental studies pertaining to the retinopathy.

Diabetic retinopathy classically has been regarded as a disease of the microvasculature of the retina. The natural history of this microvascular disease has been divided into two stages: an early, nonproliferative (or background) stage, and a later, proliferative stage [1]. Nonproliferative diabetic retinopathy currently is diagnosed ophthalmoscopically based on the presence of retinal vascular abnormalities, including microaneurysms, intraretinal microvascular abnormalities (IRMAs; which include intraretinal new vessels), areas of capillary nonperfusion, retinal hemorrhages, cotton wool spots (infarctions within the nerve fiber layer), edema, and exudates. All these signs indicate regional failure of the retinal microvascular circulation, which presumably results in ischemia. Proliferative diabetic retinopathy is diagnosed based on the presence of new vessels on the surface of the retina. The preretinal new vessels or fibrovascular membrane are major factors causing vitreous hemorrhages and visual loss in diabetes. They also can contribute to tractional retinal detachments from the accompanying contractile fibrous tissue. Retinal edema is the other major contributor to visual impairment in diabetes [2], which involves the breakdown of the blood-retinal barrier, with leakage of plasma from small blood vessels. Macula, the central portion of the retina that is responsible for the major part of visual function, is especially sensitive to this retinal thickening, leading to impaired vision.

Multiple animal models are used to investigate the pathogenesis of this ocular disease, but the value of any animal model depends in large part on how well the model reproduces some or all lesions of the human disease. This chapter will summarize the histopathology of diabetic retinopathy, describe which lesions are reproduced by the various animal models reported, and focus on the early stage retinopathy lesions reproduced by diabetic animal models. Nondiabetic models that develop the later stage retinopathy are reviewed in other chapters.

Early Stage of Diabetic Retinopathy, Histopathology

Changes in the Vascular Retina

Histologically, early stage of diabetic retinopathy in patients is characterized by the presence of saccular capillary microaneurysms, pericyte-deficient capillaries, and obliterated and acellular capillaries (fig. 1). Pericyte loss is evident as an excessive number of pericyte 'ghosts' on viable capillaries, the 'ghost' referring to a pocket in the basement membrane that was formally occupied by a pericyte. Acellular capillaries apparently were functional capillaries that degenerated until only a basement membrane tube remains. Acellular, degenerate capillaries are not perfused, and are regarded as histologic markers of nonperfused capillaries [3]. As suggested by Ashton [4], and consistent with findings of Aguilar et al. [5], microaneurysms might be abortive attempts at vascular growth or proliferation.

Capillary occlusion initially occurs early in diabetes in single, isolated capillaries, and at that early stage is of no clinical significance. As more and more capillaries become occluded, however, local areas of the retina likely become deprived of oxygen and nutrients, contributing to produce one or more growth factors, such as vascular endothelial growth factor (VEGF), a key molecule leading to retinal neovascularization. Thus, capillary vaso-obliteration represents a discrete event that progressively contributes to the development of retinal ischemia, and presumably leads to later neovascularization. Although devoid of nuclei, these degenerate vessels sometimes are not truly acellular, and may be filled with cytoplasmic processes of glial cells [6]. Whether the invasion of retinal capillaries by glia in diabetes is secondary to capillary degeneration, or whether it initiates vessel occlusion and degeneration, is not known.

The basement membrane that surrounds retinal capillaries thickens in diabetes, and had been postulated to play a role in the development of the retinopathy. This view had become less popular in recent years, but that may need to be reexamined in light of the finding that the degeneration of retinal capillaries in galactose-fed rats, a model that develops the 'diabetic-like' retinopathy, can be significantly inhibited merely by inhibiting synthesis of fibronectin, a component of the basement membrane [7].

Histologically, loss of pericytes was regarded as the first capillary lesion of the retinopathy [8], but quantitation of apoptotic capillary cells in human and animal retinas indicates that both endothelial cells and pericytes are dying in diabetes [9]. Hammes et al. [10] reported nearly a 20% reduction in the number of pericytes after 2 months of diabetes in rats, based on immunologic identification of pericytes using an antibody against vitronectin and on morphological criteria (shape, relative position in the capillary). The magnitude and rapid development of this pericyte loss is important but surprising, and needs to be confirmed. A different method used to assess pericyte loss (quantification of the number of pericyte 'ghosts') has demonstrated a significant increase in the number of these pericyte 'carcasses' after 6–8 months of diabetes in rodents [11], but shorter durations apparently have not been studied. Researchers have reported an increase in the ratio of endothelial cells to pericytes (E/P ratio) in retinas from diabetic patients or animals

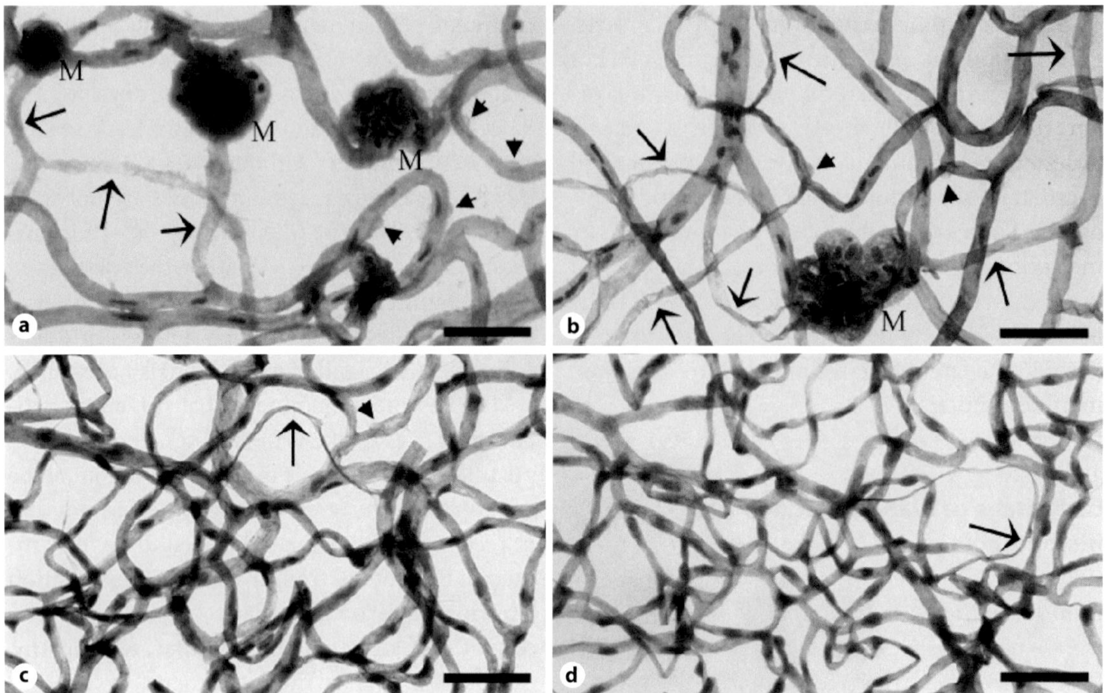

Fig. 1. Vascular lesions of diabetic retinopathy. Microaneurysm (M), acellular capillaries (arrows) and pericyte ghosts (arrowheads) in retinal capillaries from diabetic patient (**a**), diabetic dog (**b**), diabetic rat (**c**) and diabetic mouse (**d**). PAS and hematoxylin. All pictures were taken in the mid-retina and at the same magnification. Bars = 50 μm.

[8, 12, 13], and some have attributed this change to diabetes-induced pericyte loss. Two potential problems with this interpretation are that an increased E/P ratio could be due to endothelial cell proliferation, pericyte loss or both, and that an appreciable number of nuclei cannot be unambiguously attributed to endothelial cells or pericytes based on histological criteria, especially in mice [14, 15; Kern, unpubl. data], making it less favorable for current studies. Using antibodies that can specifically identify pericytes may be a better way to analyze pericyte density and loss.

Efforts to identify which lesion of the retinopathy comes first are further complicated by evidence that the capillary disease which develops in diabetes is not uniformly distributed across the retina [16, 17], and the rare lesions in early diabetes are difficult to differentiate from the occasional pericyte ghosts and obliterated capillaries found even in retinas of nondiabetic humans or animals. Thus, the mere presence of a few acellular capillaries or pericyte ghosts is not sufficient to claim that diabetic retinopathy is present; only when the numbers of lesions in diabetic subjects become statistically significantly greater than those in nondiabetic cohorts can the retinopathy be claimed to be really present.

Methods to Study the Retinal Vasculature

To investigate vascular changes in retinopathies, several methods have been developed. Those in which the vasculature bed is perfused with colored or fluorescent dye [18–21] provide information similar to that obtained by fluorescein angiography, but do not offer the opportunity to detect or quantitate pericyte loss and capillary degeneration, important histological markers of early stage of the retinopathy. Isolation of retinal vasculature allows histological as well as immunohistological analysis carried out on capillary cells. Methods in which retinal vasculature is isolated include (1) the trypsin digest method [12, 22]; (2) pepsin-trypsin digest [10]; (3) elastase method [23], and (4) osmotic isolation [14]. The first three methods involve incubation of formalin-fixed retina in a proteolytic solution. The trypsin digest method uses a crude proteolytic mixture, but surprisingly, trypsin is not the active agent in this mix (even if a trypsin inhibitor is added to this solution, the vessels still can be isolated [Kern unpubl. data]). Results achieved by the elastase method are morphologically comparable to those of the trypsin digest method, except that a purified, defined enzyme is responsible for the digestion. The osmotic isolation method uses unfixed retina. The advantage of using this method is that the isolated retinal vessels retain their metabolic activities, and thus can be used for Western blot analysis or for measuring activities of enzymes [24–28].

Changes in the Nonvascular Part of the Retina

The clinically demonstrable changes to the retinal vasculature in diabetes have led to the general assumption that the retinopathy is solely a microvascular disease. Nevertheless, it was recognized that structural and functional damage also occurred in nonvascular cells of the retina in diabetic human [29, 30]. Reduced amplitude and delayed latency of oscillatory potentials of electroretinogram are commonly found in diabetic patients [31–33]. There has been a growing appreciation of nonvascular changes that happened in the experimental diabetic animals. Loss of neuronal cells, including ganglion cells, horizontal cells, amacrine cells and photoreceptors, have been shown to undergo cell death within a few weeks after the onset of diabetes in rodents (detail description listed in sections below). Changes of neuronal function, mainly demonstrated by abnormal electroretinogram, have also been found in rodents after only several weeks of diabetes. Glia is another important component of the nonvascular part of the retina. Overexpression GFAP (glial fibrillary acidic protein), a hallmark of glial cell activation, has been reported in the retinas of diabetic rats [34] and in diabetic patients [35]. Whether or how the neurodegeneration and glial activation contribute to capillary degeneration in the retina of diabetes are still under investigation; however, glial activation and loss of ganglion cells seems not to happen in all diabetic animal models studied to date, suggesting that the changes of nonvascular components in diabetes might be regulated through different pathways from those involved in vascular lesions in diabetes [11].

Animal Models of Diabetic Retinopathy

The mechanisms of how diabetic retinopathy develops remain under investigation. Animal models of diabetic retinopathy are valuable in efforts to understand the pathogenesis of retinopathy and to identify promising therapies. Many different models have been described, and many of them have unique advantages or disadvantages which will be discussed below.

Questions occasionally arise about whether an animal model is relevant to type 1 diabetes or type 2 diabetes. This confusion seems to have arisen in part from use of the term 'noninsulin-dependent diabetes' as a description of type 2 diabetes in the past. The mere fact that diabetic animals (most commonly induced by streptozotocin) can survive without exogenous insulin is not sufficient justification to regard them as a model of type 2 diabetes. Current understanding of type 1 and type 2 diabetes suggests that the classification of type 2 diabetes should be based on the presence of insulin resistance and/or hyperinsulinemia, as well as hyperglycemia.

Type 1 Diabetes

Investigations focused on type 1 diabetes have used models in which diabetes has been experimentally induced with alloxan, streptozotocin, growth hormone or pancreatectomy. At least in dogs, the retinopathy that developed after these different diabetogenic insults was similar [Engerman and Kern, unpubl. data]. Early studies of animal models have been reviewed elsewhere [36–39].

Dogs and Cats

The anatomic features of retinopathy in diabetic dogs have been shown repeatedly to be morphologically indistinguishable from those of the nonproliferative phase of retinopathy seen in diabetic patients, including capillary microaneurysms, acellular (and nonperfused) capillaries, pericyte ghosts, varicose and dilated capillaries (or IRMAs), and dot and blot hemorrhages [6, 38, 40, 41]. Arteriolar smooth muscle cell loss also has been observed in diabetic humans and dogs [42, 43].

Microaneurysms, leukocyte and platelet plugging of aneurysms and venules, and degenerating endothelial cells likewise were observed in cats after several years of diabetes [44, 45]. These histologic abnormalities were confined to small regions, and these animals developed retinal hypoxia early in the development of diabetic retinopathy, before capillary dropout was evident. Hypoxia was correlated with endothelial cell death, leukocyte plugging of vessels, and microaneurysms.

As is true in diabetic humans, there is a long interval before retinopathy becomes manifest in diabetic dogs or cats, capillary aneurysms usually not beginning to appear in these animals until about 2–3 years after induction of elevated hexose levels. Likewise, after about 2 years of hyperglycemia in diabetic dogs, increasing numbers of retinal capillaries come to possess endothelial cells but few or no pericytes. Gradual obliteration of retinal vessels is apparent histologically from the increasing numbers of acellular capillaries that are scattered singly and in small groups on the retinal vasculature, especially in the temporal retina [16]. After 5 years of insulin-deficient diabetes, all dogs have marked vascular lesions of retinopathy. The reason for the prolonged interval before retinopathy develops is unknown, but any explanation of this latent period might offer valuable insight into the pathogenesis of the retinopathy. Improved glycemic control has been found to significantly inhibit the development and progression of retinopathy in diabetic dogs [46, 47] and in patients [48, 49]. Neovascularization has been observed to develop in diabetic dogs, albeit only within the retina and not in the preretinal vitreous [50]. However, the cost, slow development of lesions, and lack of availability of antibodies or molecular approaches have made dog and cat models less used for the study of the retinopathy in recent years.

Rats

Diabetic rats have been the most commonly used animals in studies of the retinopathy. They develop at least the early stages of the retinopathy within only months of diabetes, are inexpensive to house, easy to handle, and experimental tools (including antibodies) are widely available.

Chemically Induced Diabetic Models

During the past decade, streptozotocin-diabetic or alloxan-diabetic rats have been a primary model for research into the pathogenesis of diabetic retinopathy, especially the vascular lesions. These models reproducibly develop acellular, degenerate capillaries, pericyte loss and basement membrane thickening, which are characteristic of early stage of vascular lesions of the retinopathy. Immunohistochemical methods have demonstrated a significant loss of pericytes after 2 months of diabetes [10], whereas numbers of pericyte ghosts have not been significantly increased until about 6 months of diabetes [26, 51–53]. More advanced stages of the retinal microvascular disease (microaneurysms, IRMA, and hemorrhages) have not been reported to develop reproducibly, although some of these abnormalities have been reported at 28 months of diabetes [54]. Vascular abnormalities consistent with possible neovascularization also have been observed [54; Kern, unpubl. data], but these new vessels have been formed within the retina, and not in the preretinal vitreous.

Recently, there has been renewed appreciation of diabetes-induced damage to nonvascular cells of the retina in animals. Diabetic rats lose ganglion cells [55–66], and this neurodegeneration has been detected as early as 1 month of diabetes [59]. Thus, the retinal nonvascular abnormality seems to precede the development of the vascular cell changes in diabetes, raising a possibility that this neurodegeneration might contribute to the pathogenesis of the vascular disease. This possibility has yet to be conclusively studied, but Nepafenac, a cyclooxygenase inhibitor, was able to prevent diabetes-induced degeneration of retinal capillaries while having no effect on the loss of retinal ganglion cells [67].

Retinal glial cells also undergo changes in diabetes in rats. Müller glial cells in diabetic rats were reported to become apoptotic [58], to show an increased nuclear translocation of glyceraldehydes-3-phosphate dehydrogenase [68] (a change that has been strongly linked to apoptosis), and to change from a quiescent phenotype to an injury-associated phenotype with high levels of expressed GFAP [34, 58, 61, 63, 69–73]. In contrast, the number of retinal Müller cells and microglia in rats diabetic for 4 weeks has been reported to be significantly greater than normal [34].

Horizontal cells [61, 65], amacrine cells [74] and photoreceptors [65] also have been reported to undergo degeneration in diabetic rats. However, these changes are not known to be characteristic of retinal changes seen in diabetic patients, and the significance and reproducibility of these changes in animals remains to be learned.

Spontaneously Diabetic Models

The study of animals displaying spontaneous diabetic syndromes has contributed significantly to the understanding of the diabetic syndromes of human, but these models have been less well studied with regard to development of diabetic retinopathy, and have been focused predominantly on vascular lesions.

Diabetic BB (BioBreeding) or BBW (BioBreeding Wistar) rats were discovered in 1974, and both sexes are affected. Overt insulin-dependent diabetes occurs from 40 to 140 days of age, with a mean age at onset of glycosuria of about 90 days. Diabetic BB rats exhibit retinal lesions similar to those observed in rats having chemically induced diabetes, including pericyte loss, basement membrane thickening, 'microinfarctions with areas of nonperfusion' (i.e. capillary degeneration), and an absence of microaneurysms after 8–11 months of diabetes [75–78]. Pancreas transplantation inhibited development of the retinal microvascular lesions in this model [77].

Spontaneously diabetic Torii (SDT) is an inbred rat strain established from a colony of normal Sprague-Dawley rats in 1997. Male Torii rats exhibit spontaneous glucose intolerance with impaired insulin secretion at 14 weeks of age, and by 20 weeks of age, they develop diabetes with marked hyperglycemia and insulin deficiency, and develop severe ocular lesions [79]. This model has been originally claimed to be a model of type 2 diabetes, apparently due to the fact the hyperglycemic rats can survive for a long time without insulin therapy. However, greatly subnormal levels of insulin and loss of body weight in hyperglycemic animals suggest that this model better represents type 1 diabetes. Investigations on the ocular disorders developed in this model gave inconsistent results. The first report about this animal model demonstrated that SDT rats develop ocular complications such as cataracts (by 40 weeks of age) and retinal detachment with fibrous proliferation (by 70 weeks of age) [79]. However, fluorescein angiography and immunohistochemistry have demonstrated nonperfusion and neovascularization in the retina at the extraordinarily short duration (5–10 weeks) of diabetes, and the histopathological changes were inhibited by pancreas transplantation [80]. Actually, the data only suggest increased vascular density in the outer plexiform layer, which in our opinion is not sufficient to claim neovascularization happened in this model. In light of these original reports, it is surprising that Yamada et al. [81] claim that male SDT rats at the age of 50 weeks show proliferative retinopathy without evidence of vascular nonperfusion. The proliferations affected 50% of the animals, with all of the neovascularization originating from the optic disc. More studies need to prove these are truly new vessels, and not merely incomplete regression of the hyaloid vasculature.

Old male WBN/Kob rats are spontaneously hyperglycemic, and develop cataracts, nephropathy, neuropathy, pancreatic fibrosis and hyperlipemia at about 9 months of age. Females do not develop these abnormalities [82]. Degeneration of retinal capillaries and preretinal neovascularization has been reported at 19 and 24 months of age, respectively [83]; but photographic documentation of the new vessels has been equivocal. Transmission electron microscopy revealed thickened capillary basement membranes [84, 85], but neither microaneurysms nor arteriovenous shunts were seen [84]. Retinal degeneration (not typical histologic lesion of diabetic retinopathy) also occurred in this model [85–87]. The possible contribution of retinal degeneration or incomplete regression of the hyaloid vasculature to these vascular abnormalities remains to be demonstrated.

Mice

In the 1970s and 1980s, there were a number of attempts to determine whether or not mice developed diabetic retinopathy, but the results were controversial [88–91]. Since then, mice were little studied with respect to diabetic retinopathy until recently.

Recent studies have begun to characterize the development of retinopathy in the streptozotocin-diabetic C57Bl/6J mouse and spontaneously type 1 diabetic Akita ($Ins2^{Akita}$) mouse. C57B1/6J mice develop vascular pathology characteristic of diabetic retinopathy (acellular capillaries, pericyte ghosts and capillary cell apoptosis) beginning at about 6 months of diabetes, and the number of acellular capillaries and pericyte ghosts becomes more numerous with increasing duration of diabetes [11, 92]. Whether or not neurodegeneration occurs in the diabetic C57Bl/6J model is less clear to date; some investigators have reported a 20–25% loss of cells in the ganglion cell layer after only 14 weeks of diabetes [66], whereas others have detected no evidence of ganglion cell loss after as long as a year of diabetes [11, 93, 94]. Diabetic C57Bl/6J mice have not been found to show Müller glial cell activation (based on GFAP induction) [63, 95], other than a transient increase soon after induction of diabetes [11].

More genetically modified C57B1/6J mice have been used to explore the roles of certain molecules in the pathogenesis of diabetes-induced retinal vascular disease. Diabetic mice deficient in the genes encoding CD18 and ICAM-1 (the adhesion molecules involved in leukocyte adherence to the vessel wall) were observed to develop less degeneration of retinal capillaries, pericyte loss, as well as associated abnormalities including leukostasis, increased capillary permeability and capillary basement membrane thickening compared to the wild-type diabetic mice [53]. Diabetic mice deficient in iNOS [93] or 5-lipoxygenase [94], both key enzymes involved in the inflammatory response, also developed less capillary degeneration, pericyte ghosts, leukostasis, and superoxide compared to the wild-type diabetic mice. Diabetic mice overexpressing mitochondrial superoxide dismutase were protected from diabetes-induced loss of mitochondrial GSH and increased mitochondrial membrane permeability (swelling) in the retina, and also developed less degeneration of retinal capillaries [96]. All of these genetically modified mice provide valuable novel insights about critical molecules that involved in the pathogenesis of the retinopathy.

The $Ins2^{Akita}$ mouse contains a dominant point mutation in the insulin 2 gene that induces spontaneous type 1 diabetes with a rapid onset. Heterozygous $Ins2^{Akita}$ males show hyperglycemia and hypoinsulinemia after 4 weeks of age [97]. Compared with sibling control mice (homozygous for the wild-type insulin 2 gene), heterozygous $Ins2^{Akita}$ male mice developed increased retinal vascular permeability after 12 weeks of hyperglycemia; characteristic retinal vascular pathology markers including acellular capillaries and pericyte ghosts were also found to develop with increasing duration of diabetes [95]. In contrast to streptozotocin-diabetic C57Bl/6J mice, heterozygous $Ins2^{Akita}$ males showed significant reductions in the thickness of the inner plexiform and inner nuclear layers and loss of cell bodies in the retinal ganglion cell layer after 22 weeks of hyperglycemia [95]. Diabetes-induced ganglion cell loss in this model occurs mostly in the peripheral retina without significant change in the central retina [98]. Although alterations in the morphology of astrocytes and microglia were observed in $Ins2^{Akita}$ mice, glial cell activation was not observed in this model [95].

Compared to the other models mentioned above, mice models have the advantage in that genetic modifications are relatively easy to achieve, reagents and antibodies are readily available, housing is relatively inexpensive, and the histopathology develops relatively quickly. Whether or not there are differences among the various strains of mouse with regard to development of diabetic retinopathy remains to be explored.

Other Animal Models of Type 1 Diabetes

Species used in studies of the effect of diabetes on the retina also have included spontaneously diabetic fish [99], but these reports were only descriptive in nature, and have unclear relevance for the mammalian retina. Recently, Gleeson et al. [100] induced hyperglycemia in zebrafish by putting the fish in water containing glucose. After 28 days in this environment, blood glucose levels in treated fish were increased, and the inner plexiform and inner nuclear layers were significantly thinner in the hyperglycemic fish. Some laboratory species, including guinea pigs, rabbits and fish, are inherently of limited usefulness for the study of the vascular lesions of diabetic retinopathy. The guinea pig retina is avascular, as is much of the rabbit retina, and the retinal vessels in rabbits are tortuous and limited chiefly to the most superficial inner layers of nasal and temporal retina.

Type 2 Diabetes

Animal models of type 2 diabetes have been less utilized in studies of diabetic retinopathy, and most of those studies so far have focused on the vascular lesions of the retinopathy. Animal models of this type commonly are obese, hyperglycemic, hyperinsulinemic and in some cases, hypertensive.

Rats

The Zucker diabetic fatty rat (ZDF/Gmi-fa, formerly designated as ZDF/Drt) is a partially inbred strain in which the genetic propensity for diabetes is only found in about 50% of obese males. These obese males are born normoglycemic and normoinsulinemic but become frankly hyperglycemic at 6–7 weeks of age [101, 102]. Thereafter, they maintain blood glucose levels at around 500 mg/dl throughout life. Evaluation of the retinal vasculature in this model after approximately 5 months of diabetes revealed that retinal capillary basement membrane thickness was greater than normal, but surprisingly also that the capillary cell nuclear density (hypercellularity) in the retinas of diabetic animals was *greater* than normal compared to lean controls [15, 103], while no pericyte ghosts or acellular capillaries were observed [103]. However, Behl et al. [104] recently observed increases in pericyte ghosts and acellular capillaries in ZDF rats diabetic for about 6 months.

The Goto-Kakizaki rat represents a model of hereditary noninsulin-dependent diabetes mellitus, characterized by mild hyperglycemia, impaired glucose tolerance, and a markedly defective insulin response to glucose but no obesity. Only mild morphological retinal vascular changes were detected after 2-year study. An increase in the ratio of retinal capillary endothelial cells to pericytes was detected at 8 months of age [105]. No pericyte ghosts or increased acellular vessels were detected [105], but a recent study reported increased TUNEL-positive retinal microvascular cells in these rats [106].

The BBZDP/Wor strain is an obese, hypertensive, and insulin-resistant type 2 diabetic rat model, generated by introgressing the faulty $Lepr^{fa}$ allele from the Zucker fatty rat into the BB rat background. These animals have been reported to develop pericyte loss and retinal capillary basement thickening [107].

The Otsuka Long-Evans Tokushima fatty (OLETF) rat develops a spontaneous noninsulin-dependent diabetes mellitus, including polyuria, polydipsia and mild obesity. The blood sugar level of OLETF rats becomes higher than that of control rats after 5 months of age, and at 14 months of age, retinal capillary basement membrane has been reported to be significantly thicker, and the ratio of pericyte area to the capillary cross-section area significantly lower than that of nondiabetic controls rats [108]. In addition, the number of cells in the inner nuclear layer and photoreceptor layers of the retina decreased, endothelial cells showed ultrastructural evidence of degeneration, and vascular corrosion casts showed microaneurysm-like lesions and other vascular abnormalities [109]. In contrast, other investigators found no pericyte ghosts, no increase in number of acellular capillaries in 45-week-old OLETF rats, and the authors concluded that this strain of rat was not a good model for studying the vascular lesions of diabetic retinopathy [110]. However, the lack of the vascular degeneration in this model could be due to the short duration of diabetes that the authors had been investigated. A recent report demonstrated that there were significantly fewer ganglion cells in the retinas of 35-week-old OLETF rats compared to their nondiabetic controls [111]. Unfortunately, in this report, no vascular lesions of this model had been investigated. Whether the neurodegeneration is independent of vascular degeneration in the retinas of this model remains to be demonstrated.

Obese Koletsky (SHROB) rats [112, 113], in which an autosomal recessive mutation of the leptin receptor resulted in hypertension, obesity, hyperlipidemia, and hyperinsulinemia after 4–6 weeks of age, also have been used in studies of retinopathy. Examination of the retinal vasculature in the Koletsky rats demonstrated degeneration and loss of intramural pericytes and extensive capillary dropout after 3 months of age in lean and obese rats, with more frequent pathology observed in the obese rat [114]. Retinal capillary dropout is severe and progressive, resulting in some cases in preretinal neovascularization after 6–12 months of age [Khosrof and Benetz unpubl. data]. No microaneurysms and retinal hemorrhages were found. However, these reports were only descriptive, with no quantitative or mechanistic studies to explain the histopathology.

The spontaneously hypertensive/NIH-corpulent rat strain is another genetic model developed for the study of obesity and diabetes. This strain resulted from mating Koletsky rats (which are heterozygous for the *cp* gene) with SHR rats. Obesity and diabetes are most pronounced when the weaning rats are provided with a high-sucrose diet [115], although diabetes also occurs with chow diet at the age of 10–18 weeks [116]. Obese male rats are mildly hypertensive, and when fed with high-sucrose diet, exhibit metabolic alterations associated with noninsulin-dependent diabetes mellitus, including hyperinsulinemia, hyperlipidemia, glucose intolerance, and glycosuria [115]. After 24 weeks of consuming a 54% sucrose diet, increased numbers of pericyte ghosts were detected in the obese diabetic rats compared to lean nondiabetic controls fed with sucrose diet. Endothelial cell proliferation, capillary dilation, and varicose loop formation were noted in some of these animals [78].

The spontaneously hypertensive/McCune-corpulent rat (SHR/N:Mcc-cp) was derived by breeding the SHR/N-cp with the Koletsky rat [117]. Male rats develop glucosuria, polyuria, proteinuria, glucose intolerance, and insulin resistance in a short period of time. At 6 months of age, the males showed an increased E/P ratio, increased basement membrane thickness, and capillary obstruction [118]. Acellular capillaries and pericyte ghosts were also detected in these animals but not quantified in this study.

The nonobese, SDT rat has been claimed to be a model of type 2 diabetes, but greatly subnormal levels of insulin and loss of body weight as hyperglycemia appears strongly suggest that this model is more representative of type 1 diabetes.

Mice

Although multiple type 2 diabetic mouse models exist, few of them have been used to study the pathogenesis of diabetic retinopathy. Leptin receptor-deficient db/db mice *($Lepr^{db}$)* are spontaneous diabetes. These animals become obese at approximately 3–4 weeks of age, increase in plasma insulin at 10–14 days and elevations of blood glucose at 4–8 weeks. Homozygous mutant mice are polyphagic, polydipsic, and polyuric. Diabetic *db/db* mice have been observed to develop an increased E/P ratio compared to that in nondiabetic controls, and to develop strand-like and relatively acellular capillaries [119]. Thickening of retinal capillary basement membranes also has been detected in this diabetic mouse strain at the age of 22 weeks [120]. Fifteen-month-old *db/db* mice were reported to have blood-retinal barrier breakdown, loss of pericytes, and increased apoptosis of retinal ganglion cells and other cells of the neural retina. Glial cells showed evidence of concurrent degeneration and proliferation, and in contrast to type 1 models of diabetes in mice, also glial activation [121]. These animals also showed increased density of retinal capillaries in the inner nuclear layer, which was interpreted as evidence of vessel proliferation. To investigate whether hyperlipidemia accelerates the development of retinal vascular histopathology, both hyperglycemia and hyperlipidemia (HGHL) mouse model was made by crossing *db/db* mice with apolipoprotein E-deficient mice. The HGHL mice at 6 months of age exhibited accelerated development of acellular capillaries and pericyte ghosts compared with littermate control animals, demonstrating that hyperlipidemia can accelerate the degeneration of retinal capillaries in diabetes [122].

The KK mouse strain exhibits glucose intolerance and insulin resistance, and becomes obese with aging [123]. Pericyte ghosts, acellular capillaries with occasional microaneurysms have been reported between 20 and 64 weeks of age in this model [89]. Introduction of lethal yellow *agouti* gene (A^y) into KK mice resulted in KKA^y mice [124], which are characterized by early onset and prolongation of severe levels of hyperinsulinemia, hyperglycemia, obesity and yellow coat color [125], accompanied by pathological changes in a variety of tissues [126]. After 1 month of diabetes, the numbers of apoptotic cells in the retinal ganglion cell and inner nuclear layers were significantly greater in the diabetic KKA^y mice than in the control group, and the rate of cell death increased with the duration of diabetes [127]. After 3 months of diabetes, the major changes in the retinal capillaries involved mitochondria, with endothelial cell hyperplasia, basement membrane thickening, and some edema and vacuolar degeneration of capillary cells [127].

Other Animal Models of Type 2 Diabetes
Aging primates commonly become obese and develop insulin resistance, and in some cases, also hypertension. Retinas from these diabetic animals have been found to show hemorrhages, large areas of retinal capillary nonperfusion, cotton-wool spots, intraretinal hemorrhages, and hard exudates in the macula. Formation of small IRMAs and microaneurysms were associated with the areas of nonperfusion, and some animals developed macular edema [128–130]. As would be expected, monkeys with type 2 diabetes have many of the angiopathic changes associated with human diabetic retinopathy, but hypertension correlates with the severity of the diabetic retinopathy.

Diabetic hamsters develop the usual spectrum of lesions, including acellular capillaries, pericyte loss, endothelial proliferation, but lack microaneurysms or neovascularization [131].

Nondiabetic Models That Develop a Diabetic-Like Retinopathy

Hexose Feeding Models
Galactose Feeding
The importance of hyperglycemia per se in the pathogenesis of diabetic retinopathy was demonstrated a number of years ago by study of normal, nondiabetic dogs fed a galactose-rich diet [132]. During the 3–5 years of study, nondiabetic dogs fed a 30% galactose diet developed a retinopathy that was indistinguishable from that of diabetic dogs and patients, including microaneurysms, vaso-obliteration, pericyte ghosts, and hemorrhages [16, 41, 132–141]. Likewise, experimental galactosemia has been shown to cause diabetic-like retinal lesions also in rats and mice. Nondiabetic rats and mice fed a 50 or 30% galactose diet develop a significantly greater than normal prevalence of acellular capillaries and pericyte ghosts, excessive thickening of capillary basement membrane and, eventually, IRMA in galactose-fed rats and rare but unmistakable saccular microaneurysms in galactose-fed mice [52, 53, 138, 142–147].

The galactose retinopathy model was utilized extensively for studies of the role of aldose reductase in the pathogenesis of 'diabetic-like' retinopathy [16, 41, 133–145]. Nevertheless, biochemical sequelae of galactosemia are not merely limited to increased activity of aldose reductase, and have been found since to include increased levels of nonenzymatic glycation, protein kinase C activity, and oxidative stress [24, 148–155]. More recently, the model has been used also in studies of the role of leukostasis in the development of retinopathy [53], and the ability of aminoguanidine, antioxidants and antisense against fibronectin to inhibit the retinopathy [7, 51, 52].

As a means for producing a model of diabetic retinopathy in animals, experimental galactosemia can be advantageous because it is easily established and requires less nursing care than experimental diabetes. Not to be overlooked, however, is the expense of the galactose diet, which can be costly if animals are large or numerous. Moreover, the galactose-induced retinopathy has at least two important differences from that in diabetes. First, the galactose-induced retinopathy develops despite the absence of many of the systemic abnormalities of metabolism that are characteristic of diabetes (such as those involving concentrations of glucose, insulin, fatty acids, etc.) [132]. This is valuable, in that it demonstrates that excessive blood hexose (either glucose or galactose) is important in the initiation of retinopathy. The second difference between the retinopathies induced by diabetes and galactose feeding is a different response to at least one therapy. Aminoguanidine has been shown several times to inhibit the retinal microvascular disease in diabetic dogs and rat [51, 146, 156, 157], but has not been found to do so in galactose-fed rats [51, 158]. Moreover, caspases activated in diabetic mice differ from those induced in galactose-fed mice [92]. Thus, although the final histopathology induced by galactosemia seems morphologically identical to that in diabetes, the biochemical steps leading to that pathology apparently differ between the two models. Degeneration of retinal neurons apparently has not yet been assessed in galactosemic models.

Sucrose or Fructose Feeding

Nondiabetic rats fed very high concentrations of sucrose or fructose (approximately 70% in the diet) also have been reported to develop retinal lesions, including loss of pericytes and endothelial cells, and formation of capillary strands [159, 160].

Models with Altered Growth Factor Levels

VEGF Overexpression

VEGF 165 was injected into the eyes of normal cynomolgus monkeys, and as a result, capillaries became nonperfused, dilated, and tortuous [161]. Preretinal neovascularization was observed throughout peripheral retina, but not in the posterior pole. Arterioles demonstrated endothelial cell hyperplasia and microaneurysmal dilations. Thus, pharmacologic doses of VEGF alone were able to produce many features of nonproliferative and proliferative diabetic retinopathy.

Insulin-Like Growth Factor Overexpression

Nondiabetic mice overexpressing insulin-like growth factor-1 (IGF-1) in the retina developed several vascular alterations characteristic of diabetic retinopathy, including nonproliferative lesions (pericyte loss, thickened capillary basement membrane, intraretinal microvascular abnormalities), proliferative retinopathy, and retinal detachment [162]. Likewise, injection of a single dose of hrIGF-1 into the vitreous cavity of pigs resulted in an angiopathy that included increased endothelial density, basement membrane thickening, vascular leakage, and microaneurysms) [163]. No acellular capillaries or pericyte ghosts were detected.

Genetic Platelet-Derived Growth Factor-Modified Mice

Platelet-derived growth factor (PDGF) has major effects on pericyte activation, survival, and growth [164]. Mice with a genetic ablation of PDGF-B exhibit several vascular phenotypes characteristic of diabetic retinopathy, including microvascular leakage and hemorrhage, pericyte loss and microaneurysms in brain capillaries [165, 166]. In the retina of PDGF-B heterozygous mice, a reduction in pericyte numbers was accompanied by a slight but significant increase in the numbers of acellular capillaries compared to their wild-type littermates [167]. In chronic hyperglycemia, PDGF-B heterozygous mice developed aggravated retinopathy, including high numbers of acellular capillaries and the formation of microaneurysms. Specific ablation of PDGF-B on the endothelium also caused pericyte dropout, vessel occlusion, capillary regression and vascular proliferation [166]. Overexpression of PDGF-A under the control of the rhodopsin promoter resulted in extensive proliferation of glial cells and traction retinal detachment without vascular cell involvement, whereas overexpression of PDGF-B under the control of rhodopsin promoter resulted in tractional retinal detachment and proliferation of both vascular and nonvascular cells [168].

Other Models

Several retinal lesions consistent with diabetic retinopathy have also been detected after sympathectomy in rats [169]. Experimental elimination of sympathetic innervation to the eye by removal of the superior cervical ganglion (demonstrated by ptosis of the eyelid) has been reported to result in increased expression of basement membrane proteins, increased capillary basement membrane thickness and reduced number of capillary pericytes. Increased GFAP staining was also noted after sympathectomy in the ganglion cell layer [170]. There was a significant reduction in the number of photoreceptors due to apoptosis and changes of choroidal vascularity in the sympathectomized eye [171]. All these data raise a possibility that sympathetic nerves may play a role in diabetes-induced vascular disorders of the eye [172].

Retinal ischemia and reperfusion caused by elevated ocular pressure in nondiabetic rats and mice has been used to study the mechanism of neurodegeneration in the retina. A recent report demonstrated that after severe neuron death in the retina, increased numbers of 'diabetic retinopathy-like' acellular, degenerate capillaries were also found in this model [173]. The model can be used to study the relationship between neuronal degeneration and vascular degeneration in the retina. Fast development of 'diabetic retinopathy-like' acellular capillaries (weeks after injury) makes this model attractive for screening purposes of potential vaso- or neuroprotective agents, but how closely the cause of capillary and neural degeneration of this model matches those of diabetes remains to be established.

Neovascularization

Retinal neovascularization is the abnormal growth of new vessels, and is not merely increased vascular density of previously formed vessels or incomplete regression of the hyaloid vasculature. To date, diabetic animal models (without other genetic modifications or experimental manipulations) have not been demonstrated to reproducibly progress to preretinal neovascularization, and some have criticized the available diabetic models for this failure.

Why diabetic animals do not develop preretinal neovascularization is an important question. Vaso-obliteration and subsequent retinal ischemia are believed to be major causes of neovascularization in the retina, so one likely reason that the diabetic models have not developed preretinal neovascularization is that much less vaso-obliteration develops in the retina of the diabetic animals during the short duration of diabetes that they are studied (as compared to the more extensive vaso-obliteration that develops over many years in diabetic patients). Moreover, diabetic or galactosemic animals *have* been demonstrated to develop intraretinal vessel structures that are characteristic of intraretinal neovascularization [50]. These vessels, identified by their lack of basement membrane and 'chicken-wire' pattern that is characteristic of embryonic vessels, have developed within the retina in diabetic dogs and experimentally galactosemic dogs, but have not extended into the vitreous during the 5 years of study. New vessels extending into the vitreous have been reported in 2 of 9 dogs fed galactose for 6–7 years [137]. The diabetic Ren-2 rat has been demonstrated to develop proliferation of retinal endothelial cells, but overt neovascularization has not been demonstrated [174]. The endothelial proliferation in these rats can be attenuated by renin-angiotensin system blockade via VEGF-dependent pathways.

Conclusions

The early vascular lesions of diabetic retinopathy have been found to develop in essentially most species studied who have had diabetes for long durations. Thus, there is no evidence that the ability to develop microvascular lesions characteristic of the early stages of diabetic retinopathy is in any way unique to only some species. The relationship between neuronal injury, glial injury and vascular injury in diabetic retinopathy are still under investigation.

The use of animal models of diabetic retinopathy likely will continue to contribute on multiple fronts. Rats and genetically modified mice are likely to remain the most utilized models to study the pathogenesis of the retinopathy and in efforts to develop pharmacological therapies to inhibit it. The Animal Models of Diabetic Complications Consortium (AMDCC; www.amdcc.org) is available to facilitate the development of new animal models of diabetic complications, including retinopathy. Genetically altered mice will be a valuable resource to investigate the role of specific genes in the pathogenesis of the retinopathy. There remains considerable value, however, in the use also of larger animals as models of diabetic retinopathy, since the rate at which the retinopathy develops, the life span of the animals, and the size of eye are more comparable to that of humans. Moreover, only primates have the macula, an important site of damage in diabetic retinopathy.

Animal models of diabetic retinopathy have provided a wealth of information pertaining to biochemical, physiological, and histopathologic abnormalities that contribute to the development of diabetic retinopathy. New opportunities can be expected to arise for use of the models in increasingly sophisticated methods of investigation, but advantages and deficiencies of the various models need to be recognized in order to utilize them to their fullest potential.

References

1 Davis MD, Kern TS, Rand LI: Diabetic Retinopathy; in Alberti KGMM, Zimmet P, DeFronzo RA (eds): International Textbook of Diabetes Mellitus, ed 2. New York, John Wiley & Sons, 1997, pp 1413–1446.

2 Cunha-Vaz J, Faria de Abreu JR, Campos AJ: Early breakdown of the blood-retinal barrier in diabetes. Br J Ophthalmol 1975;59:649–656.

3 Kohner EM, Henkind P: Correlation of fluorescein angiogram and retinal digest in diabetic retinopathy. Am J Ophthalmol 1970;69:403–414.

4 Ashton N: Pathogenesis of diabetic retinopathy; in Little HLJR, Patz A, Forsham PH (ed): Diabetic Retinopathy. New York, Thieme-Stratton Inc., 1983, pp 85–106.

5 Aguilar E, Friedlander M, Gariano RF: Endothelial proliferation in diabetic retinal microaneurysms. Arch Ophthalmol 2003;121:740–741.

6 Engerman RL: Pathogenesis of diabetic retinopathy. Diabetes 1989;38:1203–1206.

7 Roy S, Sato T, Paryani G, Kao R: Downregulation of fibronectin overexpression reduces basement membrane thickening and vascular lesions in retinas of galactose-fed rats. Diabetes 2003;52:1229–1234.

8 Cogan DG, Kuwabara T: The mural cell in perspective. Arch Ophthalmol 1967;78:133–139.

9 Mizutani M, Kern TS, Lorenzi M: Accelerated death of retinal microvascular cells in human and experimental diabetic retinopathy. J Clin Invest 1996;97:2883–2890.

10 Hammes HP, Lin J, Wagner P, Feng Y, Vom Hagen F, Krzizok T, Renner O, Breier G, Brownlee M, Deutsch U: Angiopoietin-2 causes pericyte dropout in the normal retina: evidence for involvement in diabetic retinopathy. Diabetes 2004;53:1104–1110.

11 Feit-Leichman RA, Kinouchi R, Takeda M, Fan Z, Mohr S, Kern TS, Chen DF: Vascular damage in a mouse model of diabetic retinopathy: relation to neuronal and glial changes. Invest Ophthalmol Vis Sci 2005;46:4281–4287.

12 Cogan DG, Toussaint D, Kuwabara T: Retinal vascular patterns. IV. Diabetic retinopathy. Arch Ophthalmol 1961;66:366–378.

13 Kuwabara T, Cogan DG: Retinal vascular patterns. VI. Mural cells of the retinal capillaries. Arch Ophthalmol 1963;69:492–502.

14 Cuthbertson RA, Mandel TE: Anatomy of the mouse retina. Endothelial cell-pericyte ratio and capillary distribution. Invest Ophthalmol Vis Sci 1986;27:1659–1664.

15 Danis RP, Yang Y: Microvascular retinopathy in the Zucker diabetic fatty rat. Invest Ophthalmol Vis Sci 1993;34:2367–2371.

16 Kern TS, Engerman RL: Vascular lesions in diabetes are distributed non-uniformly within the retina. Exp Eye Res 1995;60:545–549.

17 Tang J, Mohr S, Du Y, Kern TS: Non-uniform distribution of lesions and biochemical abnormalities within the retina of diabetic humans. Curr Eye Res 2003;27:7–13.

18 Danis RP, Wallow IL: HRP/trypsin technique for studies of the retinal vasculature. Invest Ophthalmol Vis Sci 1986;27:434–437.

19 Penn JS, Gay CA: Computerized digital image analysis of retinal vessel density: application to normoxic and hyperoxic rearing of the newborn rat. Exp Eye Res 1992;54:329–336.

20 D'Amato R, Wesolowski E, Smith LE: Microscopic visualization of the retina by angiography with high-molecular-weight fluorescein-labeled dextrans in the mouse. Microvasc Res 1993;46:135–142.

21 Ben-nun J, Alder VA, Constable IJ: Retinal microvascular patency in the diabetic rat. Int Ophthalmol 2004;25:187–192.
22 Kuwabara T, Cogan DG: Studies of retinal vascular patterns: I. Normal architecture. Arch Ophthalmol 1960;64:904–911.
23 Laver NM, Robison WG Jr, Pfeffer BA: Novel procedures for isolating intact retinal vascular beds from diabetic humans and animal models. Invest Ophthalmol Vis Sci 1993;34:2097–2104.
24 Kowluru RA, Jirousek MR, Stramm LE, Farid NA, Engerman RL, Kern TS: Abnormalities of retinal metabolism in diabetes or experimental galactosemia. V. Relationship between protein kinase C and ATPases. Diabetes 1998;47:464–469.
25 Badr GA, Tang J, Ismail-Beigi F, Kern TS: Diabetes down-regulates Glut1 expression in retina and its microvessels, but not in cerebral cortex or its microvessels. Diabetes 2000;49:1016–1021.
26 Zheng L, Szabo C, Kern TS: Poly(ADP-ribose) polymerase is involved in the development of diabetic retinopathy via regulation of nuclear factor-kappaB. Diabetes 2004;53:2960–2967.
27 Podesta F, Romeo G, Liu WH, Krajewski S, Reed JC, Gerhardinger C, Lorenzi M: Bax is increased in the retina of diabetic subjects and is associated with pericyte apoptosis in vivo and in vitro. Am J Pathol 2000;156:1025–1032.
28 Dagher Z, Park YS, Asnaghi V, Hoehn T, Gerhardinger C, Lorenzi M: Studies of rat and human retinas predict a role for the polyol pathway in human diabetic retinopathy. Diabetes 2004;53:2404–2411.
29 Bresnick GM, Palta M: Predicting progression of severe proliferative diabetic retinopathy. Arch Ophthalmol 1987;105:810–814.
30 Bresnick GH, Palta M: Oscillatory potential amplitudes: Relation to severity of diabetic retinopathy. Arch Ophthalmol 1987;105:929–933.
31 Falsini B, Porciatti V, Scalia G, Caputo S, Minnella A, Di Leo MA, Ghirlanda G: Steady-state pattern electroretinogram in insulin-dependent diabetics with no or minimal retinopathy. Doc Ophthalmol 1989;73:193–200.
32 Caputo S, Di Leo MA, Falsini B, Ghirlanda G, Porciatti V, Minella A, Greco AV: Evidence for early impairment of macular function with pattern ERG in type I diabetic patients. Diabetes Care 1990;13:412–418.
33 Prager TC, Garcia CA, Mincher CA, Mishra J, Chu HH: The pattern electroretinogram in diabetes. Am J Ophthalmol 1990;109:279–284.
34 Rungger-Brandle E, Dosso AA, Leuenberger PM: Glial reactivity, an early feature of diabetic retinopathy. Invest Ophth Vis Sci 41:1971–1980, 2000
35 Carrasco E, Hernandez C, de Torres I, Farres J, Simo R: Lowered cortistatin expression is an early event in the human diabetic retina and is associated with apoptosis and glial activation. Mol Vis 2008;14:1496–1502.
36 Engerman RL, Meyer RK, Buesseler JA: Effects of alloxan diabetes and steroid hypertension on retinal vasculature. Am J Ophthalmol 1964;58:965–978.
37 Toussaint D: Contribution a l'etude anatomique et clinque de la retinopathie diabetique chez l'homme et chez l'animal. Pathologia Eur 1968:108–148.
38 Engerman RL, Finkelstein D, Aguirre G, Diddie K, Fox R, Frank R, Varma S: Appropriate animal models for research on human diabetes mellitus and its complications. Ocular complications. Diabetes 1982;31(suppl 1):82–88.
39 Engerman RL, Kern TS: Retinopathy in animal models of diabetes. Diabetes Metab Rev 1995;11:109–120.
40 Engerman RL, Bloodworth JMB Jr: Experimental diabetic retinopathy in dogs. Arch Ophthalmol 1965;73:205–210.
41 Engerman RL, Kern TS: Aldose reductase inhibition fails to prevent retinopathy in diabetic and galactosemic dogs. Diabetes 1993;42:820–825.
42 Ashton N: Arteriolar involvement in diabetic retinopathy. Br J Ophthalmol 1953;37:282–292.
43 Gardiner TA, Stitt AW, Anderson HR, Archer DB: Selective loss of vascular smooth muscle cells in the retinal microcirculation of diabetic dogs. Br J Ophthalmol 1994;78:54–60.
44 Hatchell DL, Braun RD, Lutty GA, McLeod DS, Toth CA: Progression of diabetic retinopathy in a cat. Invest Ophthalmol Vis Sci 1995;36:S1067.
45 Linsenmeier RA, Braun RD, McRipley MA, Padnick LB, Ahmed J, Hatchell DL, McLeod DS, Lutty GA: Retinal hypoxia in long-term diabetic cats. Invest Ophthalmol Vis Sci 1998;39:1647–1657.
46 Engerman RL, Bloodworth JMB Jr, Nelson S: Relationship of microvascular disease in diabetes to metabolic control. Diabetes 1977;26:760–769.
47 Engerman RL, Kern TS: Progression of incipient diabetic retinopathy during good glycemic control. Diabetes 1987;36:808–812.
48 Diabetes Control and Complications Trial Research Group: The effect of intensive treatment of diabetes on the development of long-term complications in insulin-dependent diabetes mellitus. N Engl J Med 1993;329:977–986.
49 United Kingdom Prospective Diabetes Study: Intensive blood-glucose control with sulphonylureas or insulin compared with conventional treatment and risk of complications in patients with type 2 diabetes. Lancet 1998;352:837–853.
50 Wallow IH, Engerman RL: Permeability and patency of retinal blood vessels in experimental diabetes. Invest Ophthalmol 1977;16:447–461.
51 Kern TS, Tang J, Mizutani M, Kowluru RA, Nagaraj RH, Romeo G, Podesta F, Lorenzi M: Response of capillary cell death to aminoguanidine predicts the development of retinopathy: comparison of diabetes and galactosemia. Invest Ophthalmol Vis Sci 2000;41:3972–3978.
52 Kowluru RA, Tang J, Kern TS: Abnormalities of retinal metabolism in diabetes and experimental galactosemia. VII. Effect of long-term administration of antioxidants on the development of retinopathy. Diabetes 200150:1938–1942.
53 Joussen AM, Poulaki V, Le ML, Koizumi K, Esser C, Janicki H, Schraermeyer U, Kociok N, Fauser S, Kirchhof B, Kern TS, Adamis AP: A central role for inflammation in the pathogenesis of diabetic retinopathy. FASEB J 2004;18:1450–1452.
54 Yu DY, Cringle SJ, Su EN, Yu PK, Jerums G, Cooper ME: Pathogenesis and intervention strategies in diabetic retinopathy. Clin Experiment Ophthalmol 2001;29:164–166.

55 Chakrabarti S, Zhang WX, Sima AA: Optic neuropathy in the diabetic BB-rat. Adv Exp Med Biol 1991;291:257–264.
56 Sima AA, Zhang WX, Cherian PV, Chakrabarti S: Impaired visual evoked potential and primary axonopathy of the optic nerve in the diabetic BB/W-rat. Diabetologia 1992;35:602–607.
57 Kamijo M, Cherian PV, Sima AAF: The preventive effect of aldose reductase inhibition on diabetic optic neuropathy in the BB/W rat. Diabetologia 1993;36:893–898.
58 Hammes HP, Federoff HJ, Brownlee M: Nerve growth factor prevents both neuroretinal programmed cell death and capillary pathology in experimental diabetes. Mol Med 1995;1:527–534.
59 Barber AJ, Lieth E, Khin SA, Antonetti DA, Buchanan AG, Gardner TW: Neural apoptosis in the retina during experimental and human diabetes. Early onset and effect of insulin. J Clin Invest 1998;102:783–791.
60 Lieth E, Gardner TW, Barber AJ, Antonetti DA: Retinal neurodegeneration: early pathology in diabetes. Clin Experiment Ophthalmol 2000;28:3–8.
61 Agardh E, Bruun A, Agardh CD: Retinal glial cell immunoreactivity and neuronal cell changes in rats with STZ-induced diabetes. Curr Eye Res 2001;23:276–284.
62 Aizu Y, Oyanagi K, Hu J, Nakagawa H: Degeneration of retinal neuronal processes and pigment epithelium in the early stage of the streptozotocin-diabetic rats. Neuropathology 2002;22:161–170.
63 Asnaghi V, Gerhardinger C, Hoehn T, Adeboje A, Lorenzi M: A role for the polyol pathway in the early neuroretinal apoptosis and glial changes induced by diabetes in the rat. Diabetes 2003;52:506–511.
64 Aizu Y, Katayama H, Takahama S, Hu J, Nakagawa H, Oyanagi K: Topical instillation of ciliary neurotrophic factor inhibits retinal degeneration in streptozotocin-induced diabetic rats. Neuroreport 2003;14:2067–2071.
65 Park SH, Park JW, Park SJ, Kim KY, Chung JW, Chun MH, Oh SJ: Apoptotic death of photoreceptors in the streptozotocin-induced diabetic rat retina. Diabetologia 2003;46:1260–1268.
66 Martin PM, Roon P, Van Ells TK, Ganapathy V, Smith SB: Death of retinal neurons in streptozotocin-induced diabetic mice. Invest Ophthalmol Vis Sci 2004;45:3330–3336.
67 Kern TS, Miller CM, Du Y, Zheng L, Mohr S, Ball SL, Kim M, Jamison JA, Bingaman DP: Topical administration of nepafenac inhibits diabetes-induced retinal microvascular disease and underlying abnormalities of retinal metabolism and physiology. Diabetes 2007;56:373–379.
68 Kusner LL, Sarthy VP, Mohr S: Nuclear translocation of glyceraldehyde-3-phosphate dehydrogenase: a role in high glucose-induced apoptosis in retinal Muller cells. Invest Ophthalmol Vis Sci 2004;45:1553–1561.
69 Lieth E, Barber AJ, Xu B, Dice C, Ratz MJ, Tanase D, Strother JM: Glial reactivity and impaired glutamate metabolism in short-term experimental diabetic retinopathy. Penn State Retina Research Group. Diabetes 1998;47:815–820.
70 Mizutani M, Gerhardinger C, Lorenzi M: Muller cell changes in human diabetic retinopathy. Diabetes 1998;47:445–449.
71 Barber AJ, Antonetti DA, Gardner TW: Altered expression of retinal occludin and glial fibrillary acidic protein in experimental diabetes. The Penn State Retina Research Group. Invest Ophthalmol Vis Sci 2000;41:3561–3568.
72 Zeng XX, Ng YK, Ling EA: Neuronal and microglial response in the retina of streptozotocin-induced diabetic rats. Visual Neurosci 2001;17:463–471.
73 Li Q, Zemel E, Miller B, Perlman I: Early retinal damage in experimental diabetes: electroretinographical and morphological observations. Exp Eye Res 2002;74:615–625.
74 Seki M, Tanaka T, Nawa H, Usui T, Fukuchi T, Ikeda K, Abe H, Takei N: Involvement of brain-derived neurotrophic factor in early retinal neuropathy of streptozotocin-induced diabetes in rats: therapeutic potential of brain-derived neurotrophic factor for dopaminergic amacrine cells. Diabetes 2004;53:2412–2419.
75 Sima AA, Garcia-Salinas R, Basu PK: The BB Wistar rat: an experimental model for the study of diabetic retinopathy. Metabolism 1983;32(suppl 1):136–140.
76 Sima AA, Chakrabarti S, Garcia-Salinas R, Basu PK: The BB-rat–an authentic model of human diabetic retinopathy. Curr Eye Res 4:1087–1092, 1985
77 Chakrabarti S, Sima AAF, Tze WJ, Tai J: Prevention of diabetic retinal capillary pericyte degeneration and loss by pancreatic islet allograft. Curr Eye Res 1987;6:649–658.
78 Robison WG Jr, McCaleb ML, Feld LG, Michaelis OE, IV, Laver N, Mercandetti M: Degenerated intramural pericytes ('ghost cells') in the retinal capillaries of diabetic rats. Curr Eye Res 1991;10:339–350.
79 Shinohara M, Masuyama T, Shoda T, Takahashi T, Katsuda Y, Komeda K, Kuroki M, Kakehashi A, Kanazawa Y: A new spontaneously diabetic non-obese Torii rat strain with severe ocular complications. Int J Exp Diabetes Res 2000;1:89–100.
80 Miao G, Ito T, Uchikoshi F, Kamei M, Akamaru Y, Kiyomoto T, Komoda H, Nozawa M, Matsuda H: Stage-dependent effect of pancreatic transplantation on diabetic ocular complications in the spontaneously diabetic Torii rat. Transplantation 2004;77:658–663.
81 Yamada H, Yamada E, Higuchi A, Matsumura M: Retinal neovascularisation without ischaemia in the spontaneously diabetic Torii rat. Diabetologia 2005;48:1663–1668.
82 Nakama K, Shichinohe K, Kobayashi K, Naito K, Uchida O, Yasuhara K, Tobe M: Spontaneous diabetes-like syndrome in WBN/KOB rats. Acta Diabetol Lat 1985;22:335–342.
83 Matsuura T, Horikiri K, Ozaki K, Narama I: Proliferative retinal changes in diabetic rats (WBN/Kob). Lab Anim Sci 1999;49:565–569.
84 Bhutto IA, Miyamura N, Amemiya T: Vascular architecture of degenerated retina in WBN/Kob rats: corrosion cast and electron microscopic study. Ophthalmic Res 1999;31:367–377.
85 Miyamura N, Amemiya T: Lens and retinal changes in the WBN/Kob rat (spontaneously diabetic strain). Electron-microscopic study. Ophthalmic Res 1998;30:221–232.
86 Ogawa T, Ohira A, Amemiya T: Superoxide dismutases in retinal degeneration of WBN/Kob rat. Curr Eye Res 1998;17:1067–1073.

87 Azuma M, Sakamoto-Mizutani K, Nakajima T, Kanaami-Daibo S, Tamada Y, Shearer TR: Involvement of calpain isoforms in retinal degeneration in WBN/Kob rats. Comp Med 2004;54:533–542.
88 Kaczurowski M: Angiopathy of retinal vessels in diabetic mice. Arch Ophthalmol 1970;84:316–320.
89 Duhault J, Lebon F, Boulanger M: KK mice as a model of microangiopathic lesions in diabetes; in Ditzel J, Lewis D (eds): 7th European Conference on Microcirculation, Aberdeen. Basel, Karger, 1972, pp 453–458.
90 Cuthbertson RA, Mandel TE: The effect of murine fetal islet transplants on renal and retinal capillary basement membrane thickness. Transplant Proc 1987;19:2919–2921.
91 Agren A, Rehn G, Naeser P: Morphology and enzyme activities of the retinal capillaries in streptozotocin-diabetic mice. Acta Ophthalmol (Copenh) 1979;57:1065–1069.
92 Mohr S, Tang J, Kern TS: Caspase activation in retinas of diabetic and galactosemic mice and diabetic patients. Diabetes 2002;51:1172–1179.
93 Zheng L, Du Y, Miller C, Gubitosi-Klug RA, Ball S, Berkowitz BA, Kern TS: Critical role of inducible nitric oxide synthase in degeneration of retinal capillaries in mice with streptozotocin-induced diabetes. Diabetologia 2007;50:1987–1996.
94 Gubitosi-Klug RA, Talahalli R, Du Y, Nadler JL, Kern TS: 5-Lipoxygenase, but not 12/15-lipoxygenase, contributes to degeneration of retinal capillaries in a mouse model of diabetic retinopathy. Diabetes 2008;57:1387–1393.
95 Barber AJ, Antonetti DA, Kern TS, Reiter CE, Soans RS, Krady JK, Levison SW, Gardner TW, Bronson SK: The Ins2Akita mouse as a model of early retinal complications in diabetes. Invest Ophthalmol Vis Sci 2005;46:2210–2218.
96 Kanwar M, Chan PS, Kern TS, Kowluru RA: Oxidative damage in the retinal mitochondria of diabetic mice: possible protection by superoxide dismutase. Invest Ophthalmol Vis Sci 2007;48:3805–3811.
97 Yoshioka M, Kayo T, Ikeda T, Koizumi A: A novel locus, Mody4, distal to D7Mit189 on chromosome 7 determines early-onset NIDDM in nonobese C57BL/6 (Akita) mutant mice. Diabetes 1997;46:887–894.
98 Gastinger MJ, Kunselman AR, Conboy EE, Bronson SK, Barber AJ: Dendrite remodeling and other abnormalities in the retinal ganglion cells of Ins2 Akita diabetic mice. Invest Ophthalmol Vis Sci 2008;49:2635–2642.
99 Yokote M: Retinal and renal microangiopathy in carp with spontaneous diabetes mellitus. Adv Metab Disord 1973;2(suppl 2):299–230.
100 Gleeson M, Connaughton V, Arneson LS: Induction of hyperglycaemia in zebrafish (Danio rerio) leads to morphological changes in the retina. Acta Diabetol 2007;44:157–163.
101 Clark JB, Palmer CJ, Shaw WN: The diabetic Zucker fatty rat. Proc Soc Exp Biol Med 1983;173:68–75.
102 Greenhose DD MO, Peterson RG: New models of genetically obese rats for studies in diabetes, heart disease, and complications of obesity; in Greenhouse DD, et al (eds): The Development of Fatty and Corpulent Rat Strains. Bethesda, NIH, Division of Research Service: Veterinary Resources Branch, 1988, pp 3–6.
103 Yang YS, Danis RP, Peterson RG, Dolan PL, Wu YQ: Acarbose partially inhibits microvascular retinopathy in the Zucker Diabetic Fatty rat (ZDF/Gmi-fa). J Ocul Pharmacol Ther 2000;16:471–479.
104 Behl Y, Krothapalli P, Desta T, DiPiazza A, Roy S, Graves DT: Diabetes-enhanced tumor necrosis factor-alpha production promotes apoptosis and the loss of retinal microvascular cells in type 1 and type 2 models of diabetic retinopathy. Am J Pathol 2008;172:1411–1418.
105 Agardh CD, Agardh E, Zhang H, Ostenson CG: Altered endothelial/pericyte ratio in Goto-Kakizaki rat retina. J Diabetes Complications 1997;11:158–162.
106 Yatoh S, Mizutani M, Yokoo T, Kozawa T, Sone H, Toyoshima H, Suzuki S, Shimano H, Kawakami Y, Okuda Y, Yamada N: Antioxidants and an inhibitor of advanced glycation ameliorate death of retinal microvascular cells in diabetic retinopathy. Diabetes Metab Res Rev 2006;22:38–45.
107 Murray F, Wachowski M, Diani A, Ellis E, Grant M: Intermediate and long term diabetic (type II) complications in the spontaneously diabetic (BBZ/Wor) rat (Abstract). Diabetes 1996;45(suppl 2):272A.
108 Miyamura N, Bhutto IA, Amemiya T: Retinal capillary changes in Otsuka Long-Evans Tokushima fatty rats (spontaneously diabetic strain). Electron-microscopic study. Ophthalmic Res 1999;31:358–366.
109 Lu ZY, Bhutto IA, Amemiya T: Retinal changes in Otsuka long-evans Tokushima Fatty rats (spontaneously diabetic rat) – possibility of a new experimental model for diabetic retinopathy. Jpn J Ophthalmol 2003;47:28–35.
110 Matsuura T, Yamagishi S, Kodama Y, Shibata R, Ueda S, Narama I: Otsuka Long-Evans Tokushima fatty (OLETF) rat is not a suitable animal model for the study of angiopathic diabetic retinopathy. Int J Tissue React 2005;27:59–62.
111 Kim YH, Kim YS, Park CH, Chung IY, Yoo JM, Kim JG, Lee BJ, Kang SS, Cho GJ, Choi WS: Protein kinase C-delta mediates neuronal apoptosis in the retinas of diabetic rats via the Akt signaling pathway. Diabetes 2008;57:2181–2190.
112 Koletsky S: Animal model: obese hypertensive rat. Am J Pathol 1975;81:463–466.
113 Koletsky S: Pathologic findings and laboratory data in a new strain of obese hypertensive rats. Am J Pathol 1975;80:129–142.
114 Huang SS, Khosrof SA, Koletsky RJ, Benetz BA, Ernsberger P: Characterization of retinal vascular abnormalities in lean and obese spontaneously hypertensive rats. Clin Exp Pharmacol Physiol 1995;22(suppl 1):S129–S131.
115 Michaelis OEI, Ellwood KC, Judge JM, Schoene NW, Hansen CT: Effect of dietary sucrose on the SHR/N-corpulent rat: a new model for insulin-independent diabetes. Am J Clin Nutr 1984;39:612–618.
116 Voyles NR, Bhathena SJ, Kennedy B, Wilkins SD, Michaelis OEt, Zalenski CM, Timmers KI, Recant L: Tissue somatostatin levels in three models of genetic obesity in rats. Proc Soc Exp Biol Med 1987;185:49–54.

117 McCune SA, Baker PB, Stills HF: SHHF/Mcc-cp rat: model of obesity, non-insulin-dependent diabetes, and congestive heart failure. ILAR News 1990;32:23–37.
118 Kim SH, Chu YK, Kwon OW, McCune SA, Davidorf FH: Morphologic studies of the retina in a new diabetic model; SHR/N:Mcc-cp rat. Yonsei Med J 1998;39:453–462.
119 Midena E, Segato T, Radin S, di Giorgio G, Meneghini F, Piermarocchi S, Belloni AS: Studies on the retina of the diabetic db/db mouse. I. Endothelial cell-pericyte ratio. Ophthalmic Res 1989;21:106–111.
120 Clements RS Jr, Robison WG Jr, Cohen MP: Anti-glycated albumin therapy ameliorates early retinal microvascular pathology in db/db mice. J Diabetes Complications 1998;12:28–33.
121 Cheung AK, Fung MK, Lo AC, Lam TT, So KF, Chung SS, Chung SK: Aldose reductase deficiency prevents diabetes-induced blood-retinal barrier breakdown, apoptosis, and glial reactivation in the retina of db/db Mice. Diabetes 2005;54:3119–3125.
122 Barile GR, Pachydaki SI, Tari SR, Lee SE, Donmoyer CM, Ma W, Rong LL, Buciarelli LG, Wendt T, Horig H, Hudson BI, Qu W, Weinberg AD, Yan SF, Schmidt AM: The RAGE axis in early diabetic retinopathy. Invest Ophthalmol Vis Sci 2005;46:2916–2924.
123 Ikeda H: KK mouse. Diabetes Res Clin Pract 1994;24(suppl):S313–S316.
124 Iwatsuka H, Shino A, Suzuoki Z: General survey of diabetic features of yellow KK mice. Endocrinol Jpn 1970;17:23–35.
125 Siracusa LD: The agouti gene: turned on to yellow. Trends Genet 1994;10:423–428.
126 Herberg L, Coleman DL: Laboratory animals exhibiting obesity and diabetes syndromes. Metabolism 1977;26:59–99.
127 Ning X, Baoyu Q, Yuzhen L, Shuli S, Reed E, Li QQ: Neuro-optic cell apoptosis and microangiopathy in KKAY mouse retina. Int J Mol Med 2004;13:87–92.
128 Laver N, Robison WG Jr, Hansen BC: Spontaneously diabetic monkeys as a model for diabetic retinopathy. (ARVO Abstract). Invest Ophthalmol Vis Sci 1994;35(suppl):1733.
129 Kim SY, Johnson MA, McLeod DS, Alexander T, Otsuji T, Steidl SM, Hansen BC, Lutty GA: Retinopathy in monkeys with spontaneous type 2 diabetes. Invest Ophthalmol Vis Sci 2004;45:4543–4553.
130 Johnson MA, Lutty GA, McLeod DS, Otsuji T, Flower RW, Sandagar G, Alexander T, Steidl SM, Hansen BC: Ocular structure and function in an aged monkey with spontaneous diabetes mellitus. Exp Eye Res 2005;80:37–42.
131 Hammes HP, Wellensiek B, Kloting I, Sickel E, Bretzel RG, Brownlee M: The relationship of glycaemic level to advanced glycation end-product (AGE) accumulation and retinal pathology in the spontaneous diabetic hamster. Diabetologia 1998;41:165–170.
132 Engerman RL, Kern TS: Experimental galactosemia produces diabetic-like retinopathy. Diabetes 1984;33:97–100.
133 Kador PF, Akagi Y, Terubayashi H, Wyman M, Kinoshita JH: Prevention of pericyte ghost formation in retinal capillaries of galactose-fed dogs by aldose reductase inhibitors. Arch Ophthalmol 1988;106:1099–1102.
134 Kador PF, Akagi Y, Takahashi Y, Ikebe H, Wyman M, Kinoshita JH: Prevention of retinal vessel changes associated with diabetic retinopathy in galactose-fed dogs by aldose reductase inhibitors. Arch Ophthalmol 1990;108:1301–1309.
135 Frank RN: The galactosemic dog. A valid model for both early and late stages of diabetic retinopathy. Arch Ophthalmol 1995;113:275–276.
136 Engerman RL, Kern TS: Retinopathy in galactosemic dogs continues to progress after cessation of galactosemia. Arch Ophthalmol 1995;113:355–358.
137 Kador PF, Takahashi Y, Wyman M, Ferris F III: Diabetes-like proliferative retinal changes in galactose-fed dogs. Arch Ophthalmol 1995;113:352–354.
138 Kern TS, Engerman RL: Galactose-induced retinal microangiopathy in rats. Invest Ophthalmol Vis Sci 1995;36:490–496.
139 Neuenschwander H, Takahashi Y, Kador PF: Dose-dependent reduction of retinal vessel changes associated with diabetic retinopathy in galactose-fed dogs by the aldose reductase inhibitor M79175. J Ocul Pharmacol Ther 1997;13:517–528.
140 Kobayashi T, Kubo E, Takahashi Y, Kasahara T, Yonezawa H, Akagi Y: Retinal vessel changes in galactose-fed dogs. Arch Ophthalmol 1998;116:785–789.
141 Kador PF, Takahashi Y, Akagi Y, Neuenschwander H, Greentree W, Lackner P, Blessing K, Wyman M: Effect of galactose diet removal on the progression of retinal vessel changes in galactose-fed dogs. Invest Ophthalmol Vis Sci 2002;43:1916–1921.
142 Robison WG Jr, Nagata M, Laver N, Hohman TC, Kinoshita JH: Diabetic-like retinopathy in rats prevented with an aldose reductase inhibitor. Invest Ophthalmol Vis Sci 1989;30:2285–2292.
143 Robison WG Jr, Nagata M, Tillis TN, Laver N, Kinoshita JH: Aldose reductase and pericyte-endothelial cell contacts in retina and optic nerve. Invest Ophthalmol Vis Sci 1989;30:2293–2299.
144 Robison WG Jr, Laver NM, Jacot JL, Glover JP: Sorbinil prevention of diabetic-like retinopathy in the galactose-fed rat model. Invest Ophthalmol Vis Sci 1995;36:2368–2380.
145 Robison WG Jr: Diabetic retinopathy: galactose-fed rat model. Invest Ophthalmol Vis Sci 1995;36:4A, 1743–1744.
146 Kern TS, Engerman RL: Pharmacologic inhibition of diabetic retinopathy: Aminoguanidine and aspirin. Diabetes 2001;50:1636–1642.
147 Kern TS, Engerman RL: A mouse model of diabetic retinopathy. Arch Ophthalmol 1996;114:986–990.
148 Chiou SH, Chylack LT Jr, Bunn HF, Kinoshita JH: Role of nonenzymatic glycosylation in experimental cataract formation. Biochem Biophys Res Commun 1980;95:894–901.
149 Monnier VM, Sell DR, Abdul-Karim FW, Emancipator SN: Collagen browning and cross-linking are increased in chronic experimental hyperglycemia: relevance to diabetes and aging. Diabetes 1988;37:867–872.
150 Kern TS, Kowluru R, Engerman RL: Abnormalities of retinal metabolism in diabetes or galactosemia. ATPases and glutathione. Invest Ophthalmol Vis Sci 1994;35:2962–2967.

151 Kowluru R, Kern TS, Engerman RL: Abnormalities of retinal metabolism in diabetes or galactosemia II. Comparison of gamma-glutamyl transpeptidase in retina and cerebral cortex, and effects of antioxidant therapy. Curr Eye Res 1994;13:891–896.
152 Xia P, Inoguchi T, Kern TS, Engerman RL, Oates PJ, King GL: Characterization of the mechanism for the chronic activation of DAG-PKC pathway in diabetes and hypergalactosemia. Diabetes 1994;43:1122–1129.
153 Kern TS, Kowluru RA, Engerman RL: Effect of antioxidants on the development of retinopathy in diabetes and galactosemia. Invest Ophthalmol Vis Sci 1996;37:S970.
154 Kowluru RA, Kern TS, Engerman RL: Abnormalities of retinal metabolism in diabetes or experimental galactosemia. IV. Antioxidant defense system. Free Radic Biol Med 1996;22:587–592.
155 Kowluru RA, Engerman RL, Kern TS: Abnormalities of retinal metabolism in diabetes or experimental galactosemia. VI. Comparison of retinal and cerebral cortex metabolism, and effects of antioxidant therapy. Free Radic Biol Med 1999;26:371–378.
156 Hammes HP, Martin S, Federlin K, Geisen K, Brownlee M: Aminoguanidine treatment inhibits the development of experimental diabetic retinopathy. Proc Natl Acad Sci USA 1991;88:11555–11558.
157 Hammes HP, Brownlee M, Edelstein D, Saleck M, Martin S, Federlin K: Aminoguanidine inhibits the development of accelerated diabetic retinopathy in the spontaneous hypertensive rat. Diabetologia 1994;37:32–35.
158 Frank RN, Amin R, Kennedy A, Hohman TC: An aldose reductase inhibitor and aminoguanidine prevent vascular endothelial growth factor expression in rats with long-term galactosemia. Arch Ophthalmol 1997;115:1036–1047.
159 Yanko L, Michaelson IC, Cohen AM: The retinopathy of sucrose-fed rats. Israel J Med Sci 1972;8:1633–1636.
160 Boot-Handford R, Heath H: Identification of fructose as the retinopathic agent associated with the ingestion of sucrose-rich diets in the rat. Metabolism 1980;29:1247–1252.
161 Tolentino MJ, Miller JW, Gragoudas ES, Jakobiec FA, Flynn E, Chatzistefanou K, Ferrara N, Adamis AP: Intravitreous injections of vascular endothelial growth factor produce retinal ischemia and microangiopathy in an adult primate. Ophthalmology 1996;103:1820–1828.
162 Ruberte J, Ayuso E, Navarro M, Carretero A, Nacher V, Haurigot V, George M, Llombart C, Casellas A, Costa C, Bosch A, Bosch F: Increased ocular levels of IGF-1 in transgenic mice lead to diabetes-like eye disease. J Clin Invest 2004;113:1149–1157.
163 Danis RP, Bingaman DP: Insulin-like growth factor-1 retinal microangiopathy in the pig eye. Ophthalmology 1997;104:1661–1669.
164 Benjamin LE, Hemo I, Keshet E: A plasticity window for blood vessel remodelling is defined by pericyte coverage of the preformed endothelial network and is regulated by PDGF-B and VEGF. Development 1998;125:1591–1598.
165 Lindahl P, Johansson BR, Leveen P, Betsholtz C: Pericyte loss and microaneurysm formation in PDGF-B-deficient mice. Science 1997;277:242–245.
166 Enge M, Bjarnegard M, Gerhardt H, Gustafsson E, Kalen M, Asker N, Hammes HP, Shani M, Fassler R, Betsholtz C: Endothelium-specific platelet-derived growth factor-B ablation mimics diabetic retinopathy. EMBO J 2002;21:4307–4316.
167 Hammes HP, Lin J, Renner O, Shani M, Lundqvist A, Betsholtz C, Brownlee M, Deutsch U: Pericytes and the pathogenesis of diabetic retinopathy. Diabetes 2002;51:3107–3112.
168 Mori K, Gehlbach P, Ando A, Dyer G, Lipinsky E, Chaudhry AG, Hackett SF, Campochiaro PA: Retina-specific expression of PDGF-B versus PDGF-A: vascular versus nonvascular proliferative retinopathy. Invest Ophthalmol Vis Sci 2002;43:2001–2006.
169 Wiley LA, Rupp GR, Steinle JJ: Sympathetic innervation regulates basement membrane thickening and pericyte number in rat retina. Invest Ophthalmol Vis Sci 2005;46:744–748.
170 Steinle JJ, Lindsay NL, Lashbrook BL: Cervical sympathectomy causes photoreceptor-specific cell death in the rat retina. Auton Neurosci 2005;120:46–51.
171 Steinle JJ, Smith PG: Sensory but not parasympathetic nerves are required for ocular vascular remodeling following chronic sympathectomy in rat. Auton Neurosci 2003;109:34–41.
172 Steinle JJ, Pierce JD, Clancy RL, P GS: Increased ocular blood vessel numbers and sizes following chronic sympathectomy in rat. Exp Eye Res 2002;74:761–768.
173 Zheng L, Gong B, Hatala DA, Kern TS: Retinal ischemia and reperfusion causes capillary degeneration: similarities to diabetes. Invest Ophthalmol Vis Sci 2007;48:361–367.
174 Moravski CJ, Skinner SL, Stubbs AJ, Sarlos S, Kelly DJ, Cooper ME, Gilbert RE, Wilkinson-Berka JL: The renin-angiotensin system influences ocular endothelial cell proliferation in diabetes: transgenic and interventional studies. Am J Pathol 2003;162:151–160.

Timothy S. Kern, PhD
Departments of Medicine and Ophthalmology
434 Biomedical Research Building, Case Western Reserve University
10900 Euclid Ave, Cleveland, OH 44106 (USA)
Tel. +1 216 368 0800, Fax +1 216 368 5824, E-Mail tsk@case.edu

Hammes H-P, Porta M (eds): Experimental Approaches to Diabetic Retinopathy.
Front Diabetes. Basel, Karger, 2010, vol 20, pp 61–78

Pericyte Loss in the Diabetic Retina

Frederick Pfister · Jihong Lin · Hans-Peter Hammes

Section of Endocrinology, 5th Medical Department, Mannheim Medical Faculty, University Hospital Mannheim, Ruprechts-Karls University Heidelberg, Mannheim, Germany

Abstract

Retinal pericytes are enigmatic cells. The lack of a pan-pericyte marker and the diversity of possible origins suggest that there is not one pericyte population recruited to the retina. The important functions of pericytes related to the specific demands of the retina are the control of endothelial survival and growth, and the tightness of the blood retinal barrier. Pericyte loss is a common early phenomenon of all diabetic mammalians. An important molecular contribution to pericyte functionality comes from the angiopoietin-Tie system that is involved in the maturation of the developing vascular network as well as in its destabilization and angiogenesis. Hyperglycemia induces upregulation of angiopoietin-2 which inhibits the pericyte-recruiting function of angiopoietin-1, suggesting a novel, active mechanism in pericyte loss, rather than a passive intoxication by glycolytic intermediates. Posttranslational modification involving intracellular methylglyoxal type advanced glycation end products and enzymatic modification of transcription factors are involved in glucose-induced transcription changes of Ang-2. Metabolic signal blockers as well as catalytic antioxidants prevent Ang-2 upregulation as well as diabetic pericyte loss in vivo.

Promoted by the observation that they are selectively lost in early diabetic retinopathy, pericytes have attracted the interest of researchers from many disciplines. Still, pericytes are enigmatic cells. Neither their origin, nor their normal function has been fully delineated, and the biological meaning and the causes and consequences of their loss in the diabetic retina are still under investigation. It is useful to review current knowledge about the cellular crosstalk between vascular cells, before adding a further level of complexity by addressing the cellular crosstalk between vascular and neuroglial cells [1, 2]. Pericytes are functionally co-dependent on endothelial cell (EC) and each cell type provides his counterpart with growth factors and contact-dependent signals that influence survival and/or proliferation [3]. Diabetic pericyte loss may represent one of the prominent examples in which the survival impact of pericytes on ECs is critically lost.

Pericyte

Origin and Differentiation

The origin, tissue and environment-dependent differentiation, and the potency of context-dependent activation and transdifferentiation of resident retinal pericytes remain obscure.

Pericytes derive from the mesoderm and from neural crest cells during development [4]. In the retina, a common pluripotent mural precursor cell has been identified giving rise to both vascular smooth muscle cells (vSMCs) and pericytes [5]. The relative contribution of common embryonic stem cell precursors which incorporate into vessels under the influence of pericyte-recruiting factors such as platelet-derived growth factor (PDGF)-B remains unclear [6]. Recently, evidence for a bone marrow origin of mural cells supporting adult angiogenesis has been presented [7]. Furthermore, EC transdifferentiation into pericytes under postnatal vascular repair conditions has been suggested [8]. Whether endothelial precursor cells of nondiabetic origin can integrate into diabetic retinal capillaries and replace functional pericytes needs further investigation.

Pericytes are able to transdifferentiate into other cell types. In vitro observations demonstrated transdifferentiation potential into adipogenic, chondrogenic, and osteogenic cells [9, 10], reflecting the heterogeneity of pericyte populations in general. Growing evidence suggests that pericytes may represent a perivascular niche of mesenchymal stem cells, and that the transition to progenitor and mature cell phenotypes is coordinated by local cues. Regarding pericytes as a reservoir of mesenchymal stem cells, it might be possible that pericytes stabilize blood vessels and contribute to tissue homeostasis under physiological conditions, but assume a more active role in the repair of focal tissue injury. For example, in the rat brain, phagocytic pericytes attain microglial functions [11]. The conversion of pericytes to tissue macrophages has been observed, suggesting an active contribution to a variety of clearance and defense functions [12]. In the brain, a transitional cell phenotype of pericytes compatible with fibroblast morphology and localization, but with a surface expression pattern of a pericyte (see below) has also been reported. In particular, pericytes can differentiate into vSMCs and fibroblasts, and the reverse transformation of vSMCs and fibroblasts into pericytes is possible [12–17]. Evidence thus far indicates that the cellular component of the perivascular compartment that is more likely to function as a stem cell in the postnatal organism is the pericyte.

Morphology and Distribution

Pericytes are the supporting cells of the microvasculature and regular components of capillaries in almost all human tissues and organs. In contrast to arteries and arterioles, where the coverage consists of single or multilayers of vSMCs, the capillary system is exclusively covered by individual pericytes. It has been suggested that vSMCs and pericytes represent phenotypic variations of a continuous cell lineage because of morphological similarities and the expression of common markers such as smooth muscle actin and desmin [3].

Scanning electron micrography shows that pericytes usually possess a cell body with a prominent nucleus and a small cytoplasmic margin from which processes extend. The body of the pericyte protrudes cellular projections away from the vessel. The primary process of pericytes parallels the axis of the capillary and the secondary processes encircle the capillary perpendicularly. Tertiary processes extend to more than one capillary [18]. The projections are thought to mediate cell-cell communications between individual pericytes, pericytes and ECs in vessels, and pericytes and the retinal neuroglia.

In capillaries, pericytes are identified by shape, orientation along the capillary wall, staining intensity with periodic acid Schiff base, and extracapillary protrusion [19, 20] (fig. 1). They form processes which vary in length, and contact different capillary branches, which suggest their mobility [21]. Pericytes in the retina are completely embedded within the capillary basement membrane [22], surrounding the ECs which form the capillary tube ('intramural pericytes').

The density of pericyte coverage in the capillary varies from organ to organ. The highest relative ratio of pericytes to ECs is found

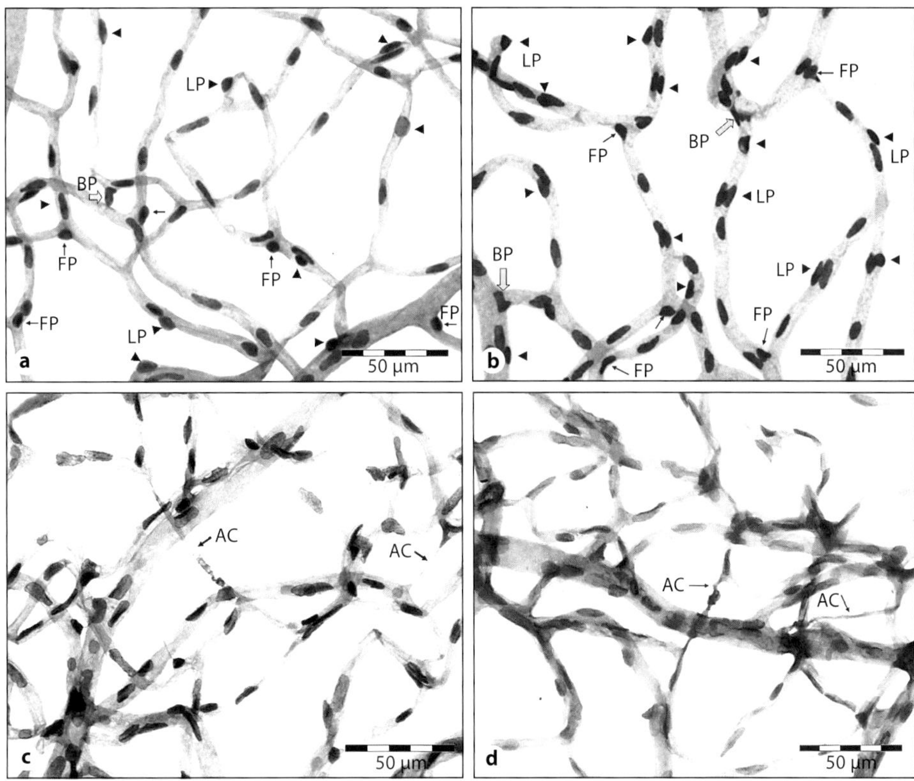

Fig. 1. Capillary network of normal mouse retina (**a**) and rat retina (**b**), as well as diabetic retinae of mouse (**c**) and rat (**d**), digested with 3% trypsin, PAS stained. **a**, **b** FP: pericyte located at fork of vessel (arrows) and FP type pericyte is about 20% of total pericyte in normal rat retina. BP: less pericytes bridged over two capillaries (thick arrow). LP: most pericytes situated on vessels in longitudinal orientation (arrowheads). Note the ratio of pericyte to EC in nondiabetic animal is approximately 1:1 (**a**, **b**), but <1 in diabetic animal (**c**, **d**). AC = Acellular capillaries (arrows). Original magnification, ×400. Scale bar = 50 μm.

in the retinal microvasculature (1:1; fig. 1a, b), followed by brain capillaries (1:5–1:3), skeletal muscle capillaries (1:5), lung and the cardiac muscle capillaries (1:10), and striated muscle (skeletal/cardiac muscle 1:100) [23]. One explanation for the exclusively high pericyte coverage of capillaries in the retina is the function of blood vessels in this specialized organ. On the one hand, blood supply to the retina is the highest among the organs of the body, as determined by perfusion/organ weight. On the other hand, the need for vessel tightness is particularly high in the retina, as any extra fluid deposition would interfere with proper visual function. The greater the number of pericytes covering the EC tube, the better the barrier function [18]. Interestingly, tissues with the slowest EC turnover show the largest pericyte coverage [24, 25]. Both notions suggest that primary pericyte functions in the retina relate to the maintenance of a tight blood-retinal barrier and the support of EC survival.

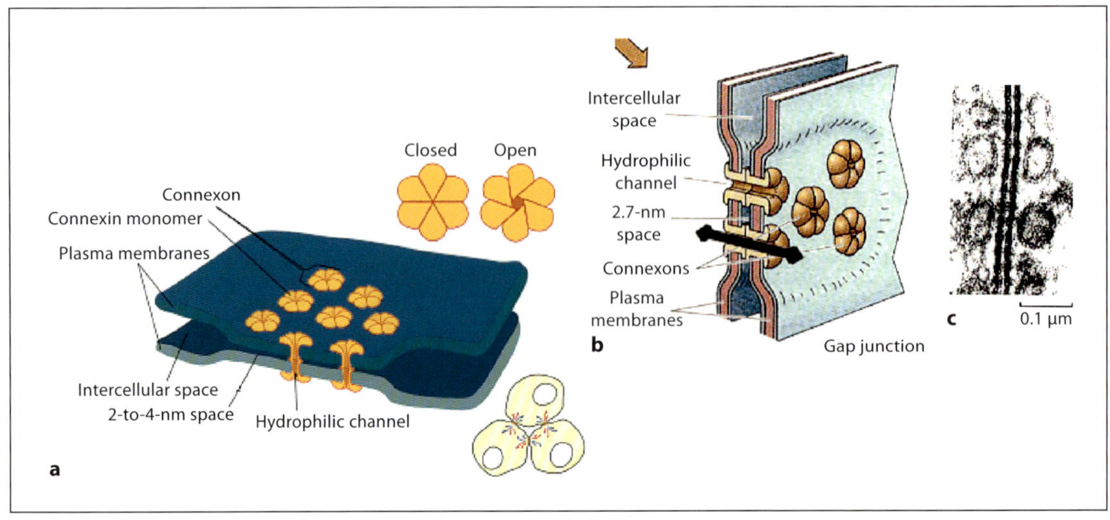

Fig. 2. Gap junction schematic. **a** Proteinaceous tubes/channels that connect adjacent cells. These tubes/channel (orange) allow material to pass from one cell to the next without having to pass through the plasma membranes of the cells. Dissolved substances such as ions or glucose can pass through the gap junctions. Intracellular calcium concentration controls the channel opening and closure. When intracellular calcium is low, the gap junctions are open; when intracellular calcium concentration is high, the channels are closed. **b** A vertical view of gap junction. **c** Gap junction image with electron microscope. http://academic.brooklyn.cuny.edu/biology/bio4fv/page/gap-junctions.html, http://images.google.com/images?um=1&hl=de&lr=&q=gap+junction

Cellular Crosstalk

Cell Contacts

The unique position of pericytes in contact with the endothelial monolayer predicts a direct interaction. This unique position within the common basement membrane and the proximity to perivascular cells renders the pericyte a privileged modulator of endothelial function under physiological and pathological conditions. Pericytes communicate with ECs via various adhesive structures, such as gap junctions, tight junctions, adhesion plaques and peg and socket contacts [26, 27]. These communications are the basis for the variety of direct or indirect consequences of pericytes on endothelial survival and proliferation.

Gap junctions between ECs and pericytes are membranous channels directly connecting the cytoplasms of both cell types (fig. 2). The concentration of intracellular calcium controls those channels to be ‘open or close’. These junctions are involved in the exchange of nucleotides and small molecules between pericytes and ECs [28]. Major components of gap junctions are the connexins of which Cx-37, -42, and -57, have been identified in the eye. Gap junctions provide a substantial role in controlling EC proliferation during physiological angiogenesis [29, 30].

Tight junctions are membrane proteins which interconnect ECs and pericytes. Pericytes are frequently located adjacent to or over tight endothelial junctions, supporting a direct barrier-promoting role. These contacts form a diffusion barrier that controls paracellular fluid transport through the capillary wall. By this, the number of pericytes determines the number of tight junction proteins. Importantly, membrane protein families of tight junctions are the claudins and the occludins. Both are transmembrane proteins which link to the actin cytoskeleton via interaction with the cytosolic proteins zona occludin-1 (ZO-1) and ZO-2. The tight junction proteins are an integral structural component of the blood-retinal barrier which breaks down in early diabetic retinopathy [31]. These EC-pericyte junctional complexes are thought to involve cell adhesion molecules that mediate interaction between EC and pericyte. Pericytes express vascular cell adhesion molecules and ECs express PCAM-1 and P-/E-selectins which mediate EC-platelet, EC-leukocyte and/or EC-EC interaction. Cell culture experiments demonstrated that pericytes induce occludin production of brain ECs and occludin expression is induced by the pericyte-derived angiopoietin-1 (Ang-1) which induces phosphorylation of the cognate receptor Tie2 and subsequent translocation to cell-cell junctions, as well as cell migration [32, 33]. In brain microvessels, the induction of occludin expression enhances the tightness of tight junctions. Further studies suggest that the attenuation or inhibition of Ang-1/Tie-2 signaling leads to dysfunction of blood brain barrier in disease [34]. These data exemplify the importance of pericytes for the maintenance of endothelial barrier function.

Another variant of cell contact between pericytes and EC are adhesion plaques which are rich in fibronectin depositions. These cell contacts anchor the pericyte to the endothelium during the transfer of contractile forces such as during contraction or during propagation of shear stress [21, 35–37].

Intercellular Signaling

Several pairs of ligands and corresponding receptors exist in EC-pericyte interaction and communication, for example PDGF-B and its receptor PBGFR-β, vascular endothelial growth factor (VEGF) and its receptors fetal liver kinase 1 (flk-1, human counterpart, KDR) and fetal liver tyrosine kinase 1 (flt-1), transforming growth factor (TGF)-β and TGF-βR and Ang-1/-2 and their receptor Tie2.

ECs produce PDGF-B which acts on PDGF receptor-β (PDGFR-β) expressed by pericytes. The most intensively studied function of this ligand-receptor system is its role in pericyte recruitment during angiogenesis (see below). VEGF is produced by pericyte and stimulates the proliferation and differentiation of ECs through its receptor flk-1. Contact between ECs and pericytes activates TGF-β1 which inhibits the proliferation and migration of ECs and induces pericytes differentiation [38]. A ligand-receptor system of special importance for the interaction of EC and pericyte is the angiopoietin-Tie system. Ang-1 is expressed mainly by pericytes and acts on endothelial Tie2-receptor. Ang-1 stabilizes the vessel by inducing pericyte attachment and reducing vascular permeability [39, 40]. Ang-2 antagonizes the role of Ang-1, thereby loosening the attachment of ECs and pericytes. In combination with VEGF, Ang-2 promotes controversial effects on microvessels. When VEGF is present, Ang-2 facilitates vessel sprouting. Otherwise, when VEGF is absent, Ang-2 promotes vessel regression [38].

Over and above, pericytes release soluble factors that are potent inhibitors of EC growth and promote microvessel constriction by upregulation of the potent vasoconstrictor and mitogen endothelin-1 (ET-1) [41] and downregulation of iNOS production by ECs [42].

Besides the interaction of EC and pericyte, the conversation between retinal neuroglia and microvascular cells (fig. 3) is of great importance in organs that feature a blood-tissue barrier, like the retina. There are two types of glial cells in the mammalian retina which contribute to the blood-retina barrier: astrocytes and Müller cells [43–45]. Müller cells are the main glial cells of the retina. While astrocytes play an important role in retinal vascular development, Müller cells maintain retinal homeostasis and participate in signal transmission. Beside their active role in retinal function, Müller cells also protect neurons and

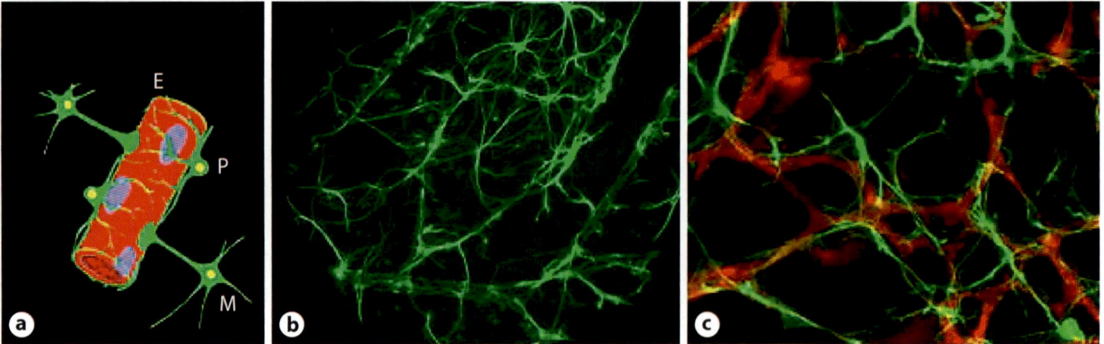

Fig. 3. Retinal neuroglia and microvessel. **a** Schematic of cell contact: EC (blue), Müller cell (green M) and pericyte (green P). **b** Adult mouse retina stained with glial fibrillary acidic protein (GFAP green). **c** Whole mount of mouse retina (postnatal day 13) stained by glial cell marker GFAP (green) and vessel marker isolectin B4 (red). Original magnification, ×200 (**b**) and ×400 (**c**).

vascular cells from injury of hyperglycemia-produced ROS [46, 47]. During the development of diabetic retinopathy, Müller cells become activated, reflected by an increased expression of glial fibrillary acidic protein, and express the angiogenic factor Ang-2, which is implicated in the development of diabetic retinopathy, probably by a direct effect on retinal pericytes (see below) [48].

Identification of Pericytes

The phenotypic nature of pericytes was largely disclosed by transmission and scanning electron microscopy. However, due to the morphological similarities of rodent retinal capillary ECs and pericytes, markers allowing for the distinction of retinal capillary cells were crucial for quantitative analysis.

As expected from the diversity of origin, and the heterogeneity of conditions, there is no 'pan pericyte marker' [27]. Besides PDGFR-β and the proteoglycan NG2, α-smooth muscle actin and desmin are the most commonly used pericyte markers. Additionally, aminopeptidase N, the identification of the expression of XlacZ gene in pericytes (and vSMCs), the regulator of G-protein signaling 5 (RGS5) and the cell membrane protein endosialin/Tem 1 are used for identification of pericytes in the different tissues [14, 49–62]. Comparison of cDNA microarrays of mouse brain of PDGF-B knockout with wild-type embryos, revealed the ATP-sensitive potassium channel complex (Kir 6.1), the sulfonylurea receptor 2 and the delta homolog 1 (45) as brain pericyte markers [63].

Common to all markers is that they fail to recognize all pericytes at all stages [26], and numerous studies demonstrated that marker expression is context dependent. Hughes and Chan-Ling [5] showed that the expression of the pericyte marker NG2 changes during retinal development, identifying juvenile and adult pericyte phenotypes in the retina. In contrast to pericytes of retinal mid-capillaries, pericytes of pre- and postcapillary vessels express the smooth muscle isoform of α-actin. The XlacZ4 mouse is used as a model to study the role of pericytes and SMC because it expresses the LacZ reporter gene under control of a pericyte/SMC-specific promoter. However, according to our analysis, only 55–65% of retinal pericytes express the LacZ reporter gene. In line with the first descriptions by Tidhar et al. [58], detachment of pericytes from capillaries is associated with transgene downregulation. Sometimes, pericytes change their expression profile during adulthood. For example, RGS-5 represents a marker that is specific for 'activated' pericytes [64], and therefore vascular maturation results in the loss of RGS5 [65]. Another marker, endosialin is expressed by pericytes during periods of embryonic angiogenesis and in tumor vessels. The analogy in the diabetic retina awaits further investigation.

Retinal Pericyte Function

Contractility and Regulation of Flow

Pericytes are the capillary counterparts to SMC on arterioles and arteries [57, 66]. One remarkable feature that pericytes have in common with SMC is their contractile phenotype. Pericytes contain both smooth muscle and nonsmooth muscle isoforms of actin and myosin; however, with an uneven distribution within the pericyte population [53]. The differential expression of smooth muscle actin in pericytes may reflect the continuum from SMC of arteries and arterioles to pericytes of true capillaries, and may correlate with the physical forces that pericytes are exposed to. These pericytes are immunolabeled with smooth muscle tropomyosin and cGK, suggestive of a contractile function [51, 67, 68]. Several paracrine factors were identified that regulate pericyte contractility in vitro. While α_2-adrenergic agonists, cholinergic agonists, histamine, serotonin, angiotensin II and ET-1 lead to vasoconstriction, β_2-adrenergic agonists, NO and atrial natriuretic peptide lead to a dilatation of the pericyte-covered capillaries [37]. As mentioned above, ET-1 binds to pericytes for vessel contraction, whereas NO promotes vessel relaxation by a cGTP-dependent mechanism. As demonstrated in in vivo studies, pericytes in brain and retinal capillaries constrict in response to increase in the extracellular Ca^{2+} concentration through electrical stimulation, superperfusion with ATP and noradrenalin. The contraction of pericyte can propagate from stimulated one to distant pericyte along the capillary [69]. Interestingly, pericytes located at branching points of capillaries (about 20% of total pericytes) express especially high concentrations of contractile proteins, suggesting an association with physiological shear stress and a subsequent stabilization function [21].

These data support the evidence that pericytes control capillary blood flow in response to local modulation by vasoactive mechanisms. However, whether the hyperglycemic milieu or the loss of pericytes has an impact on contractility, in particular when basement membrane components have changed under hyperglycemic conditions, needs further clarification.

Role of Pericytes in Vessel Formation and Stabilization

The most prominent function of pericytes is their role in vascular growth and vessel stabilization. Studies highlighted the importance of pericytes for vessel maturation in embryonic development, in vascular remodeling, and in guidance of sprouting angiogenesis [70–74].

ECs can initiate, but not complete vessel formation. After the primary network of vessels has formed during vasculogenesis (de novo formation of vessels from vascular precursor cells), maturation of the primitive network ensues. During this process, pericytes are recruited to the forming vasculature. Important molecular pathways involved in pericyte recruitment during embryonic vessel maturation are PDGF-B and its receptor PDGFR-β, TGF-β and its receptor and the angiopoietin/Tie-2 system (Ang/Tie-2). While the PDGF/PDGFR system is crucial for pericyte migration and proliferation during vascular maturation, the angiopoietin/Tie-2 system is essential for subsequent vessel stabilization, and TGF-β is involved in the interaction of vascular cells with extracellular matrix (ECM) and ECM production and further mural cell differentiation. Inhibition of pericyte recruitment to capillaries by interfering with the recruitment leads to abnormal remodeling of developing vessels, a process that is reversed by administration of endothelial survival factors [75].

The term angiogenesis describes a different process of blood vessel formation and is probably the predominant way of de novo blood vessel formation in the mature retina. In response to growth factor gradients, capillary sprouts start to evade from preexisiting vessels [76]. Recent studies demonstrated that in sprouting angiogenesis, individual ECs achieve a guiding tip cell phenotype while neighboring stalk cells proliferate and form the vascular lumen [77]. EC proliferation and migration of sprouting tip cells include the degradation and losing of ECM and is dependent on tip cell guidance [78]. To achieve a functional capillary network, pericytes are recruited to the growing vessels by a platelet-derived growth factor PDGF-B gradient which is produced by the sprouting ECs, but factors like Ang-1 also induce pericyte recruitment and the subsequent stabilization of newly formed vessels during development. Vessels are resistant to hyperoxic vasoregression when covered with pericytes. This led to the concept of the 'window of plasticity' determined by pericyte recruitment lagging behind endothelial sprouting [79]. By the use of complementary phase-specific pericyte markers outlined earlier, it was shown that pericytes play an active role in physiological and pathological angiogenesis, as they are frequently found near, at or even in front of the tips of endothelial sprouts [14, 27, 80]. Besides the PDGF-B/PDGFR-β system, other factors such as sphingosine-1-phosphate-1 and the angiopoietins and are also involved in angiogenesis [81]. For the completion of vessel maturation, active TGF-β signaling via the ALK-1 and Smad5 pathway is needed [82]. When remodeling ceases, pericytes contribute to the stabilization of vessels by the production of collagen and ECM proteins, such as fibronectin, laminin and glycosaminoglycans to the basal lamina [36, 83–86].

Once the entire vascular system has formed, the major function of pericytes is the maintenance of an intact vascular network. An important paracrine signaling pathways implicated in stabilization and survival of mature vessels is the angiopoietin/Tie-2 system; a growth factor system, known to be deregulated during diabetic retinopathy [87]. Ang-1 and Ang-2 signal via the tyrosine kinase receptor Tie-2. While Ang-1 activates Tie-2, the natural antagonist Ang-2 blocks Ang-1-induced Tie-2 phosphorylation by competitive binding. Tie-2-mediated signaling via the Akt/PKB pathway regulates cell survival, cell migration and cell-cell interactions [88]. In the retina, pericytes are a predominant source of Ang-1 [74, 89] and ECs express the Tie-2 receptor. Pericyte-derived Ang-1 might promote vessel integrity and tightness of blood-retinal barrier by controlling EC proliferation, induction of cell-contact proteins, and making ECs refractory to shifts in oxygen tension and growth factor levels. Under certain pathological conditions the expression of Ang-1, its natural antagonist Ang-2 or Tie-2 receptor may change, resulting in altered EC-pericyte interaction and capillary regression.

Pericyte Loss in Diabetic Retinopathy

Given the complex cell-cell crosstalk outlined earlier, and the specific function of pericytes in maintaining blood-retinal barrier and quiescent vasculature, their loss in diabetic retinopathy predicts profound consequences for the integrity of the affected tissue.

The complex structure of retinal microvasculature, as an integrative part of the retina, and lack of adequate animal models slowed down progress in understanding the cellular changes in diabetic retinopathy. Important insight into the histopathological changes of diabetic retinopathy dates back to the early 1960s. Cogan et al. [19]

developed a method that allowed for the direct inspection of the affected retinal vasculature liberated from neuronal and neuroglial tissues due to differential susceptibility against trypsin digestion. As a result of their work and that of others presented later, pericyte loss was identified as one of the earliest changes in the diabetic retina. Given the complex function of pericytes in the mature vasculature, their early loss in developing retinopathy would have profound consequences for the underlying endothelium and the integrity of the blood-retina barrier. In fact, pericyte loss as a hallmark of human diabetic retinopathy is accompanied by EC degeneration leading to vasoregression, vascular leakage and formation of microaneurysms as a sign of vessel destabilization and focal EC proliferation.

Animal Models of Diabetic Retinopathy

Human original material is unavailable, and data on the degree and the time course of pericyte function mostly derive from animal models as widespread as from mice to monkeys.

Hyperglycemic Animal Models of Diabetic Retinopathy

Rats are the most commonly used models of experimental diabetic retinopathy. Permanent hyperglycemia is usually achieved by chemical induction with streptozotocin. In this model, pericyte loss of over 30% after 6 months of hyperglycemia and progressive capillary regression is reproducible, depending on the strain used [90–92]. Rat models mimicking human type 2 diabetes show similar morphological characteristics, suggesting that pericyte loss and other changes characteristic for retinopathy are caused by hyperglycemia-mediated mechanisms [93–95]. As in other animal models, the addition of sucrose to the diet in genetically obese fatty fa/fa rats resulted in a pronounced decrease in pericytes and signs of pericyte degeneration.

With the widespread use of genetically manipulated mice, their use, in particular in combination with chronic hyperglycemia, has become popular, although their retinopathic phenotype is considered less severe and the identification of pericytes more difficult than rats. Like in rats, diabetic retinal capillaries of mice show a loss of pericytes of 15–25% and significantly increased formation of acellular capillaries after 6 months of diabetes duration. Spontaneous diabetic mice as well as mouse models of type 2 diabetes are available [96–100]. Exceptional animal models of diabetic retinopathy are the spontaneous diabetic Chinese hamster, diabetic dogs and diabetic monkeys. They all show morphological characteristics of diabetic retinopathy, including early pericyte loss and vasoregression [101–109]. Therefore, pericyte loss represents a universal event in diabetic retinopathy, not restricted to specific conditions or species, and it is unlikely that humans are an exception from the rule. Nevertheless, the degree of pericyte loss and the severity of hyperglycemia-induced vascular changes differ in the different specimens and animal strains. Over and above, severity of hyperglycemia and hypertension has a clear impact on the degree of pericyte loss.

Genetically Modified Models Mimicking Diabetic Retinopathy

Availability of genetically modified organisms introduced a novel approach to study pathomechanisms of diabetic retinopathy. As noted earlier, angiogenic factors like the PDGF-B/PDGFR-β, the Ang/Tie-2 system and other factors are important in the recruitment of pericytes to the vasculature during retinal development. It becomes apparent that the same growth factors play key roles in the mechanisms underlying vascular changes in diabetic retinopathy. Thus, mice with modifications of these factors are suitable to understand the vascular consequences of pericyte deficiencies.

In diabetic mouse retinas, PDGF-B mRNA is decreased when compared to nondiabetic controls, suggesting a role of PDGF-B in hyperglycemia-induced pericyte loss. Heterozygous

PDGF-B-deficient mice showed a 28% reduction in the number of retinal pericytes compared to wild-type littermates and an increase in acellular capillaries during adulthood, implying that pericytes have survival-promoting functions for established retinal capillary. Hyperglycemia further aggravates pericyte dropout in this animal model. Retina of mice with an endothelium-restricted ablation of PDGF-B showed that pericyte loss up to 50% was accompanied by vasoregression in the retina, whereas pericyte deficits exceeding 50% induced retinal vasoproliferation mimicking proliferative diabetic retinopathy [52, 110]. The effect of inhibition of PDGF-B/PDGFR signaling in either a genetic or a therapeutic approach needs to be investigated.

Another growth factor system gaining increasing attention in regard to early pericyte loss in diabetic retinopathy is the angiopoietin/Tie receptor system. The interaction of Ang-1 with Tie-2 is crucial for the timely and coordinated recruitment of pericytes to the developing vascular system. To assess the pathogenetic role of the angiopoietin-Tie system in diabetic pericyte loss, the expression of Ang-1 and -2 was studied in a diabetic rat model, in which the onset of pericyte dropout is exactly known. It was found that Ang-2 is dramatically upregulated prior to the onset of pericyte dropout. Injection of recombinant Ang-2 into the vitreous of nondiabetic rats reproduced pericyte dropout within days, and the 25% pericyte loss of diabetic C56BL6/J mice after 6 months of diabetes was abolished in a diabetic mouse with a 50% reduction of Ang-2 gene dose [87]. Furthermore, constitutive overexpression of Ang-2 in photoreceptor cells induces reduced pericyte coverage in the deep capillary layers of the retina during retinal development. Similarly to the changes in PDGF-B+/– mice, hyperglycemia aggravates pericyte loss and vascular changes in adult Ang-2 overexpressing retina over time [111].

Studies in animal models of VEGF and IGF-1/-receptor signaling revealed that VEGF may play a significant role in pericyte recruitment, but the specific and predominant mechanism working in the eye, and in particular in the capillary network under pathological condition may be difficult to dissect [112]. In contrast, overexpression of IGF-1 in the outer nuclear layer and in photoreceptors of the retina led to almost 50% reduction in pericyte numbers [113]. Interestingly, the numbers of ECs remained unexpectedly unchanged, whereas acellular capillaries were more numerous already at the observed time point.

Mechanisms of Pericyte Loss

The underlying causes and mechanisms of early pericyte dropout in diabetic retinopathy still remain unclear. It is possible that pericyte loss is a result of passive processes, such as degeneration and apoptosis. For example, streptozotocin diabetic Wistar rats showed a 2.65-fold increase in the numbers of TUNEL-positive cells (including pericytes) in retinae after 11 months of hyperglycemia [114, 115]. Pericyte death was also present in retinal vessels of diabetic patients suggesting its relevance in clinical disease [116]. Alternatively to this hypothesis, growing evidence indicates that pericyte loss in diabetic retinopathy is the result of an active elimination via altered growth factor production by the neighboring cells in the retina.

Biochemical Mechanisms

The selective damage of pericytes by chronic hyperglycemia may be explained by altered biochemical pathways which have been implicated in the pathogenesis of microvascular damage, so that pericyte loss may be the consequence of hyperglycemic toxicity. The four biochemical pathways that have been discussed over years to be involved in the pathogenesis of diabetic complications are (a) increased activity of the polyol pathway, (b) activation of protein kinase C (PKC) isoforms by de novo synthesis of diacylglycerol

(DAG), (c) increased flux through the hexosamine pathway, and (d) supply of glycolytic intermediates for the formation of advanced glycation end products (AGEs). Furthermore, a direct toxic effect of modification of LDL has been discussed.

Polyol Pathway

The first pathway to be studied in this regard, was the aldose reductase pathway, as immunological evidence had suggested the selective presence of aldose reductase in pericytes [117]. When glucose levels in cells are low, the enzyme aldose reductase functions by detoxifying aldehydes to inactive alcohols. When glucose levels in cells rise in diabetes, the enzyme starts to reduce glucose to sorbitol, and this process consumes the cofactor NADPH. Since NADPH is an essential cofactor for the regeneration of an important intracellular antioxidant, reduced glutathione, its depletion may induce a significant impact on cellular defense against oxidative stress. According to novel findings, the expression and activity of aldose reductase are increased in bovine retinal pericytes in vitro when cultured in high glucose [118], and are accompanied by elevated intracellular sorbitol levels. Whether this leads to increased pericyte death and is amenable to pharmacological inhibition has not yet been demonstrated. Overall, in line with the notion that the absolute levels of aldose reductase in the retina may be too low to contribute significantly to retinopathy development, the majority of experimental, and one large clinical trial failed to establish this pathway as playing a major role.

Activation of Protein Kinase C Isoforms

Most PKC isoforms are activated by the lipid second messenger DAG. Intracellular hyperglycemia increases the amount of DAG in cultured microvascular cells and in the retina, and the de novo synthesis DAG subsequently promotes PKC activation. The β- and δ-isoforms of PKC are activated primarily and elevate PKC-α and PKC-ε isoforms in the retina. Hyperglycemia-induced activation of PKC isoforms may mediate by the receptor of AGE and increased activity of polyol pathway (ROS). In retinal pericytes, the activation of PKC-β_2 isoform is involved in control of VEGF expression through RNA-binding protein HuR, which stabilizes mRNA [119]. Retinal pericytes express VEGF and pigment epithelium-derived factor (PEDF). VEGF promotes retinal neovascularization but PEDF suppresses ischemia-induced retinal neovascularization due to induction of apoptosis in retinal ECs. The PKC-MAPK signaling suppression by retinal pericyte-conditioned medium prevents retinal EC proliferation [120]. Hyperglycemia induces ET-1 mRNA expression in capillary bovine retinal ECs and bovine retinal pericytes. The α-, β_1- and δ-isoforms of PKC are significantly increased accompanied with ET-1 elevation in retinal pericytes [121–123]. PKC isoform activation can be inhibited by specific PKC inhibitors in the retina. The activation of PKC contributes to increased microvascular matrix protein accumulation by inducing TGF-β1, fibronectin and type IV collagen in mesangial cells of diabetic rats. The activation of NF-kB and overexpression of the fibrinolytic inhibitor plasminogen activator inhibitor (PAI-1) are also involved in hyperglycemia-induced activation of PKC in vSMCs.

Hexosamine Pathway

In diabetes, increased flux of fructose-6-phosphate diverted from glycolysis to UDP-N-acetylglucosamine promotes modification of protein by O-linked N-acetylglucosamine (GlcNac). The rate-limiting enzyme in this pathway is glutamine:fructose-6-phosphate aminotransferase (GFAT), converting glucose to glucosamine. GFAT is linked to transcription of TGF-α, TGF-β and PAI-1 promoter mediated by transcription factor Sp1 in vSMCs [124]. GlcNac covalently modifies Sp1 and regulates PAI-1 transcription. Glucosamine itself also activates the PAI-1 promoter through the Sp1 site. This pathway has a key role in fat- or glucose-induced insulin resistance. Apart from that, recent evidence suggests that GlcNac also contributes to hyperglycemia-induced upregulation of Ang-2 by Sp3 binding (see below).

AGE Formation

Chronic hyperglycemia-induced formation of reactive oxygen species and AGEs, which accumulate in pericytes in vivo [125] might be able to initiate pericyte degeneration. Methylglyoxal is the most important intracellular AGE precursor, which reacts with aminogroups of arginine in intracellular proteins to form AGEs. Interestingly, injection of exogenous AGE into nondiabetic animals resulted in a selective uptake in pericytes [126]. In principle, repeated injection of high doses of AGE-modified rat serum can induce selective pericyte loss in normal rats after 2 weeks [127]. Moreover, endogenous AGEs can form and accumulate in pericytes [125]. While the ingestion of exogenous AGEs is consistent with the propensity of phagocytosis of pericytes, the formation of endogenous AGEs in pericytes is inconsistent with the prior finding that pericytes and SMCs are able to downregulate glucose uptake to protect themselves from hyperglycemic damage [128]. It is thus speculated that pericytes take up AGEs from the circulation or from the direct vicinity, suggesting a clearing function under specific conditions. Since the tissue load with AGEs changes over time in diabetes, the role of pericytes as an AGE-removing cell compartment becomes increasingly relevant. However, the time course of AGE accumulation in pericytes (occurring over several months) is inconsistent with the time course of pericyte loss, starting after approximately 8 weeks of diabetes with a plateau after 6 months in diabetic animals.

Selective Pericyte Injury – Modification of LDL as an Example

Another piece of evidence suggests that pericytes may be injured by toxic plasma proteins which predominantly form in the diabetic milieu. Pericytes are differentially susceptible to damage by modified LDL in vitro [129]. As in vivo correlate, the combination of elevated glucose and lipids in ApoE$^{-/-}$ db/db mice led to an almost doubling of pericyte ghosts after 6 months of exposure. The majority of genes upregulated in human pericytes exposed to modifications of LDL such as oxidized-glycated LDL belong to the families of signal transduction, enzymes, and lipid metabolism [130, 131]. One interesting gene regulated by exposure of pericytes to modified lipids is TIMP-3, which controls vessel stability and maturation in vitro. Exposure of cultured human retinal pericytes to glycated-oxidized LDL repressed TIMP-3 expression 2.4-fold vs. pericytes exposed to unmodified LDL. Given the close cell-cell communication based on physical contacts between ECs and pericytes, it is conceivable that the MMP-TIMP system can play a significant role in execution of vascular stabilization by pericytes, and to the respective alteration in diabetes [132]. Although a clear clinical benefit of lipid-lowering treatment for diabetic retinopathy has not been demonstrated [133, 134], the preclinical data and evidence from associative studies suggest an association between lipoprotein profiles and the severity of retinopathy at least in type 1 diabetes [135]. It must be kept in mind that lipid-lowering drugs can have an independent effect on pericyte survival. For instance, it was recently reported that statins, in particular simvastatin, a potent HMG-CoA reductase inhibitor, can selectively induce pericyte apoptosis in vitro.

A Unifying Mechanism of Biochemical Dysregulation

As mentioned before, four pathways have been investigated over many years to explain how diabetes can affect diabetic vascular target cells: the polyol pathway, the hexosamine pathway, the PKC pathway, and increased production of AGEs. Recently, these seemingly independent biochemical pathways have been linked by the findings that one single mechanisms, hyperglycemia-induced mitochondrial overproduction of reactive oxygen species, is the underlying cause, which, mediated through the enzyme poly-ADP-ribose polymerase, blocks activities of the critical glycolytic enzyme glyceraldehyde-3-phosphate dehydrogenase [136, 137]. In normal cells, glucose is metabolized through glycolysis and the tricarbon cycle to generate electron donors for the mitochondrial respiratory chain. Here, energy (ATP) is generated in a precisely regulated way. In hyperglycemic cells, increased flux through glycolysis and the TCA cycle generates a voltage gradient of electrons surpassing a certain threshold which is then blocked inside complex III of the mitochondrial electron transport chain. From complex III, the surplus of electrons is purported to coenzyme Q together with molecular oxygen producing superoxide. The mitochondrial form of superoxide dismutase detoxifies this radical via hydrogen peroxide to water in the presence of oxygen. The link between the four biochemical pathways, and the mitochondrial overproduction of ROS was made when it became evident that an important change in hyperglycemic cells and in experimental animals was the reduced activity of the glycolytic enzyme glyceraldehyde-3-phosphate dehydrogenase. When examining for biochemical modifications of the enzyme, it was observed that hyperglycemia-induced superoxides caused polymers of ADP-ribose to attach and reduce enzyme activity. These changes were prevented with the inhibition of superoxide generation, and with the inhibition of the nuclear enzyme poly-ADP-ribose polymerase using a specific PARP inhibitor. The latter is activated upon DNA strand brakes known to form in hyperglycemic cells. Reduced GAPDH activity induced by PARP activation activates the biochemical pathways by increasing intermediates such as diacyl-glycerol (PKC pathway), glyceraldehyde-3-phosphate (AGE pathway), fructose-6-phosphate (hexosamine pathway), and intracellular glucose (sorbitol pathway). Thus, hyperglycemia links to biochemical pathway abnormalities via a common denominator, mitochondrial overproduction of reactive oxygen species.

Pericyte Loss through Active Elimination

Alternatively to early pericyte loss in diabetic retinopathy being the result of hyperglycemic injury, a different concept was proposed. It is possible that pericyte loss is an active process involving migration of pericytes away from the capillaries, driven by the angiopoietin-Tie system.

Hyperglycemia-Induced Ang-2 Transcription

As described above, gain of function experiments in nondiabetic animals revealed the induction of pericyte dropout in the vicinity of the Ang-2 overexpressing site. Superimposition of diabetes aggravated the most important vascular readout, i.e. the formation of acellular capillaries. Loss of function studies in the presence of diabetes yielded the prevention of pericyte dropout and the reduction in acellular capillary formation, accentuating the importance of Ang-2 in diabetic pericyte loss. Ang-2 is expressed in three cell types of the retina, i.e. the EC, the Müller cells, and the horizontal cells. In situ hybridization of diabetic retinae for Ang-2 yielded the expression particularly in Müller cells. Recently, the regulation of Ang-2 in chronic hyperglycemia has been delineated using renal microvascular cells as paradigm.

Yao et al. [138] proposed a mechanism by which AGEs enhance transcription of Ang-2, as a crucial factor in the development of diabetic retinopathy. It was found that increased glucose flux in renal microvascular ECs caused increased modification of the co-repressor mSin3A by the intracellular AGE methylglyoxal, resulting in recruitment of the enzyme O-GlcNAc transferase to an mSin3A-Sp3 complex. Subsequently, Sp3 modification by O-linked N-acetylglucosamine decreased its binding to the glucose-responsive GC box in the Ang-2 promoter and the activation of Ang-2 transcription [138]. The same mechanism was operative in retinal Müller cells consistent with in vivo data from retinae of diabetic rats and mice. These data are in line with the hypothesis that pericyte loss is induced by glial cells overexpressing Ang-2 in response to high glucose.

Ang-2 and Diabetic Pericyte Loss

The next question is how hyperglycemia-induced upregulation of Ang-2 contributes to retinal pericyte loss. Quantitation of pericyte subpopulation in diabetic retinas showed that a proportion of retinal pericytes are affected by hyperglycemia and that some pericytes lose contact with intact capillaries, defined as pericyte migration [100]. Overexpression of Ang-2 in the retina mimicked hyperglycemia-induced pericyte migration, whereas Ang-2-deficient mice completely lacked hyperglycemia-induced increase in pericyte migration when compared to diabetic wild-type mice. Therefore, pericyte destabilization and migration in response to Ang-2 upregulation due to increased AGE production represents a novel mechanism of pericyte loss in the diabetic retina.

Conclusions

Since the observation that pericyte loss is an early morphological change in the natural history of diabetic retinopathy, substantial progress has been made in the understanding of the factors and mechanisms involved. The central change causing pericyte loss is chronic elevation of glucose with subsequent generation of reactive oxygen species. The molecular scenery encompasses posttranslational modification of co-repressor and transcription factors finally resulting in altered expression of genes crucially involved in the cellular crosstalk of the retinal vasculature. These changes are amenable to therapeutic interventions.

References

1 Antonetti DA, et al: Diabetic retinopathy: seeing beyond glucose-induced microvascular disease. Diabetes 2006;55:2401–2411.

2 West H, Richardson WD, Fruttiger M: Stabilization of the retinal vascular network by reciprocal feedback between blood vessels and astrocytes. Development 2005;132:1855–1862.

3 Sims DE: Diversity within pericytes. Clin Exp Pharmacol Physiol 2000;27:842–846.

4 Etchevers HC, et al: The cephalic neural crest provides pericytes and smooth muscle cells to all blood vessels of the face and forebrain. Development 2001;128:1059–1068.

5 Hughes S, Chan-Ling T: Characterization of smooth muscle cell and pericyte differentiation in the rat retina in vivo. Invest Ophthalmol Vis Sci 2004;45:2795–2806.

6 Yamashita J, et al: Flk1-positive cells derived from embryonic stem cells serve as vascular progenitors. Nature 2000;408:92–96.

7 Rajantie I, et al: Adult bone marrow-derived cells recruited during angiogenesis comprise precursors for periendothelial vascular mural cells. Blood 2004;104:2084–2086.

8 DeRuiter MC, et al: Embryonic endothelial cells transdifferentiate into mesenchymal cells expressing smooth muscle actins in vivo and in vitro. Circ Res 1997;80:444–451.

9 Farrington-Rock C, et al: Chondrogenic and adipogenic potential of microvascular pericytes. Circulation 2004;110:2226–2232.

10 Schor AM, et al: Pericytes derived from the retinal microvasculature undergo calcification in vitro. J Cell Sci 1990;97(Pt 3):449–461.

11 van Deurs B: Observations on the blood-brain barrier in hypertensive rats, with particular reference to phagocytic pericytes. J Ultrastruct Res 1976;56:65–77.

12 Thomas WE: Brain macrophages: on the role of pericytes and perivascular cells. Brain Res Rev 1999;31:42–57.

13 Hirschi KK, Rohovsky SA, D'Amore PA: PDGF, TGF-beta, and heterotypic cell-cell interactions mediate endothelial cell-induced recruitment of 10T1/2 cells and their differentiation to a smooth muscle fate. J Cell Biol 1998;141:805–814.

14 Nehls V, Denzer K, Drenckhahn D: Pericyte involvement in capillary sprouting during angiogenesis in situ. Cell Tissue Res 1992;270:469–474.

15 Nicosia RF, Villaschi S: Rat aortic smooth muscle cells become pericytes during angiogenesis in vitro. Lab Invest 1995;73:658–666.

16 Sundberg C, et al: Pericytes as collagen-producing cells in excessive dermal scarring. Lab Invest 1996;74:452–466.
17 Villaschi S, Nicosia RF, Smith MR: Isolation of a morphologically and functionally distinct smooth muscle cell type from the intimal aspect of the normal rat aorta. Evidence for smooth muscle cell heterogeneity. In Vitro Cell Dev Biol Anim 1994;30A:589–595.
18 Shepro D, Morel NM: Pericyte physiology. FASEB J 1993;7:1031–1038.
19 Cogan DG, Toussaint D, Kuwabara T: Retinal vascular patterns. IV. Diabetic retinopathy. Arch Ophthalmol 1961;66:366–378.
20 Kuwabara T, Carroll JM, Cogan DG: Retinal vascular patterns. III. Age, hypertension, absolute glaucoma, injury. Arch Ophthalmol 1961;65:708–716.
21 Allt G, Lawrenson JG: Pericytes: cell biology and pathology. Cells Tissues Organs 2001;169:1–11.
22 Sims DE: The pericyte – a review. Tissue Cell 1986;18:153–174.
23 Sims DE: Recent advances in pericyte biology – implications for health and disease. Can J Cardiol 1991;7:431–443.
24 Tilton RG, et al: Pericyte degeneration and acellular capillaries are increased in the feet of human diabetic patients. Diabetologia 1985;28:895–900.
25 Wakui S, et al: Transforming growth factor-beta and urokinase plasminogen activator presents at endothelial cell-pericyte interdigitation in human granulation tissue. Microvasc Res 1997;54:262–269.
26 Armulik A, Abramsson A, Betsholtz C: Endothelial/pericyte interactions. Circ Res 2005;97:512–523.
27 Gerhardt H, Betsholtz C: Endothelial-pericyte interactions in angiogenesis. Cell Tissue Res 2003;314:15–23.
28 Larson DM, Carson MP, Haudenschild CC: Junctional transfer of small molecules in cultured bovine brain microvascular endothelial cells and pericytes. Microvasc Res 1987;34:184–199.
29 Crocker DJ, Murad TM, Geer JC: Role of the pericyte in wound healing: an ultrastructural study. Exp Mol Pathol 1970;13:51–65.
30 Fujimoto K: Pericyte-endothelial gap junctions in developing rat cerebral capillaries: a fine structural study. Anat Rec 1995;242:562–565.
31 Giebel SJ, et al: Matrix metalloproteinases in early diabetic retinopathy and their role in alteration of the blood-retinal barrier. Lab Invest 2005;85:597–607.
32 Fukuhara S, et al: Differential function of Tie2 at cell-cell contacts and cell-substratum contacts regulated by angiopoietin-1. Nat Cell Biol 2008;10:513–526.
33 Saharinen P, et al: Angiopoietins assemble distinct Tie2 signalling complexes in endothelial cell-cell and cell-matrix contacts. Nat Cell Biol 2008;10:527–537.
34 Hori S, et al: A pericyte-derived angiopoietin-1 multimeric complex induces occludin gene expression in brain capillary endothelial cells through Tie-2 activation in vitro. J Neurochem 2004;89:503–513.
35 Courtoy PJ, Boyles J: Fibronectin in the microvasculature: localization in the pericyte-endothelial interstitium. J Ultrastruct Res 1983;83:258–273.
36 Hirschi KK, D'Amore PA: Pericytes in the microvasculature. Cardiovasc Res 1996;32:687–698.
37 Rucker HK, Wynder HJ, Thomas WE: Cellular mechanisms of CNS pericytes. Brain Res Bull 2000;51:363–369.
38 Ramsauer M, D'Amore PA: Getting Tie(2)d up in angiogenesis. J Clin Invest 2002;110:1615–1617.
39 Hall AP: Review of the pericyte during angiogenesis and its role in cancer and diabetic retinopathy. Toxicol Pathol 2006;34:763–775.
40 Thurston G, et al: Leakage-resistant blood vessels in mice transgenically overexpressing angiopoietin-1. Science 1999;286:2511–2514.
41 Yamagishi S, et al: Endothelin 1 mediates endothelial cell-dependent proliferation of vascular pericytes. Biochem Biophys Res Commun 1993;191:840–846.
42 Martin AR, et al: Retinal pericytes control expression of nitric oxide synthase and endothelin-1 in microvascular endothelial cells. Microvasc Res 2000;59:131–139.
43 Newman EA: Propagation of intercellular calcium waves in retinal astrocytes and Muller cells. J Neurosci 2001;21:2215–2223.
44 Ochs M, Mayhew TM, Knabe W: To what extent are the retinal capillaries ensheathed by Muller cells? A stereological study in the tree shrew Tupaia belangeri. J Anat 2000;196(Pt 3):453–461.
45 Sarthy VP: Muller cells in retinal health and disease. Arch Soc Esp Oftalmol 2000;75:367–368.
46 Bringmann A, et al: Muller cells in the healthy and diseased retina. Prog Retin Eye Res 2006;25:397–424.
47 Busik JV, Mohr S, Grant MB: Hyperglycemia-induced reactive oxygen species toxicity to endothelial cells is dependent on paracrine mediators. Diabetes 2008;57:1952–1965.
48 Rungger-Brandle E, Dosso AA, Leuenberger PM: Glial reactivity, an early feature of diabetic retinopathy. Invest Ophthalmol Vis Sci 2000;41:1971–1980.
49 Bondjers C, et al: Transcription profiling of platelet-derived growth factor-B-deficient mouse embryos identifies RGS5 as a novel marker for pericytes and vascular smooth muscle cells. Am J Pathol 2003;162:721–729.
50 Cho H, et al: Pericyte-specific expression of Rgs5: implications for PDGF and EDG receptor signaling during vascular maturation. FASEB J 2003;17:440–442.
51 Joyce NC, et al: cGMP-dependent protein kinase is present in high concentrations in contractile cells of the kidney vasculature. J Cyclic Nucleotide Protein Phosphor Res 1986;11:191–198.
52 Lindahl P, et al: Pericyte loss and microaneurysm formation in PDGF-B-deficient mice. Science 1997;277:242–245.
53 Nehls V, Drenckhahn D: Heterogeneity of microvascular pericytes for smooth muscle type alpha-actin. J Cell Biol 1991;113:147–154.
54 Ozerdem U, et al: NG2 proteoglycan is expressed exclusively by mural cells during vascular morphogenesis. Dev Dyn 2001;222:218–227.
55 Piva TJ, Krause DR, Ellem KO: UVC activation of the HeLa cell membrane 'TGF alpha ase,' a metalloenzyme. J Cell Biochem 1997;64:353–368.
56 Ruiter DJ, et al: Angiogenesis in wound healing and tumor metastasis. Behring Inst Mitt, 1993:258–272.
57 Song S, et al: PDGFRbeta+ perivascular progenitor cells in tumours regulate pericyte differentiation and vascular survival. Nat Cell Biol 2005;7:870–879.

58 Tidhar A, et al: A novel transgenic marker for migrating limb muscle precursors and for vascular smooth muscle cells. Dev Dyn 2001;220:60–73.
59 Bagley RG, et al: Endosialin/TEM 1/CD248 is a pericyte marker of embryonic and tumor neovascularization. Microvasc Res 2008;76:180–188.
60 Christian S, et al: Endosialin (Tem1) is a marker of tumor-associated myofibroblasts and tumor vessel-associated mural cells. Am J Pathol 2008;172:486–494.
61 MacFadyen J, et al: Endosialin is expressed on stromal fibroblasts and CNS pericytes in mouse embryos and is downregulated during development. Gene Expr Patterns, 2007;7:363–369.
62 Simonavicius N, et al: Endosialin (CD248) is a marker of tumor-associated pericytes in high-grade glioma. Mod Pathol 2008;21:308–315.
63 Bondjers C, et al: Microarray analysis of blood microvessels from PDGF-B and PDGF-Rβ mutant mice identifies novel markers for brain pericytes. FASEB J 2006;20:1703–1705.
64 Berger M, et al: Regulator of G-protein signaling-5 induction in pericytes coincides with active vessel remodeling during neovascularization. Blood 2005;105:1094–1101.
65 Hamzah J, et al: Vascular normalization in Rgs5-deficient tumours promotes immune destruction. Nature 2008;453:410–414.
66 Bergers G, Song S: The role of pericytes in blood-vessel formation and maintenance. Neuro Oncol 2005;7:452–464.
67 Joyce NC, Haire MF, Palade GE: Contractile proteins in pericytes. II. Immunocytochemical evidence for the presence of two isomyosins in graded concentrations. J Cell Biol 1985;100:1387–1395.
68 Joyce NC, Haire MF, Palade GE: Contractile proteins in pericytes. I. Immunoperoxidase localization of tropomyosin. J Cell Biol 1985;100:1379–1386.
69 Peppiatt CM, et al: Bidirectional control of CNS capillary diameter by pericytes. Nature, 2006;443:700–704.
70 Balabanov R, Dore-Duffy P: Role of the CNS microvascular pericyte in the blood-brain barrier. J Neurosci Res 1998;53:637–644.
71 Bauer HC, Steiner M, Bauer H: Embryonic development of the CNS microvasculature in the mouse: new insights into the structural mechanisms of early angiogenesis. EXS 1992;61:64–68.
72 Egginton S, et al: The role of pericytes in controlling angiogenesis in vivo. Adv Exp Med Biol 2000;476:81–99.
73 Gerhardt H, Wolburg H, Redies C: N-cadherin mediates pericytic-endothelial interaction during brain angiogenesis in the chicken. Dev Dyn 2000;218:472–479.
74 Wakui S, et al: Localization of Ang-1, -2, Tie-2, and VEGF expression at endothelial-pericyte interdigitation in rat angiogenesis. Lab Invest 2006;86:1172–1184.
75 Uemura A, et al: Recombinant angiopoietin-1 restores higher-order architecture of growing blood vessels in mice in the absence of mural cells. J Clin Invest 2002;110:1619–1628.
76 Lundkvist A, et al: Growth factor gradients in vascular patterning. Novartis Found Symp 2007;283:194–201; discussion 201–206, 238–241.
77 Hellstrom M, et al: Dll4 signalling through Notch1 regulates formation of tip cells during angiogenesis. Nature 2007;445:776–780.
78 Anderson CR, Ponce AM, Price RJ: Immunohistochemical identification of an extracellular matrix scaffold that microguides capillary sprouting in vivo. J Histochem Cytochem 2004;52:1063–1072.
79 Benjamin LE, Hemo I, Keshet E: A plasticity window for blood vessel remodelling is defined by pericyte coverage of the preformed endothelial network and is regulated by PDGF-B and VEGF. Development 1998;125:1591–1598.
80 Ozerdem U, Stallcup WB: Early contribution of pericytes to angiogenic sprouting and tube formation. Angiogenesis 2003;6:241–249.
81 Kono M, et al: The sphingosine-1-phosphate receptors S1P1, S1P2, and S1P3 function coordinately during embryonic angiogenesis. J Biol Chem 2004;279:29367–29373.
82 Weinstein M, Yang X, Deng C: Functions of mammalian Smad genes as revealed by targeted gene disruption in mice. Cytokine Growth Factor Rev 2000;11:49–58.
83 Cohen MP, Frank RN, Khalifa AA: Collagen production by cultured retinal capillary pericytes. Invest Ophthalmol Vis Sci 1980;19:90–94.
84 Weibel ER: On pericytes, particularly their existence on lung capillaries. Microvasc Res 1974;8:218–235.
85 Schor AM, et al: Differentiation of pericytes in culture is accompanied by changes in the extracellular matrix. In Vitro Cell Dev Biol 1991;27A:651–659.
86 Kennedy A, Frank RN, Mancini MA: In vitro production of glycosaminoglycans by retinal microvessel cells and lens epithelium. Invest Ophthalmol Vis Sci 1986;27:746–754.
87 Hammes HP, et al: Angiopoietin-2 causes pericyte dropout in the normal retina: evidence for involvement in diabetic retinopathy. Diabetes 2004;53:1104–1110.
88 Kim I, et al: Angiopoietin-2 at high concentration can enhance endothelial cell survival through the phosphatidylinositol 3′-kinase/Akt signal transduction pathway. Oncogene 2000;19:4549–4552.
89 Sundberg C, et al: Stable expression of angiopoietin-1 and other markers by cultured pericytes: phenotypic similarities to a subpopulation of cells in maturing vessels during later stages of angiogenesis in vivo. Lab Invest 2002;82:387–401.
90 Hammes HP, et al: Aminoguanidine does not inhibit the initial phase of experimental diabetic retinopathy in rats. Diabetologia 1995;38:269–273.
91 Hoffmann J, et al: Tenilsetam prevents early diabetic retinopathy without correcting pericyte loss. Thromb Haemost 2006;95:689–695.
92 Lin J, et al: Effect of R-(+)-alpha-lipoic acid on experimental diabetic retinopathy. Diabetologia 2006;49:1089–1096.
93 Agardh CD, et al: Altered endothelial/pericyte ratio in Goto-Kakizaki rat retina. J Diabetes Complications 1997;11:158–162.
94 Dosso A, et al: Ocular complications in the old and glucose-intolerant genetically obese (fa/fa) rat. Diabetologia 1990;33:137–144.
95 Kim SH, et al: Morphologic studies of the retina in a new diabetic model; SHR/N:Mcc-cp rat. Yonsei Med J 1998;39:453–462.

96 Barber AJ, et al: The Ins2Akita mouse as a model of early retinal complications in diabetes. Invest Ophthalmol Vis Sci 2005;46:2210–2218.
97 Feit-Leichman RA, et al: Vascular damage in a mouse model of diabetic retinopathy: relation to neuronal and glial changes. Invest Ophthalmol Vis Sci 2005;46:4281–4287.
98 Midena E, et al: Studies on the retina of the diabetic db/db mouse. I. Endothelial cell-pericyte ratio. Ophthalmic Res 1989;21:106–111.
99 Obrosova IG, et al: Early diabetes-induced biochemical changes in the retina: comparison of rat and mouse models. Diabetologia 2006;49:2525–2533.
100 Pfister F, et al: Pericyte migration: a novel mechanism of pericyte loss in experimental diabetic retinopathy. Diabetes 2008;57:2495–2502.
101 Buchi ER, Kurosawa A, Tso MO: Retinopathy in diabetic hypertensive monkeys: a pathologic study. Graefes Arch Clin Exp Ophthalmol 1996;234:388–398.
102 Engerman RL, Kern TS: Experimental galactosemia produces diabetic-like retinopathy. Diabetes 1984;33:97–100.
103 Gardiner TA, et al: Selective loss of vascular smooth muscle cells in the retinal microcirculation of diabetic dogs. Br J Ophthalmol 1994;78:54–60.
104 Hammes HP, et al: The relationship of glycaemic level to advanced glycation end-product (AGE) accumulation and retinal pathology in the spontaneous diabetic hamster. Diabetologia 1998;41:165–170.
105 Kador PF, et al: Age-dependent retinal capillary pericyte degeneration in galactose-fed dogs. J Ocul Pharmacol Ther 2007;23:63–69.
106 Kador PF, et al: Effect of galactose diet removal on the progression of retinal vessel changes in galactose-fed dogs. Invest Ophthalmol Vis Sci 2002;43:1916–1921.
107 Kador PF, et al: Amelioration of diabetes-like retinal changes in galactose-fed dogs. Prev Med 1994;23:717–721.
108 Kador PF, et al: Diabetes-like proliferative retinal changes in galactose-fed dogs. Arch Ophthalmol 1995;113:352–354.
109 Kim SY, et al: Retinopathy in monkeys with spontaneous type 2 diabetes. Invest Ophthalmol Vis Sci 2004;45:4543–4553.
110 Hammes HP, et al: Pericytes and the pathogenesis of diabetic retinopathy. Diabetes 2002;51:3107–3112.
111 Feng Y, et al: Impaired pericyte recruitment and abnormal retinal angiogenesis as a result of angiopoietin-2 overexpression. Thromb Haemost 2007;97:99–108.
112 Stalmans I, et al: Arteriolar and venular patterning in retinas of mice selectively expressing VEGF isoforms. J Clin Invest 2002;109:327–336.
113 Ruberte J, et al: Increased ocular levels of IGF-1 in transgenic mice lead to diabetes-like eye disease. J Clin Invest 2004;113:1149–1157.
114 Kowluru RA: Diabetic retinopathy: mitochondrial dysfunction and retinal capillary cell death. Antioxid Redox Signal 2005;7:1581–1587.
115 Kowluru RA, Odenbach S: Effect of long-term administration of alpha-lipoic acid on retinal capillary cell death and the development of retinopathy in diabetic rats. Diabetes 2004;53:3233–3238.
116 Mizutani M, Kern TS, Lorenzi M: Accelerated death of retinal microvascular cells in human and experimental diabetic retinopathy. J Clin Invest 1996;97:2883–2890.
117 Akagi Y, et al: Aldose reductase localization in human retinal mural cells. Invest Ophthalmol Vis Sci 1983;24:1516–1519.
118 Berrone E, et al: Regulation of intracellular glucose and polyol pathway by thiamine and benfotiamine in vascular cells cultured in high glucose. J Biol Chem 2006;281:9307–9313.
119 Amadio M, et al: PKCbetaII/HuR/VEGF: a new molecular cascade in retinal pericytes for the regulation of VEGF gene expression. Pharmacol Res 2008;57:60–66.
120 Kondo T, et al: PKC/MAPK signaling suppression by retinal pericyte conditioned medium prevents retinal endothelial cell proliferation. J Cell Physiol 2005;203:378–386.
121 Lee TS, et al: Endothelin stimulates a sustained 1,2-diacylglycerol increase and protein kinase C activation in bovine aortic smooth muscle cells. Biochem Biophys Res Commun 1989;162:381–386.
122 Lee TS, et al: Characterization of endothelin receptors and effects of endothelin on diacylglycerol and protein kinase C in retinal capillary pericytes. Diabetes 1989;38:1643–1646.
123 Park JY, et al: Induction of endothelin-1 expression by glucose: an effect of protein kinase C activation. Diabetes 2000;49:1239–1248.
124 Chen YQ, et al: Sp1 sites mediate activation of the plasminogen activator inhibitor-1 promoter by glucose in vascular smooth muscle cells. J Biol Chem 1998;273:8225–8231.
125 Yamagishi S, et al: Advanced glycation endproducts accelerate calcification in microvascular pericytes. Biochem Biophys Res Commun 1999;258:353–357.
126 Stitt AW, et al: Advanced glycation end products (AGEs) co-localize with AGE receptors in the retinal vasculature of diabetic and of AGE-infused rats. Am J Pathol 1997;150:523–531.
127 Xu X, et al: Exogenous advanced glycosylation end products induce diabetes-like vascular dysfunction in normal rats: a factor in diabetic retinopathy. Graefes Arch Clin Exp Ophthalmol 2003;241:56–62.
128 Kaiser N, et al: Differential regulation of glucose transport and transporters by glucose in vascular endothelial and smooth muscle cells. Diabetes 1993;42:80–89.
129 Lyons TJ, et al: Aminoguanidine and the effects of modified LDL on cultured retinal capillary cells. Invest Ophthalmol Vis Sci 2000;41:1176–1180.
130 Song W, et al: Effects of modified low-density lipoproteins on human retinal pericyte survival. Ann N Y Acad Sci 2005;1043:390–395.
131 Song W, et al: Effects of oxidized and glycated LDL on gene expression in human retinal capillary pericytes. Invest Ophthalmol Vis Sci 2005;46:2974–2982.
132 Barth JL, et al: Oxidised, glycated LDL selectively influences tissue inhibitor of metalloproteinase-3 gene expression and protein production in human retinal capillary pericytes. Diabetologia 2007;50:2200–2208.
133 Keech AC, et al: Effect of fenofibrate on the need for laser treatment for diabetic retinopathy (FIELD study): a randomised controlled trial. Lancet 2007;370:1687–1697.

134 Colhoun HM, et al: Primary prevention of cardiovascular disease with atorvastatin in type 2 diabetes in the Collaborative Atorvastatin Diabetes Study (CARDS): multicentre randomised placebo-controlled trial. Lancet 2004;364:685–696.
135 Lyons TJ, et al: Diabetic retinopathy and serum lipoprotein subclasses in the DCCT/EDIC cohort. Invest Ophthalmol Vis Sci 2004;45:910–918.
136 Brownlee M: Biochemistry and molecular cell biology of diabetic complications. Nature 2001;414:813–820.
137 Hammes HP: Pathophysiological mechanisms of diabetic angiopathy. J Diabetes Complications 2003;17(2 suppl):16–19.
138 Yao D, Taguchi T, Matsumura T, Pestell R, Edelstein D, Giardino I, Suske G, Rabbani N, Thornalley PJ, Sarthy VP, Hammes HP, Brownlee M: High glucose increases angiopoietin-2 transcription in microvascular endothelial cells through methylglyoxal modification of mSin3A. J Biol Chem 2007;282:31038–31045.

Prof. Hans-Peter Hammes
Section of Endocrinology, 5th Medical Department, Mannheim Medical Faculty
University Hospital Mannheim, Ruprechts-Karls University Heidelberg
Theodor-Kutzer-Ufer 1–3, DE–68167 Mannheim (Germany)
Tel./Fax +49 621 383 2663, E-Mail hp.hammes@umm.de

Hammes H-P, Porta M (eds): Experimental Approaches to Diabetic Retinopathy.
Front Diabetes. Basel, Karger, 2010, vol 20, pp 79–97

Neuroglia in the Diabetic Retina

A. Bringmann[a] · A. Reichenbach[b]

[a]Department of Ophthalmology and Eye Clinic, and [b]Paul Flechsig Institute of Brain Research, Medical Faculty of the University of Leipzig, Leipzig, Germany

Abstract

In addition to vascular changes, alterations in retinal neurons and glial cells occur early during diabetic retinopathy. The glial reactivity includes all three types of retinal glial cells (microglia, astrocytes, and Müller cells) and is both a consequence of and a contributor to vascular abnormalities and neuronal dysfunction in the diabetic retina. Activated microglial cells and astrocytes contribute to neuronal apoptosis. Reactive astrocytes and Müller cells are implicated in the breakdown of the blood-retinal barrier and in neovascularization. Furthermore, glial cells are important constituents of the fibrovascular scar tissues formed during proliferative diabetic retinopathy. A crucial aspect is that activated Müller cells display a dysregulation of various neuron-supportive functions. This results in disturbances of retinal glutamate metabolism and K^+ homeostasis and in the development of retinal edema, and finally aggravates the dysfunction and loss of neurons.

Although diabetic retinopathy is primarily a microangiopathy, reactive changes in retinal neurons and glia occur early in the course of the disease and precede the onset of clinically evident vascular injury. Loss of color [1] and contrast sensitivity [2], and abnormalities in the electroretinogram [3, 4] have been found in patients before vascular changes became obvious as established diagnostic key features of diabetic retinopathy. Similar early neuronal and glial alterations, indicative of a widespread retinal dysfunction, are present in rats with chemically induced diabetes. Decreases in components of the electroretinogram [5], increased apoptosis of retinal neurons [6], and reactivity of retinal glial cells [7–9] occur early in the course of experimental diabetic retinopathy, caused by glucose-induced hypoxic and oxidative stress conditions. These observations suggest that diabetic retinopathy is a multifactorial disease involving vasculature, neurons, and glia of the retina, and that glial dysfunction may be both a consequence of, and a contributor to vascular abnormalities and neuronal dysfunction.

The mammalian retina contains three types of glial cells: microglial cells and two species of neuron-supporting macroglial cells, astrocytes and Müller cells. Astrocytes and microglial cells are normally located in the innermost retinal layers (nerve fiber and ganglion cell layers). Astrocytes are stellate cells which invade the retina mainly from the optic nerve during ontogenesis [10]. During this invasion, the astrocytes respond to tissue hypoxia by secretion of the vascular endothelial growth factor (VEGF) that guides the developing vessels towards the macula [11]. In the adult tissue, astrocytes remain in contact

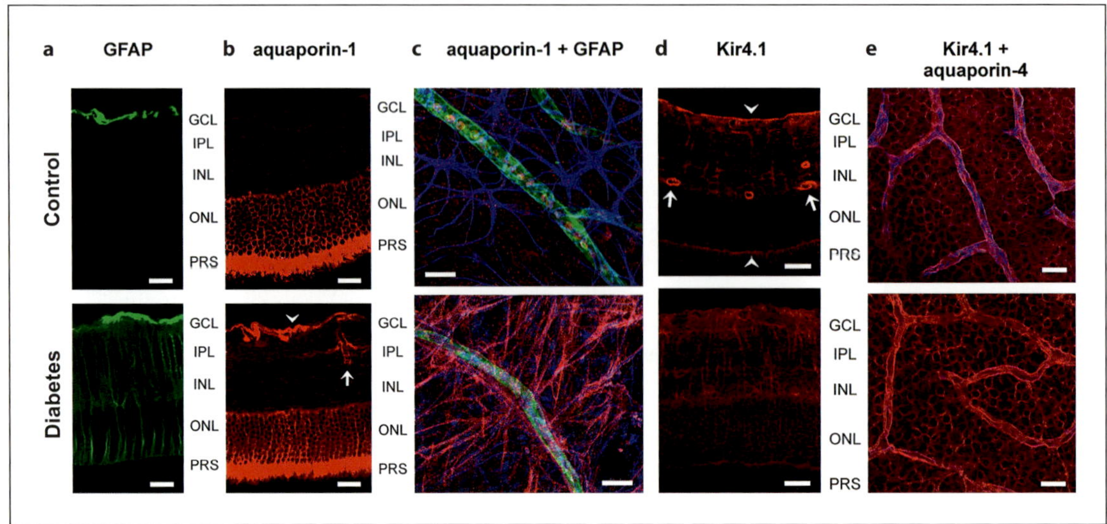

Fig. 1. Experimental diabetes alters the expression of proteins expressed by glial cells in the rat retina. The retinal slices (**a**, **b**, **d**) and flat-mounts (**c**, **e**) were derived from diabetic animals at 6 months after injection of streptozotocin and from age-matched control animals. **a** In the slice of a control retina, the immunoreactivity for GFAP is restricted to the astrocytes in the nerve fiber layer. In the diabetic retina, GFAP immunoreactivity is also expressed by the Müller cell fibers that span the whole retinal tissue. **b** The immunoreactivity for the water channel protein, aquaporin-1, is predominantly expressed by photoreceptor cells in the control retina, and is additionally expressed by astrocytes in the nerve fiber layer (arrowhead) and around vessels (arrow) in the diabetic retina. **c** The views onto the nerve fiber layer display green-stained blood vessels, and GFAP (blue) and aquaporin-1 (red) immunoreactivities in astrocytes. In the control retina, red blood cells within the capillaries express immunoreactivity for aquaporin-1. In the diabetic retina, aquaporin-1 is strongly expressed by astrocytes. **d** In the control retina, the immunoreactivity for Kir4.1 is prominently expressed around vessels (arrows) and at both limiting membranes (arrowheads). In the diabetic retina, the immunoreactivity for Kir4.1 displays a redistribution with absence of the prominent stainings around vessels and at the limiting membranes. **e** The views onto blood vessels within the inner nuclear layer display immunoreactivities for Kir4.1 (blue) and aquaporin-4 (red). Whereas the staining pattern for aquaporin-4 did not change in the course of diabetes, the prominent perivascular expression of Kir4.1 was absent in the diabetic retina. Scale bars = 20 μm. GCL = Ganglion cell layer; INL = inner nuclear layer; IPL = inner plexiform layer; ONL = outer nuclear layer; PRS = photoreceptor segments. Adapted from Pannicke et al. [54].

with the superficial vascular plexus via cellular processes which wrap around the vessels (fig. 1c). Microglial cells are the blood-derived resident immune cells within the retina; they originate from hemopoietic cells and invade the tissue from the retinal margin and the optic disc during ontogenesis, and from the vessels in the adult tissue where they form the perivascular microglia. Microglial cells have an important role in the host defense against invading microorganisms, in the initiation of inflammatory processes, and in tissue repair. In response to pathogenic stimuli, they become activated and migrate through the whole retinal tissue, to kill bacteria, release cytotoxic agents, and phagocytize cellular debris. In addition, several factors released by activated microglial cells – such as VEGF, nitric oxide, and metalloproteinases – may dissolve the blood-retinal barrier and thus facilitate the infiltration of leukocytes into the retina.

The Müller cell is the principal glial cell of the mammalian retina; it is a specialized radial glial cell spanning the entire thickness of the retina and contacting virtually all retinal neurons. Müller cells constitute an anatomic and functional link between retinal neurons and blood vessels, and play a wealth of crucial roles in supporting neuronal information processing [12, 13]. They are involved in retinal glucose metabolism and provide metabolic substrates to neurons [14]; they maintain the ion and water homeostasis of the retinal tissue [15], regulate the retinal blood flow [16], and contribute to the formation and maintenance of the blood-retinal barrier [17]. Müller cells contribute to the neuronal signaling processes, particularly by fast uptake and recycling of neurotransmitters and by providing precursors of neurotransmitters to neurons. The rapid termination of the postsynaptic action of glutamate is caused by the fast uptake of the transmitter into the Müller cells [18].

Müller cells become activated upon virtually all pathogenic stimuli. Müller cell gliosis is characterized by both nonspecific and specific responses to pathogenic factors. The former are stereotypical responses of Müller cells, independent on the type of the stimulus. The upregulation of the glial fibrillary acidic protein (GFAP) is such a nonspecific response to pathophysiological conditions [19] which is also observed early in diabetic retinopathy (fig. 1a) [8, 9, 20, 21]. One of the specific gliotic responses of Müller cells is an alteration of the expression of glutamine synthetase. After a loss of the major glutamate-releasing neurons, e.g. after photoreceptor degeneration evoked by excess light or by retinal detachment, the expression of the glutamine synthetase in Müller cells is reduced; an enhanced expression was observed during hepatic retinopathy when its activity is necessary to detoxify the tissue from elevated levels of ammonia [19]. On the other hand, no alteration of the glutamine synthetase expression by Müller cells was observed in diabetic retinopathy [20, 22]. This finding has led to the suggestion that Müller cell gliosis in the diabetic retina is not a specific response to neuronal degeneration but rather a response to more general changes occurring in the diabetic retinal milieu, caused by pathogenic factors such as oxidative stress [23, 24] and chronic inflammation [22, 25, 26].

Müller cells are targets of and players in diabetic changes in the retina. It is now well established that gliosis in the neural tissue is Janus-faced, contributing to both damage and protection of neurons [19]. Early after injury, gliosis is thought to be neuroprotective, as a cellular attempt to limit the extent of injury, e.g. by release of neurotrophic factors. However, at later stages, the formation of glial scars and the expression of inhibitory molecules on the surface of reactive glial cells inhibit tissue repair as well as regular neuroregeneration [27]. Moreover, functional changes of reactive glial cells (which in some aspects reflect a de-differentiation of the cells) may more directly contribute to further tissue damage, e.g. via disturbance of ion and water homeostasis, and dysregulation of neurotransmitter removal. It is noteworthy that the same gliotic reaction may exert biphasic effects, depending on time and/or amplitude. For instance, the induction of acute-phase proteins (e.g. proteins with antioxidant activity) in Müller cells of diabetic rats, may represent an adaptive response to restore homeostasis and to protect neurons [22]. On the other hand, persistent overexpression of acute-phase proteins may cause tissue damage, including endothelial dysfunction and angiogenesis [28, 29]. As another example, in response to ischemia and early in diabetic retinopathy, Müller cells increase the expression of inducible nitric oxide synthase [30, 31]. Though nitric oxide increases the local retinal perfusion (which is a desirable effect), higher concentrations of nitric oxide can be toxic to the retina [32]. Likewise, VEGF is one of the factors released by activated glial cells; it may have, on the one hand, neuroprotective effects [33] but, on the other hand, may exacerbate disease progression by inducing vascular leakage and neovascularization.

Activation of microglia benefits surviving cells by removing cellular debris that may be toxic. However, it is assumed that activated microglial cells may also contribute to neuronal degeneration, by release of neurotoxins such as tumor necrosis factor (TNF), reactive oxygen intermediates, nitrogen oxides, proteases, and excitatory amino acids [34, 35]. Inhibition of microglia activation slows hereditary photoreceptor degeneration and ganglion cell death after axotomy in rats [36, 37]. In vitro, retina-derived microglial cells kill neurons and photoreceptor cells [38, 39]. A proper understanding of the network of gliotic responses in the diabetic retina, and of their protective vs. damaging effects, appears to be essential for the development of novel therapeutic strategies to treat diabetic retinopathy.

Microglial Cells

Various molecular and cellular abnormalities such as leukocyte adhesion to the vascular endothelium [40], complement deposition [41], and microglial activation [39], suggest that diabetic retinopathy involves a chronic, low-grade retinal inflammation. Increased levels of the proinflammatory cytokines interleukin (IL)-1β and TNF have been measured in the retinas of rats early during diabetes [22, 39, 42, 43]. In addition, the retinal expression of the cyclooxygenase-2 (an enzyme important in prostaglandin synthesis, and a marker of inflammation) is increased in diabetes [43]. This inflammatory component may cause several of the hallmark features of diabetic retinopathy.

Retinal microglia becomes activated early during experimental diabetes in rats, before the onset of neuronal cell death [39, 44]. The main histological markers of microglial cell activation are cell proliferation, migration, and changes of the cellular phenotype [45]. The density of microglial cells increases already at 4 weeks of experimental diabetes in rats [9]. At this time, the microglia activation occurs more locally, in a patchy-like pattern, within the inner retina. The activated microglial cells display an altered morphology characteristic of their differentiation towards phagocytes capable of clearing cell debris (i.e. hypertrophy of the cell bodies and shortening and thickening of the cell processes) [39]. In the further course of diabetes, migrating microglial cells invade the outer retina [44]. Elevated cytokines activate microglial cells; the activated cells initiate an inflammatory process that may involve a direct induction of neuronal cell death through the release of cytotoxic factors. It has been shown that IL-1β and TNF induce the expression of cyclooxygenase-2 in microglial cultures, and that TNF-activated microglial cells kill retinal neurons in vitro [39]. The authors suggest that early inhibition of microglia activity should have protective effects on the diabetic retina. However, whether activated microglial cells contribute, directly or indirectly, to the neuronal apoptosis in the diabetic retina in vivo, remains to be established.

Astrocytes

Retinal astrocytes are located in the nerve fiber layer, and the processes of astrocytes establish contact to blood vessels (fig. 1c). The number of astrocytes, or the staining of astrocytes with GFAP, is reduced in the diabetic retina compared to controls [9, 8]. Both astrocytes and Müller cells contribute to endothelial cell differentiation and to the formation of the blood-retinal barrier [46, 47]. Therefore, glial malfunction may play an important role in the pathogenesis of vasogenic edema. In culture, astrocytes secrete factors that increase the transendothelial electrical resistance and the expression of tight junction proteins in retinal endothelial cells [48]. Diabetes reduces and redistributes tight junction proteins in the retinal vessels, in concert with an altered GFAP expression in glial cells [8, 49]. In addition to Müller cells, astrocytes of the optic nerve strongly express VEGF in human nonproliferative diabetic retinopathy

[50]. In the diabetic retina and under hypoxic conditions in vitro, cyclooxygenase-2 is induced in retinal astrocytes, and inhibition of this enzyme was shown to prevent neovascularization via upregulation of thrombospondin-1 [51].

It has been suggested that astrocytes play a role in the induction of apoptosis in retinal ganglion cells [52]. Whereas ganglion cells in the human diabetic retina express proapoptotic molecules such as caspase-3, Fas, and Bax, the astrocytes express antiapoptotic molecules such as Bcl-2, in addition to the cytotoxic effector molecule Fas ligand [52].

Astrocytes of diabetic retinas upregulate the expression of the water channel protein, aquaporin-1 (fig. 1b, c). In control retinas, the aquaporin-1 immunoreactivity is predominantly expressed by photoreceptor cells in the outer retina [53]. After few months of experimental diabetes, immunoreactivity for aquaporin-1 is also expressed by astrocytes which are located within the nerve fiber layer and around the vessels [own unpubl. data]. Furthermore, the contact of astrocytes with the vessels of the superficial vessel plexus changes in the course of experimental diabetes. Whereas astrocytic processes have contact only to the innermost aspects of the vessel walls in control retinas (while the other parts are surrounded by Müller cell membranes), they fully surround these vessels in the diabetic retina of the rat [54]. The functional consequences of the elevated aquaporin-1 expression, and of the altered contact of astrocytes with the superficial vessels, remain to be determined. In the brain, an elevation of aquaporin-1 expression by astrocytes has been suggested to be implicated in the development or resolution of edema [55].

Müller Cells

Müller cells become abnormal early during diabetes, and it has been suggested that the functional loss and the death of neurons can be attributed to the alterations of Müller cells [56]. Because Müller cells constitute the functional link between vasculature and neurons, changes in Müller cell function could be a key event in the development of diabetic retinopathy. Furthermore, an impairment in the supportive functions of Müller cells may increase the susceptibility of retinal neurons to additional stressful stimuli present in the diabetic retina, such as oxidative stress and inflammatory conditions.

One hallmark of reactive gliosis of Müller cells is the upregulation of the intermediate filament GFAP; it has been observed both in retinas of diabetic patients [20] and in experimental diabetes (fig. 1a). GFAP expression in Müller cells is elevated at 6 weeks and is prominent at 3 months of experimental diabetes in rats, i.e. well before overt vascular changes become demonstrable [7–9]. The upregulation of GFAP in Müller cells in the retina of diabetic rats is inhibited by the aldose reductase inhibitor, sorbinil, as well as by melatonin, suggesting that both the polyol pathway and oxidative stress contribute to the progression of Müller cell gliosis [24, 57].

Müller cells in the diabetic retina display both proliferation and apoptosis. The density of Müller cells is increased at 4 weeks of experimental diabetes [9]. During early hyperglycemia in rats, apoptosis occurs primarily in ganglion and Müller cells [58]. This is associated with the upregulation of the GFAP content in Müller cells and with an increased expression of the p75 receptor on both cell types [20, 58]. Treatment of diabetic rats with nerve growth factor prevented apoptosis in ganglion and Müller cells as well as pericyte loss and the development of acellular occluded capillaries [58]. In the rat retina, nerve growth factor is expressed by ganglion, Müller, and pigment epithelial cells, while only pigment epithelial and Müller cells express receptors for this factor [59]. Hyperglycemia induces Müller cell apoptosis in vitro, by inactivation of the Akt survival pathway [60]. A similar inactivation of Akt may contribute to the Müller cell apoptosis in the diabetic retina [60].

Vascular Leakage and Neovascularization

Retinal capillaries are endowed with endothelial cells and pericytes which are covered by a basement membrane, and are ensheathed by glial cell processes ('end feet') arising from both astrocytes and Müller cells. During diabetes, acellular vessels cause a hypoxia which stimulates abnormal angiogenesis. Müller cell processes grow into the lumen of occluded vessels where they form a glial scar; these glial scars within vessels have even been suggested to cause (further) vessel occlusion [61]. In hyperglycemic rats, a disruption of the inner blood-retinal barrier – which is formed by the tight junctions between the vascular endothelial cells – is one of the earliest observable events, occurring at 2 weeks of hyperglycemia [62, 63], i.e. before Müller cell reactivity is morphologically apparent by enhanced expression of GFAP [7, 9]. The disruption of the blood-retinal barrier before glial reactivity suggests that glial cells are early targets of vascular hyperpermeability [9]. Simultaneously, Müller cells which participate in the establishment of the normal blood-retinal barrier [17] are assumed to contribute to vessel leakage in the diabetic retina. In vitro, Müller cells enhance the endothelial cell barrier function under normoxic conditions but impair the barrier function under hypoxic conditions [64].

Among the various vasoactive factors that have been found to cause vascular leakage in the retina (e.g. prostaglandins, IL-1β, TNF [65]), VEGF (the 'vascular permeability factor') is a major mediator of the clinical manifestations in diabetic retinopathy. VEGF is a signaling molecule that stimulates not only revascularization and vessel permeability but is generally involved in neural tissue repair after injury, by actions that include vasodilatation, inflammation, glial cell proliferation, neuroprotection and neurogenesis [33, 66]. VEGF is an important survival factor for endothelial and neuronal cells; this pro-survival signaling of VEGF is likely the cause for its upregulation early in diabetes. The cellular effects of VEGF are elicited by activation of two receptors, VEGF-R1 (flt-1) and VEGF-R2 (flk-1/KDR). In the neural retina, VEGF-R1 has been localized to pericytes [67], while VEGF-R2 is expressed by blood vessels, astrocytes, Müller cells, and ganglion cells [11]. In the human retina, immunoreactivity for VEGF is expressed, in addition to vascular endothelial cells, by all major classes of retinal neurons and by Müller glial cells [50, 68]. Upregulation of VEGF depends directly on tissue hypoxia [69]; various ischemic and inflammatory ocular diseases cause an upregulation of retinal VEGF [70].

Müller cells produce various factors capable of modulating blood flow and vascular permeability. Glial cell line-derived neurotrophic factor, neurturin, and pigment epithelium-derived growth factor (PEDF), which all are secreted by Müller cells, decrease the permeability of the barrier [71], while TNF and VEGF, also secreted by Müller cells [72–75], open the blood-retinal barrier. Various different growth factors and cytokines stimulate the secretion of VEGF by Müller cells [76–78]. Müller cells produce increased levels of VEGF in diabetes, and the elevated VEGF expression in Müller cells precedes neovascularization in the diabetic human retina, at times when there is no anatomical evidence of retinal malperfusion [50]. In addition to hypoxia, glucose deprivation induces VEGF expression in Müller cells [79, 80], and it has been shown that elevated glucose inhibits hypoxia-induced VEGF expression in Müller cells in vitro, suggesting that the metabolic effects of hypoxia can be compensated by a surplus of glucose [80]. The high glucose-induced formation of advanced glycation end-products (AGEs) in diabetic retinas may contribute to the induction of VEGF production [81] via an activation of AGE receptors on Müller cells [82]. PEDF, which is expressed in the neural retina by neurons and glial cells [74, 83, 84], acts as an anti-angiogenic factor that downregulates the expression of VEGF. PEDF expression is reduced under hypoxic conditions in the retina and Müller cells [74, 85], and a lowered PEDF level is a strong predictor of progression of diabetic retinopathy [86].

After creation of poorly perfused acellular capillaries and large areas of hypoxia within the retina, the expression of angiogenic growth factors that initiate vascular growth determine further progression of the disease toward a proliferative retinopathy. In addition to the basic fibroblast growth factor, VEGF is the major angiogenic factor in the retina promoting pathological neovascularization [87, 88]. In the healthy retina, Müller cells provide a permanent antiproliferative condition for vascular endothelial cells, by the release of antiangiogenic factors such as PEDF and thrombospondin-1 [89]. The elevated expression of VEGF by Müller cells has been related to the induction of retinal neovascularization during diabetic retinopathy [50]. The balance between pro- and antiangiogenic factors, such as VEGF and PEDF, is thought to be essential for angiogenic homeostasis in the retina. However, in spite of the observation that hypoxia enhances the expression of VEGF and downregulates the expression of PEDF in cultured Müller cells, conditioned media of Müller cells failed to stimulate additional proliferation of retinal endothelial cells in vitro [74, 90]. This may suggest that hypoxia-stimulated Müller cells release (in addition to VEGF) other angiogenesis-inhibiting factor(s), and points to the importance of additional signals for the triggering of neovascularization in the hypoxic retina; the nature of these signals remains to be identified.

VEGF and other angiogenic cytokines released by Müller cells, e.g. transforming growth factor-β, basic fibroblast growth factor, and TNF, increase the release of matrix metalloproteinases by endothelial cells [91, 92]. Moreover, Müller cells themselves secrete matrix metalloproteinases, e.g. upon stimulation of purinergic receptors [93]. High glucose levels increase the production of matrix metalloproteinases in retinal cells [94]. Matrix metalloproteinases impair the tight junction function in retinal endothelial and pigment epithelial cells, by proteolytic degradation of the tight junction protein, occludin [94], and thus may facilitate vascular leakage. Moreover, the secretion of metalloproteinases allows endothelial cells to penetrate their underlying basement membrane, and eliminates the contact inhibition which normally blocks endothelial cell proliferation [91]. A further way for Müller cells to stimulate vasculogenesis may involve the renin-angiotensin system which has been implicated in diabetes. Müller cells express angiotensin II and renin, with the expression being most obvious in the end feet closely apposed to retinal blood vessels, while the angiotensin receptors are expressed by neurons and by the vasculature [56, 95].

The progression of proliferative retinopathy may lead to the formation of fibrovascular scar tissues. Such scar tissues form periretinal membranes which are connected with the sensory retina via hypertrophied Müller cell fibers, and which may become contractile, resulting in traction detachment of the retina. Müller cells are the principal glial cells in the fibrovascular scar tissue [96]. Müller cells de-differentiate, migrate within and out of the neural retina, and display cellular hypertrophy. The hypertrophied Müller cell fibers form intraretinal bridges between cystic spaces, and cause subretinal fibrosis [96, 97]. Müller cells in fibrovascular membranes may transdifferentiate into myofibroblasts that generate tractional forces in response to growth factors in the vitreous, thus causing traction detachment [98]. Glial cells in fibrovascular membranes express growth factors and cytokines which may drive uncontrolled cell proliferation and neovascularization. In addition, they express receptors for various growth factors. Among these factors, the hepatocyte growth factor (HGF), which has been implicated in ocular angiogenesis and has been found to be elevated in the vitreous of patients with proliferative diabetic retinopathy [99], was shown to stimulate chemotaxis and VEGF secretion by cultured Müller cells [77]. Since

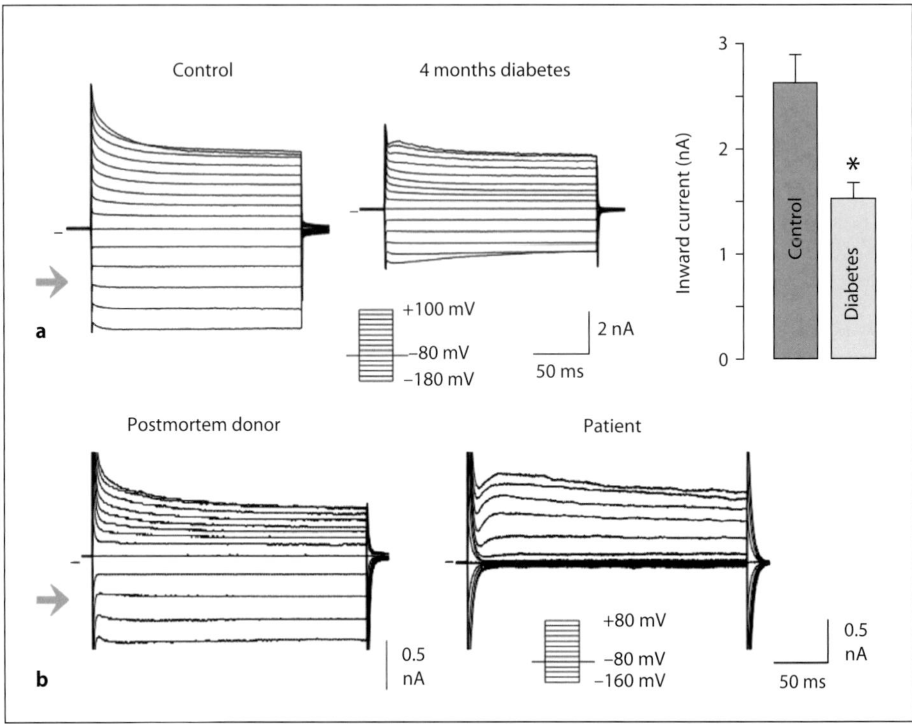

Fig. 2. Diabetes causes a decrease in the membrane K⁺ conductance of Müller glial cells. **a** Müller cells of diabetic rats display a reduced K⁺ conductance of their plasma membrane. Left: Original records of the transmembrane K⁺ currents in representative cells from a control and a diabetic animal. Right: Mean amplitude of the inward K⁺ currents in Müller cells of control and 4-month diabetic animals. * $p < 0.01$. **b** In comparison to the cell from a human postmortem donor, the Müller cell isolated from retinectomy material obtained from a patient with proliferative diabetic retinopathy displayed a strongly reduced inward K⁺ conductance (arrow). Adapted from Bringmann et al. [97] and Pannicke et al. [54].

distinct growth factors and serum stimulate the secretion of HGF by Müller cells, an autocrine/paracrine signaling pathway has been suggested that promotes glial cell responses in the diabetic retina [77]. Particularly, vessel leakage-induced serum entry into the retinal tissue may cause a strong stimulus for HGF secretion by glial cells.

Müller cells from surgically excised retinal tissue of patients with proliferative diabetic retinopathy display physiological alterations similar to those of Müller cells from patients with proliferative vitreoretinopathy [100]. Such cells show a strong hypertrophy, an almost complete absence of currents through inwardly rectifying K⁺ channels (fig. 2b), and a decreased membrane potential [97]. This current pattern suggests a de-differentiation of the cells, reminiscent of the pattern characteristic for nondifferentiated glial cells early in the ontogenesis [101]. It has been proposed that the downregulation of the K⁺ channels is a prerequisite for the re-entry of gliotic Müller cells into the proliferation cycle [102]. The strong downregulation of the K⁺ channels in Müller cells may also suggest that the retinal K⁺

homeostasis is largely disturbed during proliferative diabetic retinopathy (see section 'Retinal K^+ Homeostasis').

Glutamate Metabolism

'Neurotransmitter recycling' is a major function of Müller cells. The cells express uptake systems for various amino acid transmitters such as glutamate [103, 104] and γ-aminobutyric acid (GABA) [105, 106]. The glutamate/aspartate transporter GLAST is expressed by Müller cells, and is the predominant transporter for the removal of glutamate within the retina [107, 108] maintaining the extracellular glutamate level below neurotoxic levels. Malfunction of glutamate transport into Müller cells results in an increased extracellular level of glutamate which may contribute to neuronal dysfunction and apoptosis in the diabetic retina [109]. After experimental inhibition of glutamate uptake by Müller cells, even low concentrations of extracellular glutamate become neurotoxic, via an activation of ionotropic glutamate receptors [110, 111]. After glutamate has been taken up by Müller cells, it is intracellularly converted into glutamine, which is transported back to neurons as a precursor for neuronal synthesis of glutamate and GABA.

Retinas of diabetic animals have been found to display an impaired glutamate metabolism, manifested by an increased level of glutamate and a reduced ability to convert glutamate into glutamine [7, 21]. Both glutamate and GABA levels are elevated in the vitreous of diabetic animals and human patients [112, 113]. These alterations have been proposed to be caused by a malfunction of the glial uptake of neurotransmitter molecules. Indeed, a decrease in the currents evoked by the GLAST transporter has been observed in isolated Müller cells already at 2–4 weeks of experimental diabetes [114]. Since a reducing agent restored the activity of the glutamate transporter, it was suggested that the dysfunction of the glutamate transport is caused by oxidative stress present in the diabetic retina [114]. However, a recent study showed no alteration, or even an enhancement, of glutamate uptake in diabetic retinas [115]. The plasma membrane expression and -localization of transporter molecules in Müller cells does not change in the course of diabetes [54, 114, 115]. Moreover, the retinal expression of the glutamine synthetase protein is not different between diabetic and control retinas [20, 22]. Thus, an involvement of Müller cells in the disturbance of the glutamate turnover in diabetic retinas – if any – remains to be clarified by future investigations. Another possible explanation for the increased vitreal and retinal glutamate content is the breakdown of the blood-retinal barrier which may cause a leakage of plasma glutamate into the tissues.

The uptake of glutamate is also important for the retinal defense against free radicals mediated by Müller cells. Müller cells synthesize the tripeptide glutathione from glutamate, cysteine, and glycine. Reduced glutathione is provided to neurons and acts as a scavenger of free radicals and reactive oxygen compounds. Müller cells from aged animals contain less glutathione than cells from young animals [116]. An age-dependent decrease in Müller cell-mediated defense against free radicals may accelerate the pathogenesis of diabetic retinopathy in elderly patients.

Finally, it should be mentioned that Müller cells are the 'communicators' between vessels and neurons: they take up glucose from the circulation, metabolize glucose, and transfer energy substrates such as lactate and pyruvate to neurons [117]. Generally, the uptake and metabolization of glucose in glial cells are closely linked to the release of glutamate from neurons and its uptake by glia [118, 119]. The limiting factor in glutamate and glucose uptake by glial cells is the activity of the Na,K-ATPase which decreases very rapidly in the hyperglycemic tissue [120, 121]. An impairment of the glial sodium pump causes a depolarization of the plasma membrane that lowers the efficiency of the electrogenic glutamate uptake. This has been related to enhanced oxidative stress, e.g. via a decrease in the synthesis of glutathione.

Retinal K^+ Homeostasis

Müller cells are crucially involved in retinal K^+ homeostasis, by mediating transcellular 'spatial buffering' K^+ currents which counterbalance the changes in extracellular K^+ concentration associated with neuronal activity [13, 122, 123]. A dysregulation of the K^+ homeostasis causes K^+-evoked neuronal hyper-excitation and, therefore, glutamate toxicity. Normally, Müller cells take up neuron-derived excess K^+ particularly from the plexiform (synaptic) layers, and release a similar amount of K^+ into fluid-filled spaces outside the neural retina (blood, vitreous, and subretinal space). Though also the Na,K-ATPase and transporter molecules contribute to Müller cell-mediated K^+ homeostasis, it is now well-established that passive K^+ currents through inwardly rectifying K^+ channels play a major role in counteracting extracellular K^+ imbalances. Among the various subtypes of K^+ channels expressed by Müller cells [124, 125], the inwardly rectifying K^+ channel of the Kir4.1 subtype has been specifically implicated in mediating the K^+ buffering currents [126, 127]. The Kir4.1 channel protein is expressed in a polarized fashion in the plasma membrane of Müller cells, with a strong enrichment in such membrane domains across which the cells can dispose excess K^+, i.e. in perivascular membrane sheets, and at the inner and outer limiting membranes (fig. 1d, e) [125, 127, 128].

The K^+ conductance of rat Müller cells is significantly reduced at 4 and 6 months of experimental diabetes (fig. 2a). This decreased K^+ conductance is associated with a mislocation of the Kir4.1 protein [54]. Though the Kir4.1 protein is still expressed within the retinal tissue, the prominent expression at both limiting membranes and around the vessels is absent (fig. 1d, e). This suggests that the decrease in the K^+ currents in cells from diabetic retinas (fig. 2a) is caused by an alteration in the expression pattern of Kir4.1 channels. The downregulation of Kir4.1 channels should cause an impairment of the transglial K^+ currents and, therefore, a disturbance of the retinal K^+ homeostasis that may contribute to neuronal cell death in the diabetic retina. A similar mislocation of the Kir4.1 protein has been described in retinas of mice which carry a genetic inactivation of the dystrophin gene product Dp71 proposed to be involved in the plasma membrane clustering of Kir4.1 channels [129]. In these mice, the mislocation of Kir4.1 protein is associated with an enhanced vulnerability of retinal ganglion cells during ischemic stress [130]. Glial cells are crucially implicated in activity-dependent regulation of the local blood flow, and it has been suggested that the release of K^+ ions from perivascular end feet plays a role in the local dilation of arterioles [16]. A decrease in the activity-dependent K^+ efflux in the diabetic tissue may result in a decrease in the local blood flow, thus exacerbating hypoxic insults. Since the gating of Kir4.1 channels is dependent on intracellular ATP [131, 132], a functional inactivation of these channels may disturb retinal K^+ homeostasis in ischemic tissue areas even already before a mislocation of the channel proteins is observable.

The reason for the diabetes-induced downregulation of the prominent Kir4.1 expression in end feet and perivascular membranes of Müller cells is unclear. As similar changes were observed during experimental retinal ischemia-reperfusion and uveoretinitis, respectively [133, 134], a causative effect of oxidative stress and/or chronic inflammation is very likely. It has been shown that glial cells surrounding ischemic brain lesions display a reduction in their K^+ currents, and that a similar reduction can be observed in cultured astrocytes in the presence of TNF [135]. Activated microglial cells or blood-derived leukocytes release nitric oxide, reactive oxygen species, and proinflammatory cytokines such as TNF, which may be implicated in the altered expression of glial K^+ channels during diabetes.

It has been shown that Müller cells of patients with proliferative diabetic retinopathy display a strong reduction in their K^+ conductance (fig. 2b) [97], suggesting that the downregulation of K^+ channels may represent a characteristic feature also of glial cells of the diabetic human retina. Müller cells of the human retina display an age-dependent decrease in their K^+ conductance [136]; this age-related downregulation should contribute to retinal complications of diabetes in elderly patients.

Cytotoxic Cell Swelling and Retinal Edema

Diabetic retinopathy is the leading cause of reduced visual acuity and acquired blindness in working-age adults. Most frequently, the presence of a macular edema is responsible for the impaired vision [137]. The macular edema may be diffuse or cystic. In cystic edema, the fluid-filled cysts are predominantly located in two retinal layers, the inner nuclear and the Henle fiber layers [138, 139]. The fluid accumulation causes cell displacement and splitting of the perifoveal neuroretina within these two layers, and the fluid-filled compartments are spanned by the trunks of Müller's fibers. Additional fluid accumulation can occur in the subretinal space. By compression of retinal neurons, nerve fibers, and capillaries, edema contributes to photoreceptor degeneration and neuronal cell death, and exacerbates the ischemic conditions. Generally, an edema may develop by fluid accumulation within the interstitial spaces (extracellular edema, characterized by cell compression) caused by vascular leakage (vascular edema), or by fluid accumulation within the cells (intracellular or cytotoxic edema, characterized by cell swelling). In the preclinical stage of diabetic retinopathy, there are two types of increased retinal thickness that may be associated or not with angiographic vascular leakage [140]. Also the presence of cysts is associated or not with vascular leakage, suggesting that both vasogenic edema and cell swelling may contribute to cystoid macular edema. It has been suggested that swelling of glial cells is involved in the development of cystoid edema, with the cysts being formed by swollen and dying Müller cells [141, 142]. Both hypoxic-ischemic conditions and/or inflammatory alterations of the microvasculature have been suggested as causative factors for the development of macular edema [79, 137, 143–146]. In an animal model of retinal hypoxia, the breakdown of the blood-retinal barrier was associated with an intracellular edema of Müller cells [147].

Generally, the development of chronic edema depends on two parameters: the rate of fluid entry into the retinal parenchyma through (leaky) vessel walls and the rate of fluid reabsorption from the retinal tissue back into the blood. The development of macular edema is thought to be primarily caused by a breakdown of the blood-retinal barrier, resulting in retinal vascular leakage [139, 144, 148]. However, it has been shown that clinically significant diabetic macular edema occurs only when (in addition to vascular leakage) also the active transport mechanisms of the blood-retinal barriers are dysfunctional [149], suggesting that a disturbance of the fluid (re-)absorption from the retinal tissue is a necessary step in edema formation. In the retina, the fluid absorption is carried out by pigment epithelial cells that dehydrate the subretinal space, and by Müller cells that dehydrate the inner retina by transcellular water transport [15]. It is suggested that the water transport through Müller cells is coupled to the extrusion of osmolytes from the perivascular glial cell processes into the blood. In particular, the spatial buffering K^+ currents which flow through Müller cells into the blood (see the previous section) are associated with a water flow that dehydrates the retina in dependence on the neuronal activity [15, 128]. The co-localization of the Kir4.1 channel protein and of the glial water channel, aquaporin-4, in perivascular (fig. 1e) and vitreous-abutting membrane domains of Müller cells is suggested to facilitate this process of activity-dependent water transport from Müller cells

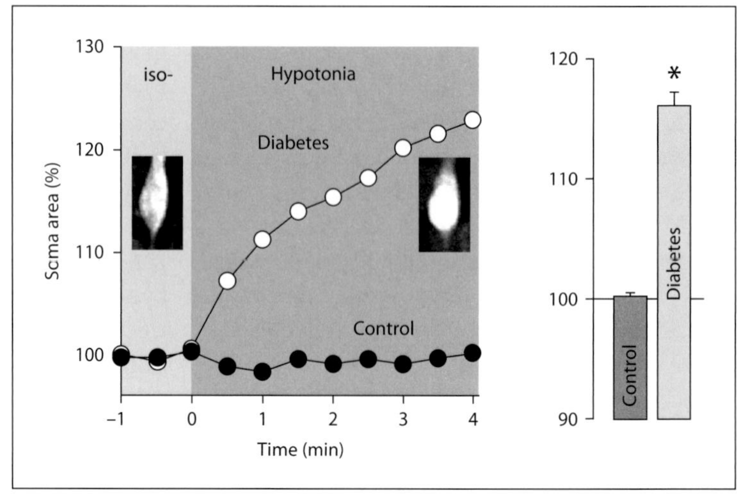

Fig. 3. Diabetes alters the osmotic swelling characteristics of Müller glial cells in the rat retina. Left: Exposure of retinal slices to hypotonic solution induced a time-dependent swelling of Müller cell bodies in a retina from a 6-month diabetic animal but had no effect on the soma volume of Müller cells in an age-matched control retina. Insets: Original records of a Müller cell body before and during hypotonic conditions. Right: Mean cross-sectional area of the Müller cell bodies in control and diabetic retinas under hypotonic conditions. The values are given in percent before hypotonic challenge (100%). * $p < 0.001$. Adapted from Pannicke et al. [54].

into the blood and vitreous [128]. However, in the course of experimental diabetes in rats, Müller cells downregulate the expression of Kir4.1 protein in these membrane domains (fig. 1d, e) [54]; the disruption of the spatial buffering K^+ currents through Müller cells should cause an impairment of the water transport through the cells. This may cause the swelling of Müller cells [134], as well as an impairment of the resolution of vasogenic and extracellular edema. Moreover, an increase in the osmotic pressure of the Müller cell interior – which must result from accumulation of K^+ ions and other osmolytes within the cells – may drive water from the blood and vitreous into the cells [15].

Experimental diabetes in rats causes a significant alteration of the swelling characteristics of Müller cells in situ. Müller cells in diabetic retinas show a swelling of their cell bodies during hypotonic stress, while Müller cells in control retinas do not alter their cell volume in response to changes in osmotic conditions (fig. 3). A similar alteration of the swelling characteristics has been observed in rat retinas during ischemia-reperfusion and uveoretinitis, respectively [133, 134], implicating oxidative stress and inflammation as causative factors for osmotic Müller cell swelling. This assumption is supported by the observations that H_2O_2 or inflammatory mediators such as arachidonic acid and prostaglandin E_2 cause osmotic Müller cell swelling in control retinas, and that inhibition of the phospholipase A_2 or of the cyclooxygenase, or the presence of a reducing agent, prevents the swelling in diabetic retinas [54]. The swelling is apparently induced by endogenous formation of arachidonic acid and prostaglandins that causes intracellular Na^+ overload; an inhibition or closure of K^+ channels prevents a compensatory K^+ efflux, and eventually results in cell swelling [150].

Diabetic retinopathy is associated with the increased production of nitric oxide, and with glucose-mediated oxidative stress [24, 23, 151–153]. Müller cells express the inducible nitric oxide synthase in diabetic retinas [31]; Müller cell-derived nitric oxide may induce neuronal cell death [32]. The expression of the inducible nitric oxide synthase and of the cyclooxygenase-2 in the retina increases during diabetes [154], and both enzymes are assumed to be involved in the retinal cell death under hyperglycemic conditions. It has been shown that hyperglycemia-simulating conditions increase the expression of both enzymes in Müller cells in vitro; the hyperglycemia-induced increase in nitric oxide in Müller cells stimulates the production of cytotoxic prostaglandins by cyclooxygenase-2 [154]. The altered swelling characteristics may represent one of the responses of Müller cells to the oxidative stress [23, 24] and to chronic inflammation in the diabetic retina [25, 26]. Other responses of Müller cells to inflammation include the upregulation of gene transcripts for inflammation-related proteins, e.g. for acute phase and antioxidant proteins [22]. It has been suggested that the strong enhancement of the proinflammatory cytokine IL-1β in the diabetic retina [42] may be a dominant cause of altered gene expression in Müller cells [22].

In recent years, intravitreal injection of anti-inflammatory corticosteroids such as triamcinolone acetonide has been increasingly used clinically for the rapid resolution of diabetic macular edema [155–157]. Generally, therapeutic agents may act at two different levels: (a) at the vascular level, they should reduce vascular leakage, and (b) at the level of glial cells, they may cause a stimulation of the fluid-absorbing function as well as an inhibition of cytotoxic edema. Anti-inflammatory agents may act at both levels. Triamcinolone inhibits both vascular and cytotoxic edema. It attenuates the vascular leakage in the diabetic retina [158] and reduces the vitreal level of VEGF in patients with diabetic retinopathy [159]. Furthermore, triamcinolone inhibits the osmotic Müller cell swelling in the ischemic, inflamed, and diabetic rat retina [54, 150]. The inhibitory effect of triamcinolone on osmotic Müller cell swelling is mediated by a stimulation of the release of endogenous adenosine and subsequent A1 receptor activation, resulting in an opening of K^+ and Cl^- channels [150]. It is conceivable but remains to be proven that triamcinolone stimulates the absorption of K^+ and, therefore, of water from the retinal parenchyma, and their subsequent clearance into the blood and vitreous. A pharmacological stimulation of fluid absorption by glial cells may thus be a promising approach to the development of novel edema-resolving drugs.

Conclusions

All three types of retinal glial cells exhibit an early reactivity to hyperglycemia in the diabetic retina. This reactivity is probably triggered by (a) blood-derived factors which diffuse into the retina due to the early vascular leakage; (b) the oxidative stress, and (c) inflammatory mediators. The dysfunction of glial cells may contribute to the progression of the retinopathy, as it exacerbates vascular abnormalities, macular edema, and neuronal dysfunction, and occurs prior to or in concomitance with the loss of endothelial and neuronal cells. Since there is a network of pathological changes in diabetes including vascular anomalies, glial cell changes, and neuronal dysfunction, it appears desirable to strive for therapeutical agents that affect all three compartments. Examples for that may be inhibitors of the angiotensin-converting enzyme [56] or anti-inflammatory steroids. Any hypothetical therapy aimed at an inhibition of gliosis is hampered by the Janus-face of gliosis, i.e. by the observation that the same factors or alterations may have both protective and damaging effects. Thus, an anti-VEGF therapy, for example, inhibits vascular leakage and neovascularization, but also extinguishes the neuroprotective effects of this factor. A better understanding of the molecular mechanisms of gliosis in the diabetic retina would help to develop therapeutic agents that support the protective, and diminish the damaging, effects of gliosis.

Acknowledgements

Some of the work presented in this review was conducted with grants from the Deutsche Forschungsgemeinschaft (BR 1249/2-1; GRK 1097/1), and from the Interdisziplinäres Zentrum für Klinische Forschung at the Faculty of Medicine of the University of Leipzig (projects C5 and C21).

References

1 Terasaki H, Hirose H, Miyake Y: S-cone pathway sensitivity in diabetes measured with threshold versus intensity curves on flashed backgrounds. Invest Ophthalmol Vis Sci 1996;37:680–684.
2 Della Sala S, Bertoni G, Somazzi L, Stubbe F, Wilkins AJ: Impaired contrast sensitivity in diabetic patients with and without retinopathy: a new technique for rapid assessment. Br J Ophthalmol 1985;69:136–142.
3 Bresnick GH, Palta M: Oscillatory potential amplitudes: relation to severity of diabetic retinopathy. Arch Ophthalmol 1987;105:929–933.
4 Juen S, Kieselbach GF: Electrophysiological changes in juvenile diabetics without retinopathy. Arch Ophthalmol 1990;108:372–375.
5 Sakai H, Tani Y, Shirasawa E, Shirao Y, Kawasaki K: Development of electroretinographic alterations in streptozotocin-induced diabetes in rats. Ophthalmic Res 1995;27:57–63.
6 Barber A, Lieth E, Khin S, Antonetti D, Buchanan A, Gardner T: Neural apoptosis in the retina during experimental and human diabetes: early onset and effect of insulin. J Clin Invest 1998;102:783–791.
7 Lieth E, Barber A, Xu B, Dice C, Ratz MJ, Tanase D, Strother JM: Glial reactivity and impaired glutamate metabolism in short-term experimental diabetic retinopathy. Diabetes 1998;47:815–820.
8 Barber AJ, Antonetti DA, Gardner TW: Altered expression of retinal occludin and glial fibrillary acidic protein in experimental diabetes. Invest Ophthalmol Vis Sci 2000;41:3561–3568.
9 Rungger-Brändle E, Dosso AA, Leuenberger PM: Glial reactivity, an early feature of diabetic retinopathy. Invest Ophthalmol Vis Sci 2000;4:1971–1980.
10 Ling T, Stone J: The development of astrocytes in the cat retina: evidence of migration from the optic nerve. Dev Brain Res 1988;44:73–85.
11 Stone J, Itin A, Alon T, Pe'er J, Gnessin H, Chan-Ling T, Keshet E: Development of retinal vasculature is mediated by hypoxia-induced vascular endothelial growth factor (VEGF) expression by neuroglia. J Neurosci 1995;15:4738–4747.
12 Reichenbach A, Stolzenburg J-U, Eberhardt W, Chao TI, Dettmer D, Hertz L: What do retinal Müller (glial) cells do for their neuronal small siblings? J Chem Neuroanat 1993;6:201–213.
13 Newman EA, Reichenbach A: The Müller cell: a functional element of the retina. Trends Neurosci 1996;19:307–317.
14 Tsacopoulos M, Magistretti PJ: Metabolic coupling between glia and neurons. J Neurosci 1996;16:877–885.
15 Bringmann A, Reichenbach A, Wiedemann P: Pathomechanisms of cystoid macular edema. Ophthalmic Res 2004;36:241–249.
16 Paulson OB, Newman EA: Does the release of potassium from astrocyte endfeet regulate cerebral blood flow ? Science 1987;237:896–898.
17 Tout S, Chan-Ling T, Hollander H, Stone J: The role of Müller cells in the formation of the blood-retinal barrier. Neuroscience 1993;55:291–301.
18 Matsui K, Hosoi N, Tachibana M: Active role of glutamate uptake in the synaptic transmission from retinal nonspiking neurons. J Neurosci 1999;19:6755–6766.
19 Bringmann A, Reichenbach A: Role of Müller cells in retinal degenerations. Front Biosci 2001;6:E77-E92.
20 Mizutani M, Gerhardinger C, Lorenzi M: Müller cell changes in human diabetic retinopathy. Diabetes 1998;47:445–449.
21 Lieth E, LaNoue KF, Antonetti DA, Ratz M: Diabetes reduces glutamate oxidation and glutamine synthesis in the retina. Exp Eye Res 2000;70:723–730.
22 Gerhardinger C, Costa MB, Coulombe MC, Toth I, Hoehn T, Grosu P: Expression of acute-phase response proteins in retinal Muller cells in diabetes. Invest Ophthalmol Vis Sci 2005;46:349–357.
23 van Dam PS: Oxidative stress and diabetic neuropathy: pathophysiological mechanisms and treatment perspectives. Diabetes Metab Res Rev 2002;18:176–184.

24 Baydas G, Tuzcu M, Yasar A, Baydas B: Early changes in glial reactivity and lipid peroxidation in diabetic rat retina: effects of melatonin. Acta Diabetol 2004;41:123–128.
25 Gardner TW, Antonetti DA, Barber AJ, LaNoue KF, Levison SW: Diabetic retinopathy: more than meets the eye. Surv Ophthalmol 2002;47:S253–S262.
26 Joussen AM, Poulaki V, Le ML, Koizumi K, Esser C, Janicki H, Schraermeyer U, Kociok N, Fauser S, Kirchhof B, Kern TS, Adamis AP: A central role for inflammation in the pathogenesis of diabetic retinopathy. FASEB J 2004;18:1450–1452.
27 Fawcett JW, Asher RA: The glial scar and central nervous system repair. Brain Res Bull 1999;49:377–391.
28 Cappelli-Bigazzi M, Ambrosio G, Musci G, Battaglia C, Bonaccorsi di Patti MC, Golino P, Ragni M, Chiariello M, Calabrese L: Ceruloplasmin impairs endothelium-dependent relaxation of rabbit aorta. Am J Physiol 1997;273:H2843–H2849.
29 Carlevaro MF, Albini A, Ribatti D, Gentili C, Benelli R, Cermelli S, Cancedda R, Cancedda FD: Transferrin promotes endothelial cell migration and invasion: implication in cartilage neovascularization. J Cell Biol 1997;136:1375–1384.
30 Goureau O, Hicks D, Courtois Y, De Kozak Y: Induction and regulation of nitric oxide synthase in retinal Müller glial cells. J Neurochem 1994;63:310–317.
31 Abu-El-Asrar AM, Desmet S, Meersschaert A, Dralands L, Missotten L, Geboes K: Expression of the inducible isoform of nitric oxide synthase in the retinas of human subjects with diabetes mellitus. Am J Ophthalmol 2001;132:551–556.
32 Goureau O, Regnier-Ricard F, Courtois Y: Requirement for nitric oxide in retinal neuronal cell death induced by activated Muller glial cells. J Neurochem 1999;72:2506–2515.
33 Yasuhara T, Shingo T, Date I: The potential role of vascular endothelial growth factor in the central nervous system. Rev Neurosci 2004;15:293–307.
34 Banati RB, Gehrmann J, Shubert P, Kreutzberg GW: Cytotoxicity of microglia. Glia 1993;7:111–118.
35 De Kozak Y, Cotinet A, Goureau O, Hicks D, Thillaye-Goldenberg B: Tumor necrosis factor and nitric oxide production by resident glial cells from rats presenting hereditary degeneration. Ocular Immunol Inflamm 1997;5:85–94.
36 Thanos S, Mey J, Wild M: Treatment of the adult retina with microglia-suppressing factors retards axotomy-induced neuronal degradation and enhances axonal regeneration in vivo and in vitro. J Neurosci 1993;13:455–466.
37 Thanos S, Richter W, Thiel HJ: The protective role of microglia-inhibiting factor in the retina suffering of hereditary photoreceptor degeneration; in Pleyer U, Schmidt K, Thiel HJ (eds): Cell and Tissue Protection in Ophthalmology. Hippokrates Verlag, Stuttgart, 1995, pp 195–203.
38 Roque RS, Rosales AA, Jingjing L, Agarwal N, Al-Ubaidi MR: Retina-derived microglial cells induce photoreceptor death in vitro. Brain Res 1999;836:110–119.
39 Krady JK, Basu A, Allen CM, Xu Y, LaNoue KF, Gardner TW, Levison SW: Minocycline reduces proinflammatory cytokine expression, microglial activation, and caspase-3 activation in a rodent model of diabetic retinopathy. Diabetes 2005;54:1559–1565.
40 Miyamoto K, Khosrof S, Bursell S-E, Rohan R, Murata T, Clermont AC, Aiello LP, Ogura Y, Adamis AP: Prevention of leukostasis and vascular leakage in streptozotocin-induced diabetic retinopathy via intercellular adhesion molecule-1 inhibition. Proc Natl Acad Sci USA 1999;96:10836–10841.
41 Zhang J, Gerhardinger C, Lorenzi M: Early complement activation and decreased levels of glycosylphosphatidylinositol-anchored complement inhibitors in human and experimental diabetic retinopathy. Diabetes 2002;51:3499–3504.
42 Carmo A, Cunha-Vaz JG, Carvalho AP, Lopes MC: L-arginine transport in retinas from streptozotocin diabetic rats: correlation with the level of IL-1β and NO synthase activity. Vision Res 1999;39:3817–3823.
43 Joussen AM, Murata T, Tsujikawa A, Kirchhof B, Bursell SE, Adamis AP: Leukocyte-mediated endothelial cell injury and death in the diabetic retina. Am J Pathol 2001;158:147–152.
44 Zeng XX, Ng YK, Ling EA: Neuronal and microglial response in the retina of streptozotocin-induced diabetic rats. Vis Neurosci 2000;17:463–471.
45 Kreutzberg GW: Microglia: a sensor for pathological events in the CNS. Trends Neurosci 1996;19:312–318.
46 Chan-Ling T, Stone J: Degeneration of astrocytes in feline retinopathy of prematurity causes failure of the blood-retinal barrier. Invest Ophthalmol Vis Sci 1992;33:2148–2159.
47 Jiang B, Bezhadian MA, Caldwell RB: Astrocytes modulate retinal vasculogenesis: effects on endothelial cell differentiation. Glia 1995;15:1–10.
48 Gardner TW, Lieth E, Khin SA, Barber AJ, Bonsall DJ, Lesher T, Rice K, Brennan WA Jr: Astrocytes increase barrier properties and ZO-1 expression in retinal vascular endothelial cells. Invest Ophthalmol Vis Sci 1997;38:2423–2427.
49 Antonetti DA, Barber AJ, Khin S, Lieth E, Tarbell JM, Gardner TW: Vascular permeability in experimental diabetes is associated with reduced endothelial occludin content: vascular endothelial growth factor decreases occludin in retinal endothelial cells. Diabetes 1998;47:1953–1959.
50 Amin RH, Frank RN, Kennedy A, Eliott D, Puklin JE, Abrams GW: Vascular endothelial growth factor is present in glial cells of the retina and optic nerve of human subjects with nonproliferative diabetic retinopathy. Invest Ophthalmol Vis Sci 1997;38:36–47.
51 Sennlaub F, Valamanesh F, Vazquez-Tello A, El-Asrar AM, Checchin D, Brault S, Gobeil F, Beauchamp MH, Mwaikambo B, Courtois Y, Geboes K, Varma DR, Lachapelle P, Ong H, Behar-Cohen F, Chemtob S: Cyclooxygenase-2 in human and experimental ischemic proliferative retinopathy. Circulation 2003;108:198–204.
52 Abu-El-Asrar AM, Dralands L, Missotten L, Al-Jadaan IA, Geboes K: Expression of apoptosis markers in the retina of human subjects with diabetes. Invest Ophthalmol Vis Sci 2004;45:2760–2766.

53 Iandiev I, Pannicke T, Reichel MB, Wiedemann P, Reichenbach A, Bringmann A: Expression of aquaporin-1 immunoreactivity by photoreceptor cells in the mouse retina. Neurosci Lett 2005;388:96–99.
54 Pannicke T, Iandiev I, Wurm A, Uckermann O, vom Hagen F, Reichenbach A, Wiedemann P, Hammes H-P, Bringmann A: Diabetes alters osmotic swelling and membrane characteristics of glial cells in rat retina. Diabetes 2006;55:633–639.
55 Badaut J, Brunet JF, Grollimund L, Hamou MF, Magistretti PJ, Villemure JG, Regli L: Aquaporin 1 and aquaporin 4 expression in human brain after subarachnoid hemorrhage and in peritumoral tissue. Acta Neurochir Suppl 2003;86:495–498.
56 Fletcher EL, Phipps JA, Wilkinson-Berka JL: Dysfunction of retinal neurons and glia during diabetes. Clin Exp Optom 2005;88:132–145.
57 Asnaghi V, Gerhardinger C, Hoehn T, Adeboje A, Lorenzi M: A role for the polyol pathway in the early neuroretinal apoptosis and glial changes induced by diabetes in the rat. Diabetes 2003;52:506–511.
58 Hammes HP, Federoff HJ, Brownlee M: Nerve growth factor prevents both neuroretinal programmed cell death and capillary pathology in experimental diabetes. Mol Med 1995;1:527–534.
59 Chakrabarti S, Sima AA, Lee J, Brachet P, Dicou E: Nerve growth factor (NGF), proNGF and NGF receptor-like immunoreactivity in BB rat retina. Brain Res 1990;523:11–15.
60 Xi X, Gao L, Hatala DA, Smith DG, Codispoti MC, Gong B, Kern TS, Zhang JZ: Chronically elevated glucose-induced apoptosis is mediated by inactivation of Akt in cultured Muller cells. Biochem Biophys Res Commun 2005;326:548–553.
61 Bek T: Immunohistochemical characterization of retinal glial cell changes in areas of vascular occlusion secondary to diabetic retinopathy. Acta Ophthalmol Scand 1997;75:388–392.
62 Corbett JA, Tilton RG, Chang K, Hasan KS, Ido Y, Wang JL, Sweetland MA, Lancaster JR Jr, Williamson JR, McDaniel ML: Aminoguanidine, a novel inhibitor of nitric oxide formation, prevents diabetic vascular dysfunction. Diabetes 1992;41:552–556.
63 Do Carmo A, Ramos P, Reis A, Proenca R, Cunha-vaz JG: Breakdown of the inner and outer blood retinal barrier in streptozotocin-induced diabetes. Exp Eye Res 1998;67:569–575.
64 Tretiach M, Madigan MC, Wen L, Gillies MC: Effect of Muller cell co-culture on in vitro permeability of bovine retinal vascular endothelium in normoxic and hypoxic conditions. Neurosci Lett 2005;378:160–165.
65 Derevjanik NL, Vinores SA, Xiao WH, Mori K, Turon T, Hudish T, Dong S, Campochiaro PA: Quantitative assessment of the integrity of the blood-retinal barrier in mice. Invest Ophthalmol Vis Sci 2002;43:2462–2467.
66 Krum JM, Khaibullina A: Inhibition of endogenous VEGF impedes revascularization and astroglial proliferation: roles for VEGF in brain repair. Exp Neurol 2003;181:241–257.
67 Witmer AN, Blaauwgeers HG, Weich HA, Alitalo K, Vrensen GF, Schlingemann RO: Altered expression patterns of VEGF receptors in human diabetic retina and in experimental VEGF-induced retinopathy in monkey. Invest Ophthalmol Vis Sci 2002;43:849–857.
68 Famiglietti EV, Stopa EG, McGookin ED, Song P, LeBlanc V, Streeten BW: Immunocytochemical localization of vascular endothelial growth factor in neurons and glial cells of human retina. Brain Res 2003;969:195–204.
69 Caldwell RB, Bartoli M, Behzadian MA, El-Remessy AE, Al-Shabrawey M, Platt DH, Caldwell RW: Vascular endothelial growth factor and diabetic retinopathy: pathophysiological mechanisms and treatment perspectives. Diabetes Metab Res Rev 2003;19:442–455.
70 Vinores SA, Youssri AI, Luna JD, Chen YS, Bhargave S, Vinores MA, Schoenfeld CL, Peng B, Chan CC, LaRochelle W, Green WR, Campochiaro PA: Upregulation of vascular endothelial growth factor in ischemic and non-ischemic human and experimental retinal disease. Histol Histopathol 1997;12:99–109.
71 Igarashi Y, Chiba H, Utsumi H, Miyajima H, Ishizaki T, Gotoh T, Kuwahara K, Tobioka H, Satoh M, Mori M, Sawada N: Expression of receptors for glial cell line-derived neurotrophic factor (GDNF) and neurturin in the inner blood-retinal barrier of rats. Cell Struct Funct 2000;25:237–241.
72 Aiello LP, Northrup JM, Keyt BA, Takagi H, Iwamoto MA. Hypoxic regulation of vascular endothelial growth factor in retinal cells. Arch Ophthalmol 1995;113:1538–1544.
73 Drescher KM, Whittum-Hudson JA: Herpes simplex virus type 1 alters transcript levels of tumor necrosis factor-alpha and interleukin-6 in retinal glial cells. Invest Ophthalmol Vis Sci 1996;37:2302–2312.
74 Eichler W, Yafai Y, Keller T, Wiedemann P, Reichenbach A: PEDF derived from glial Muller cells: a possible regulator of retinal angiogenesis. Exp Cell Res 2004;299:68–78.
75 Yafai Y, Iandiev I, Wiedemann P, Reichenbach A, Eichler W: Retinal endothelial angiogenic activity: effects of hypoxia and glial (Müller) cells. Microcirculation 2004;11:577–586.
76 Behzadian MA, Wang XL, Shabrawy M, Caldwell RB: Effects of hypoxia on glial cell expression of angiogenesis regulating factors VEGF and TGF-β. Glia 1998;24:216–225.
77 Hollborn M, Kraußβ C, Iandiev I, Yafai Y, Tenckhoff S, Bigl M, Schnurrbusch UEK, Limb GA, Reichenbach A, Kohen L, Wolf S, Wiedemann P, Bringmann A: Glial cell expression of hepatocyte growth factor in vitreoretinal proliferative disease. Lab Invest 2004;84:963–972.
78 Hollborn M, Jahn K, Limb GA, Kohen L, Wiedemann P, Bringmann A: Characterization of the basic fibroblast growth factor-evoked proliferation of the human Müller cell line, MIO-M1. Graefes Arch Clin Exp Ophthalmol 2004;242:414–422.
79 Aiello LP: The potential role of PKCβ in diabetic retinopathy and macular edema. Surv Ophthalmol 2002;47:S263–S269.
80 Eichler W, Kuhrt H, Hoffmann S, Wiedemann P, Reichenbach A: VEGF release by retinal glia depends on both oxygen and glucose supply. Neuroreport 2000;11:3533–3537.
81 Hirata C, Nakano K, Nakamura N, Kitagawa Y, Shigeta H, Hasegawa G, Ogata M, Ikeda T, Sawa H, Nakamura K, Ienaga K, Obayashi H, Kondo M: Advanced glycation end products induce expression of vascular endothelial growth factor by retinal Muller cells. Biochem Biophys Res Commun 1997;236:712–715.

82 Hammes HP, Alt A, Niwa T, Clausen JT, Bretzel RG, Brownlee M, Schleicher ED: Differential accumulation of advanced glycation end products in the course of diabetic retinopathy. Diabetologia 1999;42:728–736.
83 Aymerich MS, Alberdi EM, Martinez A, Becerra SP: Evidence for pigment epithelium-derived factor receptors in the neural retina. Invest Ophthalmol Vis Sci 2001;42:3287–3293.
84 Ogata N, Wada M, Otsuji T, Jo N, Tombran-Tink J, Matsumura M: Expression of pigment epithelium-derived factor in normal adult rat eye and experimental choroidal neovascularization. Invest Ophthalmol Vis Sci 2002;43:1168–1175.
85 Duh EJ, Yang HS, Suzuma I, Miyagi M, Youngman E, Mori K, Katai M, Yan L, Suzuma K, West K, Davarya S, Tong P, Gehlbach P, Pearlman J, Crabb JW, Aiello LP, Campochiaro PA, Zack DJ: Pigment epithelium-derived factor suppresses ischemia-induced retinal neovascularization and VEGF-induced migration and growth. Invest Ophthalmol Vis Sci 2002;43:821–829.
86 Boehm BO, Lang G, Volpert O, Jehle PM, Kurkhaus A, Rosinger S, Lang GK, Bouck N: Low content of the natural ocular anti-angiogenic agent pigment epithelium-derived factor (PEDF) in aqueous humor predicts progression of diabetic retinopathy. Diabetologia 2003;46:394–400.
87 D'Amore PA: Mechanisms of retinal and choroidal neovascularization. Invest Ophthalmol Vis Sci 1994;35:3974–3979.
88 Miller JW, Adamis AP, Shima DT, D'Amore PA, Moulton RS, O'Reilly MS, Folkman J, Dvorak HF, Brown LF, Berse B, et al: Vascular endothelial growth factor/vascular permeability factor is temporally and spatially correlated with ocular angiogenesis in a primate model. Am J Pathol 1994;145:574–584.
89 Eichler W, Yafai Y, Wiedemann P, Reichenbach A: Angiogenesis-related factors derived from retinal glial (Muller) cells in hypoxia. Neuroreport 2004;15:1633–1637.
90 Eichler W, Yafai Y, Kuhrt H, Grater R, Hoffmann S, Wiedemann P, Reichenbach A: Hypoxia: modulation of endothelial cell proliferation by soluble factors released by retinal cells. Neuroreport 2001;12:4103–4108.
91 Behzadian MA, Wang XL, Windsor LJ, Ghaly N, Caldwell RB: TGF-β increases retinal endothelial cell permeability by increasing MMP-9: possible role of glial cells in endothelial barrier function. Invest Ophthalmol Vis Sci 2001;42:853–859.
92 Majka S, McGuire PG, Das A: Regulation of matrix metalloproteinase expression by tumor necrosis factor in a murine model of retinal neovascularization. Invest Ophthalmol Vis Sci 2002;43:260–266.
93 Milenkovic I, Weick M, Wiedemann P, Reichenbach A, Bringmann A: P2Y receptor-mediated stimulation of Muller glial cell DNA synthesis: dependence on EGF and PDGF receptor transactivation. Invest Ophthalmol Vis Sci 2003;44:1211–1220.
94 Giebel SJ, Menicucci G, McGuire PG, Das A: Matrix metalloproteinases in early diabetic retinopathy and their role in alteration of the blood-retinal barrier. Lab Invest 2005;85:597–607.
95 Berka JL, Stubbs AJ, Wang DZ, DiNicolantonio R, Alcorn D, Campbell DJ, Skinner SL: Renin-containing Muller cells of the retina display endocrine features. Invest Ophthalmol Vis Sci 1995;36:1450–1458.
96 Nork TM, Wallow IHL, Sramek SJ, Anderson G: Müller's cell involvement in proliferative diabetic retinopathy. Arch Ophthalmol 1987;105:1424–1429.
97 Bringmann A, Pannicke T, Uhlmann S, Kohen L, Wiedemann P, Reichenbach A: Membrane conductance of Müller glial cells in proliferative diabetic retinopathy. Can J Ophthalmol 2002;37:221–227.
98 Guidry C: The role of Muller cells in fibrocontractive retinal disorders. Prog Retin Eye Res 2005;24:75–86.
99 Umeda N, Ozaki H, Hayashi H, Kondo H, Uchida H, Oshima K: Non-paralleled increase of hepatocyte growth factor and vascular endothelial growth factor in the eyes with angiogenic and nonangiogenic fibroproliferation. Ophthalmic Res 2002;34:43–47.
100 Bringmann A, Francke M, Pannicke T, Biedermann B, Faude F, Enzmann V, Wiedemann P, Reichelt W, Reichenbach A: Human Müller glial cells: altered potassium channel activity in proliferative vitreoretinopathy. Invest Ophthalmol Vis Sci 1999;40:3316–3323.
101 Bringmann A, Biedermann B, Reichenbach A: Expression of potassium channels during postnatal differentiation of rabbit Müller glial cells. Eur J Neurosci 1999b;11:2883–2896.
102 Bringmann A, Francke M, Pannicke T, Biedermann B, Kodal H, Faude F, Reichelt W, Reichenbach A: Role of glial K^+ channels in ontogeny and gliosis: A hypothesis based upon studies on Müller cells. Glia 2000;29:35–44.
103 Barbour B, Brew H, Attwell D: Electrogenic glutamate uptake in glial cells is activated by intracellular potassium. Nature 1988;335:433–435.
104 Derouiche A, Rauen T: Coincidence of L-glutamate/L-aspartate transporter (GLAST) and glutamine synthetase (GS) immunoreactions in retinal glia: evidence for coupling of GLAST and GS in transmitter clearance. J Neurosci Res 1995;42:131–143.
105 Qian H, Malchow RP, Ripps H: The effects of lowered extracellular sodium on gamma-aminobutyric acid (GABA)-induced currents of Müller (glial) cells of the skate retina. Cell Mol Neurobiol 1993;13:147–158.
106 Biedermann B, Bringmann A, Reichenbach A: High-affinity GABA uptake in retinal glial (Müller) cells of the guinea pig: electrophysiological characterization, immunohistochemical localization, and modeling of efficiency. Glia 2002;39:217–228.
107 Harada T, Harada C, Watanabe M, Inoue Y, Sakagawa T, Nakayama N, Sasaki S, Okuyama S, Watase K, Wada K, Tanaka K: Functions of the two glutamate transporters GLAST and GLT-1 in the retina. Proc Natl Acad Sci USA 1998;95:4663–4666.
108 Rauen T, Taylor WR, Kuhlbrodt K, Wiessner M: High-affinity glutamate transporters in the rat retina: a major role of the glial glutamate transporter GLAST-1 in transmitter clearance. Cell Tissue Res 1998;291:19–31.
109 Barnett NL, Pow DV: Antisense knockdown of GLAST, a glial glutamate transporter, compromises retinal function. Invest Ophthalmol Vis Sci 2000;41:585–591.
110 Kashii S, Mandai M, Kikuchi M, Honda Y, Tamura Y, Kaneda K, Akaike A: Dual actions of nitric oxide in N-methyl-D-aspartate receptor-mediated neurotoxicity in cultured retinal neurons. Brain Res 1996;711:93–101.

111 Izumi Y, Kirby CO, Benz AM, Olney JW, Zorumski CF: Müller cell swelling, glutamate uptake, and excitotoxic neurodegeneration in the isolated rat retina. Glia 1999;25:379–389.

112 Ambati J, Chalam KV, Chawla DK, D'Angio CT, Guillet EG, Rose SJ, Vanderlinde RE, Ambati BK: Elevated γ-aminobutyric acid, glutamate, and vascular endothelial growth factor levels in the vitreous of patients with proliferative diabetic retinopathy. Arch Ophthalmol 1997;115:1161–1166.

113 Kowluru RA, Engerman RL, Case GL, Kern TS: Retinal glutamate in diabetes and effect of antioxidants. Neurochem Int 2001;38:385–390.

114 Li Q, Puro DG: Diabetes-induced dysfunction of the glutamate transporter in retinal Müller cells. Invest Ophthalmol Vis Sci 2002;43:3109–3116.

115 Ward MM, Jobling AI, Kalloniatis M, Fletcher EL: Glutamate uptake in retinal glial cells during diabetes. Diabetologia 2005;48:351–360.

116 Paasche G, Huster D, Reichenbach A: The glutathione content of retinal Müller (glial) cells: the effects of aging and of application of free-radical scavengers. Ophthalmic Res 1998;30:351–360.

117 Poitry-Yamate CL, Poitry S, Tsacopoulos M: Lactate released by Muller glial cells is metabolized by photoreceptors from mammalian retina. J. Neurosci 1995;15:5179–5191.

118 Westergaard N, Sonnewald U, Schousboe A: Metabolic trafficking between neurons and astrocytes: the glutamate/glutamine cycle revisited. Dev Neurosci 1995;17:203–211.

119 Sonnewald U, Westergaard N, Schousboe A: Glutamate transport and metabolism in astrocytes. Glia 1997;21:56–63.

120 MacGregor LC, Matschinsky FM: Altered retinal metabolism in diabetes. II: measurement of sodium-potassium ATPase and total sodium and potassium in individual retinal layers. J Biol Chem 1986;261:4052–4058.

121 Ottlecz A, Garcia CA, Eichberg J, Fox DA: Alterations in retinal Na^+,K^+-ATPase in diabetes: streptozotocin-induced and Zucker diabetic fatty rats. Curr Eye Res 1993;12:1111–1121.

122 Newman EA, Frambach DA, Odette LL: Control of extracellular potassium levels by retinal glial cell K^+ siphoning. Science 1984;225:1174–1175.

123 Reichenbach A, Henke A, Eberhardt W, Reichelt W, Dettmer D: K^+ ion regulation in retina. Can J Physiol Pharmacol 1992;70:S239–S247.

124 Raap M, Biedermann B, Braun P, Milenkovic I, Skatchkov SN, Bringmann A, Reichenbach A: Diversity of Kir channel subunit mRNA expressed by retinal glial cells of the guinea-pig. Neuroreport 2002;13:1037–1040.

125 Kofuji P, Biedermann B, Siddharthan V, Raap M, Iandiev I, Milenkovic I, Thomzig A, Veh RW, Bringmann A, Reichenbach A: Kir potassium channel subunit expression in retinal glial cells: implications for spatial potassium buffering. Glia 2002;39:292–303.

126 Ishii M, Horio Y, Tada Y, Hibino H, Inanobe A, Ito M, Yamada M, Gotow T, Uchiyama Y, Kurachi Y: Expression and clustered distribution of an inwardly rectifying potassium channel, K_{AB}-2/Kir4.1, on mammalian retinal Müller cell membrane: their regulation by insulin and laminin signals. J Neurosci 1997;17:7725–7735.

127 Kofuji P, Ceelen P, Zahs KR, Surbeck LW, Lester HA, Newman EA: Genetic inactivation of an inwardly rectifying potassium channel (Kir4.1 subunit) in mice: phenotypic impact in retina. J Neurosci 2000;20:5733–5740.

128 Nagelhus EA, Horio Y, Inanobe A, Fujita A, Haug FM, Nielsen S, Kurachi Y, Ottersen OP: Immunogold evidence suggests that coupling of K^+ siphoning and water transport in rat retinal Müller cells is mediated by a coenrichment of Kir4.1 and AQP4 in specific membrane domains. Glia 1999;26:47–54.

129 Connors NC, Kofuji P: Dystrophin Dp71 is critical for the clustered localization of potassium channels in retinal glial cells. J Neurosci 2002;22:4321–4327.

130 Dalloz C, Sarig R, Fort P, Yaffe D, Bordais A, Pannicke T, Grosche J, Mornet D, Reichenbach A, Sahel J, Nudel U, Rendon A: Targeted inactivation of dystrophin gene product Dp71:phenotypic impact in mouse retina. Hum Mol Genet 2003;12:1543–1554.

131 Takumi T, Ishii T, Horio Y, Morishige K, Takahashi N, Yamada M, Yamashita T, Kiyami H, Sohmiya K, Nakanishi S, Kurachi Y: A novel ATP-dependent inward rectifier potassium channel expressed predominantly in glial cells. J Biol Chem 1995;270:16339–16346.

132 Kusaka S, Puro DG: Intracellular ATP activates inwardly rectifying K^+ channels in human and monkey retinal Müller (glial) cells. J Physiol (Lond) 1997;500:593–604.

133 Pannicke T, Uckermann O, Iandiev I, Wiedemann P, Reichenbach A, Bringmann A: Ocular inflammation alters swelling and membrane characteristics of rat Müller glial cells. J Neuroimmunol 2005;161:145–154.

134 Pannicke T, Iandiev I, Uckermann O, Biedermann B, Kutzera F, Wiedemann P, Wolburg H, Reichenbach A, Bringmann A: A potassium channel-linked mechanism of glial cell swelling in the postischemic retina. Mol Cell Neurosci 2004;26:493–502.

135 Köller H, Allert N, Oel D, Stoll G, Siebler M: TNFalpha induces a protein kinase C-dependent reduction in astroglial K^+ conductance. Neuroreport 1998;9:1375–1378.

136 Bringmann A, Kohen L, Wolf S, Wiedemann P, Reichenbach A: Age-related decrease of potassium currents in human retinal glial (Müller) cells. Can J Ophthalmol 2003;38:464–468.

137 Bresnick GH: Diabetic maculopathy: A critical review highlighting diffuse macular edema. Ophthalmology 1983;90:1301–1317.

138 Wolter JR: The histopathology of cystoid macular edema. Graefes Arch Clin Exp Ophthalmol 1981;216:85–101.

139 Antcliff RJ, Marshall J: The pathogenesis of edema in diabetic maculopathy. Semin Ophthalmol 1999;14:223–232.

140 Lobo CL, Bernardes RC, Cunha-Vaz JG: Alterations of the blood-retinal barrier and retinal thickness in preclinical retinopathy in subjects with type 2 diabetes. Arch Ophthalmol 2000;118:1364–1369.

141 Fine BS, Brucker AJ: Macular edema and cystoid macular edema. Am J Ophthalmol 1981;92:466–481.

142 Yanoff M, Fine BS, Brucker AJ, Eagle RC: Pathology of human cystoid macular edema. Surv Ophthalmol 1984;28:S505–S511.

143 Tso MOM: Pathology of cystoid macular edema. Ophthalmology 1982;89:902–915.

144 Marmor MF: Mechanisms of fluid accumulation in retinal edema. Doc Ophthalmol 1999;97:239–249.

145 Guex-Crosier Y: The pathogenesis and clinical presentation of macular edema in inflammatory diseases. Doc Ophthalmol 1999;97:297–309.
146 Miyake K, Ibaraki N: Prostaglandins and cystoid macular edema. Surv Ophthalmol 2002;47:S203–S218.
147 Stepinac TK, Chamot SR, Rungger-Brändle E, Ferrez P, Munoz JL, van den Bergh H, Riva CE, Pournaras CJ, Wagnieres GA: Light-induced retinal vascular damage by Pd-porphyrin luminescent oxygen probes. Invest Ophthalmol Vis Sci 2005;46:956–966.
148 Murata T, Nakagawa K, Khalil A, Ishibashi T, Inomata H, Sueishi K: The relation between expression of vascular endothelial growth factor and breakdown of the blood-retinal barrier in diabetic rat retinas. Lab Invest 1996;74:819–825.
149 Mori F, Hikichi T, Takahashi J, Nagaoka T, Yoshida A: Dysfunction of active transport of blood-retinal barrier in patients with clinically significant macular edema in type 2 diabetes. Diabetes Care 2002;25:1248–1249.
150 Uckermann O, Kutzera F, Wolf A, Pannicke T, Reichenbach A, Wiedemann P, Wolf S, Bringmann A: The glucocorticoid triamcinolone acetonide inhibits osmotic swelling of retinal glial cells via stimulation of endogenous adenosine signaling. J Pharmacol Exp Ther 2005;315:1036–1045.
151 Trotti D, Rossi D Gjesdal O, Levy LM, Racagni G, Danbolt NC, Volterra A: Peroxynitrite inhibits glutamate transporter subtypes. J Biol Chem 1996;271:5976–5979.
152 Kowluru RA, Kennedy A: Therapeutic potential of anti-oxidants and diabetic retinopathy. Expert Opin Investig Drugs 2001;10:1665–1676.
153 Du Y, Smith MA, Miller CM, Kern TS: Diabetes-induced nitrative stress in the retina, and correction by aminoguanidine. J Neurochem 2002;80:771–779.
154 Du Y, Sarthy VP, Kern TS: Interaction between NO and COX pathways in retinal cells exposed to elevated glucose and retina of diabetic rats. Am J Physiol 2004;287:R735–R741.
155 Martidis A, Duker JS, Greenberg PB, Rogers AH, Puliafito CA, Reichel E, Baumal C: Intravitreal triamcinolone for refractory diabetic macular edema. Ophthalmology 2002;109:920–927.
156 Jonas JB, Kreissig I, Sofker A, Degenring RF: Intravitreal injection of trimacinolone for diffuse diabetic macular edema. Arch Ophthalmol 2003;121:57–61.
157 Massin P, Audren F, Haouchine B, Erginay A, Bergmann JF, Benosman R, Caulin C, Gaudric A: Intravitreal triamcinolone acetonide for diabetic diffuse macular edema: preliminary results of a prospective controlled trial. Ophthalmology 2004;111:218–224.
158 Tamura H, Miyamoto K, Kiryu J, Miyahara S, Katsuta H, Hirose F, Musashi K, Yoshimura N: Intravitreal injection of corticosteroid attenuates leukostasis and vascular leakage in experimental diabetic retina. Invest Ophthalmol Vis Sci 2005;46:1440–1444.
159 Brooks HL Jr, Caballero S Jr, Newell CK, Steinmetz RL, Watson D, Segal MS, Harrison JK, Scott EW, Grant MB: Vitreous levels of vascular endothelial growth factor and stromal-derived factor 1 in patients with diabetic retinopathy and cystoid macular edema before and after intraocular injection of triamcinolone. Arch Ophthalmol 2004;122:1801–1807.

Prof. Dr. A. Reichenbach
Paul Flechsig Institute of Brain Research
Medical Faculty of the University of Leipzig
Jahnallee 59, DE–04109 Leipzig (Germany)
Tel. +49 341 9725 731, Fax +49 341 9725 739, E-Mail reia@medizin.uni-leipzig.de

Hammes H-P, Porta M (eds): Experimental Approaches to Diabetic Retinopathy.
Front Diabetes. Basel, Karger, 2010, vol 20, pp 98–108

Regulatory and Pathogenic Roles of Müller Glial Cells in Retinal Neovascular Processes and Their Potential for Retinal Regeneration

G. Astrid Limb · Hari Jayaram

UCL Institute of Ophthalmology, London, UK

Abstract

Müller glial cells are known to play a very important role in retinal homeostasis, and many metabolic functions have been ascribed to these cells not only in the normal but in the diseased retina. This chapter addresses a wide variety of activities attributed to Müller glial cells. It describes how activation of Müller glia by pro-inflammatory and pro-angiogenic factors may contribute to the development of neovascularisation and fibrosis, the characteristic pathological features of diabetic retinopathy. The chapter also highlights the regulatory role that Müller glia exert in various retinal functions, including the prevention of neural damage due to their production of neurotrophins in response to inflammatory and angiogenic signals. Recent findings that a sub-population of Müller glia have the ability to regenerate retinal neurons in adult life are described, and the implications for the potential use of Müller stem cells for cell-based therapies to regenerate diabetic retina are discussed.

Müller cells constitute the major glial cell population of the retina. They expand across the whole width of the retina and are in direct contact with all retinal cell types. They stabilize the complex retinal architecture, provide structural support to retinal neurons and blood vessels, and prevent aberrant photoreceptor migration into the subretinal space [1]. The mammalian retina harbours between 10^6 to 10^7 Müller cells [2] and their morphology varies according to their location within the retina. Müller glia in the retinal periphery comprise short thick cells with big end feet, whereas the thicker central retina is occupied by long slender cells with small end feet [2]. Independent of their location, Müller glia are sensitive to their environment and adapt to local surroundings. Within the nuclear layers of the retina, they ensheath local neurons and within the plexiform layers they extend out numerous cytoplasmic processes.

Müller glial cells promote neural survival in the retina due to their ability to remove metabolic waste from the retina and to produce trophic factors. They perform functions that astrocytes, oligodendrocytes and ependymal cells effect in other regions of the central nervous system [1]. In vitro, Müller cells promote extensive neurite outgrowth from rods [3], express several neurotransmitter receptors, including γ-aminobutyric acid type B receptors [4], and various types of glutamate transporters which facilitate glutamate uptake in order to keep its extracellular concentration below neurotoxic levels. Müller cells also express glutamine synthetase, an enzyme involved in detoxification of ammonia and glutamate that operates in concert with the L-glutamate/L-aspartate transporter to terminate the neurotransmitter action of glutamate [5]. They express K^+ channels on their plasma membrane, specially inwardly rectifying K^+ (Kir) channels, that makes them highly permeable to K^+ [6].

Changes in Müller cell membrane conductance have been extensively reported in proliferative diabetic retinopathy (PDR). It has been suggested that downregulation of active Kir channels and membrane depolarization are likely to disturb voltage-dependent Müller cell functions, such as regulation of local ion concentrations and uptake of neurotransmitters. In addition, it has been thought that enhanced entry of calcium ions from the extracellular space and the subsequent stimulation of calcium-activated potassium channels may support the Müller cell proliferation observed in this complication of diabetes mellitus [7].

In addition to the above metabolic functions, Müller cells are known to produce multiple cytokines, growth factors and neurotrophic factors in response to inflammatory and angiogenic signals, retinal hypoxia and advanced glycation end products [7]. Although the metabolic and structural functions of Müller glia in the adult eye have been known for a long time, it was not until recently that a new function for these cells as a source of retinal neurons was identified in the adult mammalian eye, including humans [8–10].

There is considerable evidence that neural degeneration observed in the diabetic retina is due to reactive changes in Müller glial cells. Neural cell damage and death have been observed prior to the onset of neovascularisation in animal models of diabetic retinopathy (DR), and accumulating evidence shows that during the diabetic process, Müller cells become gliotic and display altered potassium siphoning, glutamate and γ-aminobutyric acid uptake and express various modulators of angiogenesis [11]. Müller glia have been thought to operate as a means of communication between the neural retina and the vasculature. Microscopic studies of primate retinae have demonstrated that the Müller cell end feet completely encircle the retinal blood vessels [12]. This close anatomical apposition suggests that Müller glia form an essential part of the blood retinal barrier and changes in this structure caused by Müller cell damage are believed to contribute to vessel leakage in DR.

Role of Müller Glia in Inflammation and Angiogenesis

Several studies have implicated inflammation as a contributing factor in the microvascular and glial changes observed in DR, a common ocular complication in patients with diabetes mellitus. This evidence is derived from studies that show that fibrovascular membranes from eyes with PDR contain high levels of pro-inflammatory cytokines such as TNF-α, IL-1, IL-6, IL-8, monocyte chemotactic protein-1, and macrophage colony-stimulating factor [13–15].

Vascular endothelial growth factor (VEGF), a potent pro-angiogenic mediator which has been implicated in the pathogenesis of DR [16], has been shown to be present in the vitreous of patients with PDR, along with another pro-angiogenic factor, the hepatocyte growth factor [17]. Levels of these two factors in the vitreous of diabetic patients have been shown to correlate with the severity of the condition. Müller glial cells are thought to play an important role in the pathogenesis of this complication as they have been shown to produce most factors found in the vitreous of diabetic patients complicated by PDR. Advanced glycation end products are known to induce production of IL-6 [18] and VEGF [19] by Müller cells in vitro, whilst pro-inflammatory cytokines such as IL-1 can also activate these cells to release IL-6 [20]. High glucose levels induce production of TNF-α and IL-1β by Müller

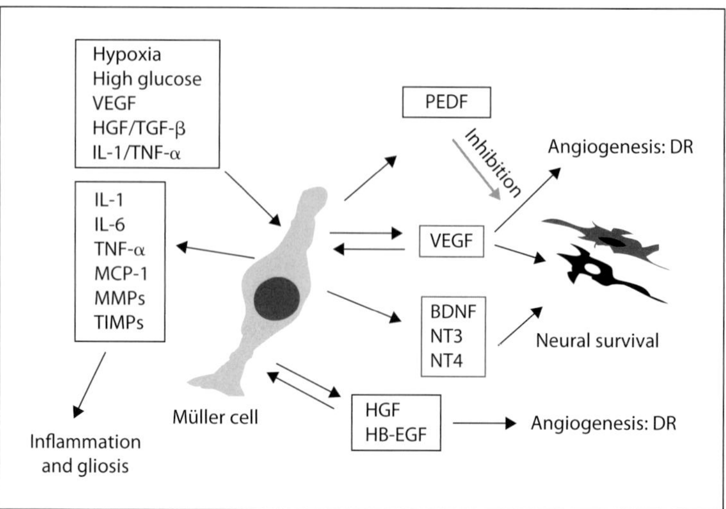

Fig. 1. Multiple metabolic and cellular functions of Müller glial cells. Illustration of the multiple functions and cell-ECM interactions of Müller glia that lead to activation of several pathways and to the release of pro-angiogenic, anti-angiogenic and neuroprotective factors implicated in the pathogenesis of DR. HB-EGF = Heparin-binding epidermal growth factor-like growth factor; MCP-1 = monocyte chemotactic protein; HGF = hepatocyte growth factor.

glia in culture [21], whilst activation of these cells with lipopolysaccharide and interferon-γ promotes release of TNF-α by these cells [22]. There is also evidence that human Müller cells express the isoform variant $VEGF_{183}$ [23] and that gene upregulation and production of VEGF by these cells may be induced by hypoxia [24], bFGF [25] and heparin-binding epidermal growth factor-like growth factor [26]. In addition to their production of pro-angiogenic factors, Müller cells have been shown to release an important anti-angiogenic factor known as pigment epithelium-derived factor (PEDF) [27]. This is of special interest as it has been recognized that the balance between VEGF and PEDF and their reciprocal interaction are important for the regulation of vascular permeability and angiogenesis. PEDF has been demonstrated to significantly decrease VEGF expression by Müller cells, whilst silencing of the PEDF gene by siRNA in Müller cells has resulted in significant upregulation of VEGF expression at both RNA and protein levels [27]. These observations suggest that PEDF is an endogenous negative regulator of VEGF in Müller cells, and that regulatory Müller glial functions are important for adjusting the balance between pro-angiogenic and anti-angiogenic mediators during retinal neovascular processes that characterise the development of DR.

Figure 1 attempts to summarize the major events that lead to activation of Müller glia within the diabetic retina, and the contribution of various factors released by Müller cells to the activation of cellular functions responsible for neovascularization, fibrosis and neural survival.

Control of Extracellular Matrix Deposition by Müller Cells

Early events leading to the development of PDR involve local cell migration and proliferation followed by extracellular matrix (ECM) deposition [28]. These cellular processes eventually lead to the formation of new vessels and fibrovascular complexes. Cell migration and matrix deposition are controlled by ECM degradation by proteolytic enzymes known as matrix metalloproteinases (MMPs) [29]. These enzymes, also known as matrixins, constitute a family of zinc-binding, calcium-dependent molecules, whose activity is regulated by natural inhibitors known as tissue inhibitors of metalloproteinases (TIMPs) [29].

Two major matrix degrading enzymes, known as MMP-2 (collagenase A) and MMP-9 (collagenase B) are found in the vitreous of eyes with PDR [30], whilst characteristic staining for active MMP-9 has been observed within the perivascular matrix of neovascular membranes with this condition [31]. The inactive forms of MMP-2 and MMP-9 have also been shown to be significantly elevated in the neovascular membranes in comparison with normal retinas [32]. Although the main source of these two MMPs in vivo has been thought to be the retinal pigment epithelial cells, which are well known to produce these molecules in vitro [33], evidence has been presented that Müller cells produce both MMP-2 and MMP-9 in vitro, and that cytokines such as TNF-α either in soluble form or bound to the ECM may induce upregulation of MMP-9 expression by these cells [34].

Despite extensive studies demonstrating the production of several MMPs and TIMPs by retinal pigment epithelial cells, there are very few investigations on the production of TIMPs by Müller glia. At present, there is limited evidence for the Müller cell expression of TIMP-2 in vivo, as demonstrated by studies showing Müller glia staining with antibodies to TIMP-2 within the degenerating retina of the rd1 mouse [35]. At the intracellular level, Müller cells have been shown to contain abundant mitochondria which are reflective of their active metabolic role within the retina. It is of interest that MMP-1, which has been shown to associate to mitochondria and to protect cells from apoptosis, is abundant within these organelles in Müller cells [36].

That Müller cells have the ability to release MMPs that promote the degradation of ECM, together with the evidence that MMPs promote cell migration and proliferation, strongly suggests that these cells play a very important role in the control of cell-ECM interactions that lead to the development of retinal neovascular processes.

Neuroprotective Role of Müller Glia

As part of their neuroprotective role within the retina, Müller glia produce a group of proteins that signal for neural survival, growth and differentiation. These proteins, known as neurotrophins (NTs), constitute a group of four structurally related factors known as nerve growth factor (NGF), brain-derived neurotrophic factor (BDNF), NT3 and NT4. NTs effect their functions by binding to two different surface receptors: the tropomyosin-related kinase receptors and the p75 NT receptor (p75NTR). NT binding to their receptors leads to phosphorylation of tyrosine residues in the receptor cytoplasmic domain. This causes activation of signalling pathways such as Ras, Rap and PI3K that in turn lead to the induction of cell survival and neurite outgrowth [37]. BDNF has been recognized to play an important role in the development, differentiation, connectivity and survival of retinal neurons [38], and Müller glial cells have been shown to constitute an important source of BDNF in vivo [39] and in vitro [40, 41]. There is evidence that BDNF promotes photoreceptor survival following experimental retinal detachment [42], and that it exerts trophic and neuroprotective effects on retinal ganglion cells during development and after optic nerve injury [43]. In addition, BDNF can rescue photoreceptors from the damaging effects of constant light, protect the retina from ischaemic injury, and modulate the morphology and the neurochemical phenotypes of amacrine cells [44]. Neural cell damage induced by cytotoxic factors such as glutamate, result in an enhanced production of BDNF by Müller glia [41] and intravitreal injection of BDNF in eyes from rodents susceptible to retinal degeneration increases expression of NT receptors on Müller glia but not on photoreceptors, although there is increased photoreceptor survival, suggesting that neurotrophic factors act indirectly through Müller cells to promote this phenomenon [45]. In addition, BDNF causes activation of intracellular signalling pathways in Müller cells [45], implicating the existence of autocrine functions mediated by this NT.

Müller glia can be induced to release NGF upon inflammatory stimulation with interferon-γ and lipopolysaccharides [46]. As seen with other NTs and growth factors, NGF has autocrine activities, as illustrated by the fact that whilst Müller glial cells are able to produce this factor, they are also receptive to its activity. This is supported by observations that programmed cell death of retinal ganglion cells and Müller glia observed in diabetic rats can be prevented by treatment with NGF [47].

Evidence for the expression of NT4 by Müller glia mainly derives from in situ observations of retina from eyes with proliferative vitreoretinopathy, a common complication of retinal detachment [48]. Presence of NTs in Müller cells within degenerated retina suggests that pro-inflammatory events that lead to the local production of NTs may reflect the mechanisms by which Müller glia exert their neuroprotective functions.

Müller Glial Cells as a Source of Retinal Neurons in the Adult Eye

The ability of fish and amphibians to regenerate retinal tissue throughout life has been known for many years. These species harbour a population of stem cells that are located at the peripheral margin of the retina adjacent to the ciliary epithelium, known as the ciliary margin zone [49]. A similar population of retinal stem cells has been identified in birds and small mammals [50] during early postnatal life, and although a population of retinal progenitor cells has been identified in the ciliary body of adult mice [51], pigs [52] and humans [53], these appear to constitute a different progenitor cell population to that observed in the ciliary margin zone of the neural retina.

During development, Müller glia and retinal neurons share a common progenitor that is multipotent at all stages of retinal histogenesis [54]. This evidence derives from examination of the progeny of a single mouse retinal progenitor cell transfected with a retrovirus, which generated clones containing up to three types of neurons, while others contained Müller glia alone, a combination of neurons and Müller glia, or a single neuron type. Markers of glial progenitors are therefore shared with retinal neural progenitors, and these can be used to identify Müller glia with stem cell characteristics, and to modulate the ability of these cells to differentiate into specified neurons in vitro and in vivo. Figure 2 summarizes the main developmental pathways that lead to Müller cell maturation and differentiation from the neural lineage.

One of the markers expressed by neural stem cells before they differentiate into the glial pathway is the bone morphogenetic protein-4 (BMP-4), a member of the transforming growth factor-β (TGF-β) family. It has been implicated as a regulator of neural and glial differentiation. Work in mouse embryonic stem cells suggested that BMP-4 acts in an inhibitory manner to prevent the neural differentiation of progenitors, directing them instead to a mesodermal fate [55]. Studies in the postnatal chick retina have demonstrated the ability of Müller glia to de-differentiate and become neurogenic in nature following chemically induced injury of the retina [56]. In the adult rat retina, they have been shown to proliferate and differentiate into bipolar cells and photoreceptors following neurotoxic injury to the adult retina [10].

Dividing Müller glia, as identified by Brd-U uptake, have been shown to express Cash-1, Chx-10 and Pax-6, which are characteristic markers of multipotent retinal progenitors. During the ensuing period, the majority of these cells remained as undifferentiated progenitors expressing Chx-10 and Pax-6, whilst the others differentiated into either Müller glia or retinal neurons. Other factors such as the basic loop-helix-loop (bHLH) transcription factors also play a key role in the regulation of multipotent progenitor

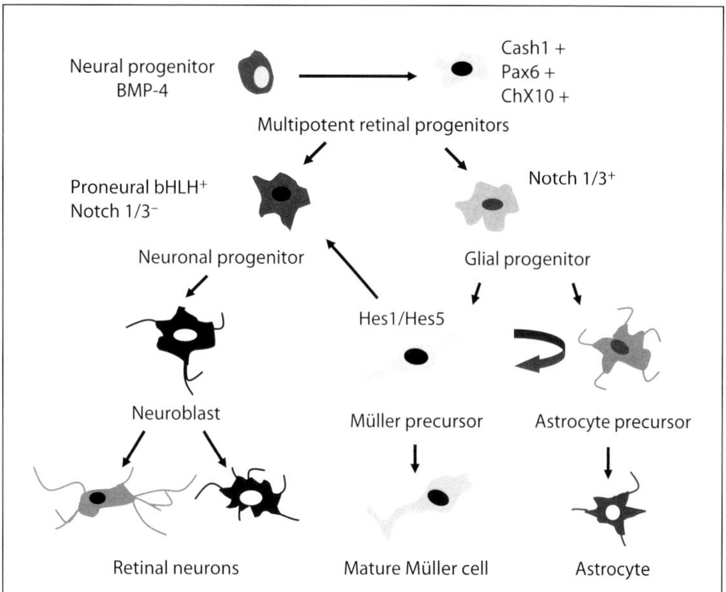

Fig. 2. Ontogenesis of Müller glial cells. Summary of the major developmental pathways that lead to the development of Müller glia from a common progenitor that is shared with retinal neurons.

differentiation into either neural or glial cells. The proneural bHLH factors have been also demonstrated to possess an intrinsic activity to induce the generation of neurons, whereas the inhibitory type has been shown to stimulate the production of astrocytes [57].

Müller glial stem cells express the transcription factor Notch, whose signalling pathway involves a cascade of activation and repression of various transcription factors that lead to specific neuronal differentiation within the eye. The Hes1/Hes5 genes, known as Notch effectors, are activated by induction of the Notch pathway. These lead to downstream inhibition of further genes that in turn lead to inhibition of neural differentiation. Therefore, inhibition of the Notch pathway induces the differentiation of neural progenitors to differentiate into neurons, in particular into retinal ganglion cells. Upregulation of the Notch pathway permits the proliferation of progenitor cell populations whilst permitting the differentiation of sub-group towards a glial fate [58].

Several studies have elucidated the possibility of Müller glia being a source of progenitor cells over the past decade. Müller cells have been described as a source of retinal progenitors in the postnatal chick retina [56], and have been shown to proliferate and differentiate into bipolar cells and photoreceptors following neurotoxic injury to the adult rat retina [10]. The neurogenic capacity of Müller glia has been clearly demonstrated in the zebrafish, where they form the retinal stem cell niche, and also show an ability to regenerate retinal neurons following injury [59].

Recent studies have identified a population of Müller glia with neural stem cell characteristics in the adult human eye, independent of sex or age [9]. These cells become spontaneously immortalized in vitro, an important characteristic of stem cells, and can be frozen and thawed without losing their progenitor ability for many passages in culture. Under normal culture conditions, they express neural stem cell markers such as nestin, βIII tubulin, Sox-2, Pax-6, Chx10 and Notch-1 [9]. In vitro differentiation studies of

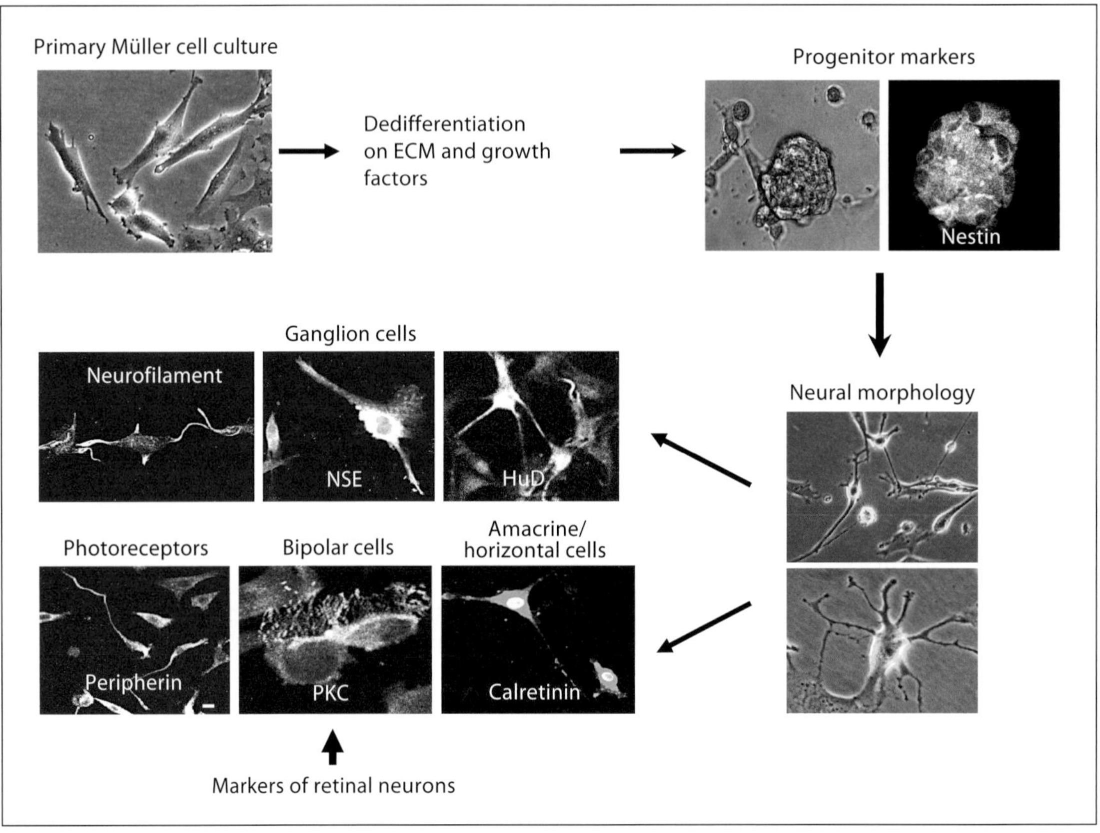

Fig. 3. In vitro characteristics of Müller stem cells isolated from the adult human retina. Müller stem cells grow as adherent monolayers in vitro. Upon culture with growth and differentiation factors, these cells form neurospheres and acquire neural morphology. Cells that acquire neural morphology express markers of different retinal neurons.

these Müller stem cells in the presence of growth factors provided further evidence of the pluripotency of this cell population. Under specific conditions in vitro they can be induced to express markers of post-mitotic retinal neurons, including peripherin, S-opsin and recoverin (markers of photoreceptor cells), calretinin and neurofilament protein (markers of ganglion, horizontal and amacrine cells), and HuD and Brn3 (markers of ganglion cells; fig. 3) [9].

Transplantation of Müller stem cells into the subretinal space of the dystrophic RCS rat and the neonatal and adult Lister hood rats has been performed to investigate the in vivo potential of these cells to migrate and differentiate into the retina and to restore damaged retina function. Initial experiments showed that only a small proportion of these cells were able to migrate into the retina. However, they expressed neural markers characteristic of the retinal cell layer to which they migrate. Transplanted cells found within the outer nuclear layer of the retina, where photoreceptors are present, expressed markers of photoreceptor cells such as recoverin and rhodopsin. Those cells that migrated into the ganglion cell layer expressed calretinin and HuD, characteristic markers of ganglion cells [9]. These findings suggest that although Müller stem cells have the ability to differentiate and repopulate damaged retinal neurons, there are barriers that prevent a successful integration of transplanted cells into the retina.

Potential Barriers for Stem Cell Transplantation to Regenerate Retinal Neurons in the Diabetic Retina

Investigations have shown that the limited migration and integration of grafted Müller stem cells into the degenerated retina of the RCS rat are partly due to the accumulation of a group of ECM proteins produced during reactive gliosis [60]. These proteins, known as chondroitin sulphate proteoglycans (CSPGs), are known to prevent axonal regeneration and synapse formation following injury [61]. Remodelling of the retina following a pathological process similar to that seen elsewhere in the central nervous system often results in the deposition of glial scar rich in CSPGs [61]. The diabetic retina exhibits all the characteristics of reactive gliosis, which in addition to neovascularization, presents with accumulation of abnormal extracellular proteins and glial cell proliferation [7]. In addition, abnormalities of retinal pericytes and endothelial cells observed in the DR have been associated with increased expression of CSPGs [62]. Based on this evidence, methodologies designed to facilitate migration and integration of transplanted Müller stem cells into other experimental models of retinal degeneration may be applied to transplantation into the diabetic retina.

In eyes with DR, microglia have been shown to be markedly increased in number and display hypertrophic features at different stages of the disease [63]. These cells accumulate around the retinal vasculature, especially the dilated veins, microaneurysms, intraretinal haemorrhages, cotton-wool spots, and areas of retinal neovascularisation. Microglia have also been observed in the outer retina and subretinal space of retinae with cystoid macular oedema, and in epiretinal membranes of PDR [63]. These observations present with another potential barrier for retinal regeneration of the diabetic retina, due to evidence that microglia prevent a successful integration of transplanted cells [64] In addition, microglia have been shown to produce the inhibitory CSPGs described above, both in vitro and in vivo, which potentiates the deposition of abnormal ECM in the diabetic retina. In this context, the demonstration of breakdown of the ECM with chondroitinase ABC in conjunction with strong microglial suppression [60] has provided major knowledge that can be applied to facilitate the development of cell-based therapies to restore retinal function lost by diseases such as DR. Further work to optimise transplantation strategies and to identify the most appropriate cell sources for retinal therapies are at present being developed in many laboratories across the world.

Potential of Müller Stem Cells for the Development of Human Therapies to Restore Retinal Function Damaged by Disease

Death of retinal neurons is the major cause of blindness in neovascular and inflammatory retinal conditions such as PDR. Current treatments currently offer a palliative role in the prevention of visual loss, but in the long term it is difficult to prevent loss of vision in many individuals. The only realistic expectation for restoration of retinal function is the development of stem-cell based therapies to replace and integrate lost neurons into the neural network.

Müller stem cells have a potential advantage over other stem cells in that they can be derived from adult human retina and can be potentially isolated from the same individual to avoid problems arising from lack of histocompatibility and crossed infections. Although Müller glial cell proliferation (reactive gliosis) has been shown to occur during degenerative retinal processes, neurogenesis occurring in these conditions has not been demonstrated in the adult human retina.

It is possible to speculate that if neural progenitors are harboured in the adult retina, these may have the potential to regenerate neurons. However, as there is no evidence that post-developmental neurogenesis may occur in the human eye, the possibility arises that this process is suppressed in vivo by unidentified factors present in the adult eye. It has been suggested that the mitotic quiescence of Müller cells within the postnatal mammalian retina is mediated by a TGF-β signal released by the cells themselves [65]. This raises the possibility that modulation of TGF-β-mediated processes may facilitate the activation of the endogenous retinal stem cell niche and may therefore facilitate strategies aimed at regeneration of the retina.

Investigations into the feasibility of activating neurogenesis mediated by Müller progenitors in vivo may have the potential to develop into treatments for endogenous replacement of dysfunctional neurons. This is suggested by recent studies that show that sonic hedgehog, a protein that plays an important role in regulating neurogenesis during retinal development, is able to induce in vitro proliferation of rat Müller cells [66]. This factor also showed to induce photoreceptor differentiation of Müller cells in culture, as well as proliferation and differentiation of these cells into rod photoreceptors in vivo following intravitreal injection into the rat eye [66]. Additional studies have also shown that following neurotoxic damage to the mice retina, Wnt3a, a transcription factor also involved in neurogenesis, is able to induce proliferation of Müller glia and generation of photoreceptors derived from these cells [67]. Based on these studies and our observations that Müller glia with stem cell characteristics are present in the adult human eye, it might be possible to explore the possibility of using these factors as adjuvant therapies to promote in situ proliferation and photoreceptor differentiation of Müller glia in order to regenerate neural retina damaged by disease.

Considering the multiple roles of Müller glia in the normal and the diabetic eye, it may be possible that either Müller stem cell transplantation or adjuvant induction of Müller stem cell proliferation in situ may not only serve as a source of neurons, but also as a source of neurotrophic and anti-angiogenic factors that may help restore retinal function in the diabetic eye.

References

1 Newman E, Reichenbach A: The Muller cell: a functional element of the retina. Trends Neurosci 1996;19:307–312.

2 Robinson SR, Dreher Z: Muller cells in adult rabbit retinae: morphology, distribution and implications for function and development. J Comp Neurol 1990;292:178–192.

3 Kljavin IJ, Reh TA: Muller cells are a preferred substrate for in vitro neurite extension by rod photoreceptor cells. J Neurosci 1991;11:2985–2994.

4 Zhang J, Yang XL: GABA(B) receptors in Muller cells of the bullfrog retina. Neuroreport 1999;10:1833–1836.

5 Derouiche A, Rauen T: Coincidence of L-glutamate/L-aspartate transporter (GLAST) and glutamine synthetase (GS) immunoreactions in retinal glia: evidence for coupling of GLAST and GS in transmitter clearance. J Neurosci Res 1995;42:131–143.

6 Newman EA: Inward-rectifying potassium channels in retinal glial (Muller) cells. J Neurosci 1993;13:3333–3345.

7 Bringmann A, Pannicke T, Grosche J, et al: Muller cells in the healthy and diseased retina. Prog Retin Eye Res 2006;25:397–424.

8 Das AV, Mallya KB, Zhao X, et al: Neural stem cell properties of Muller glia in the mammalian retina: regulation by Notch and Wnt signaling. Dev Biol 2006;299:283–302.

9 Lawrence JM, Singhal S, Bhatia B, et al: MIO-M1 cells and similar Muller glial cell lines derived from adult human retina exhibit neural stem cell characteristics. Stem Cells 2007;25:2033–2043.

10 Ooto S, Akagi T, Kageyama R, et al: Potential for neural regeneration after neurotoxic injury in the adult mammalian retina. Proc Natl Acad Sci USA 2004;101:13654–13659.

11 Fletcher EL, Phipps JA, Ward MM, Puthussery T, Wilkinson-Berka JL: Neuronal and glial cell abnormality as predictors of progression of diabetic retinopathy. Curr Pharm Des 2007;13:2699–2712.
12 Distler C, Dreher Z: Glia cells of the monkey retina. II. Muller cells. Vision Res 1996;36:2381–2394.
13 Funatsu H, Yamashita H, Mimura T, Noma H, Nakamura S, Hori S: Risk evaluation of outcome of vitreous surgery based on vitreous levels of cytokines. Eye 2007;21:377–382.
14 Limb GA, Soomro H, Janikoun S, Hollifield RD, Shilling J: Evidence for control of tumour necrosis factor-alpha (TNF-alpha) activity by TNF receptors in patients with proliferative diabetic retinopathy. Clin Exp Immunol 1999;115:409–414.
15 Limb GA, Webster L, Soomro H, Janikoun S, Shilling J: Platelet expression of tumour necrosis factor-alpha (TNF-alpha), TNF receptors and intercellular adhesion molecule-1 (ICAM-1) in patients with proliferative diabetic retinopathy. Clin Exp Immunol 1999;118:213–218.
16 Witmer AN, Vrensen GF, Van Noorden CJ, Schlingemann RO: Vascular endothelial growth factors and angiogenesis in eye disease. Prog Retin Eye Res 2003;22:1–29.
17 Murugeswari P, Shukla D, Rajendran A, Kim R, Namperumalsamy P, Muthukkaruppan V: Proinflammatory cytokines and angiogenic and anti-angiogenic factors in vitreous of patients with proliferative diabetic retinopathy and Eales' disease. Retina 2008;28:817–824.
18 Nakamura N, Hasegawa G, Obayashi H, et al: Increased concentration of pentosidine, an advanced glycation end product, and interleukin-6 in the vitreous of patients with proliferative diabetic retinopathy. Diabetes Res Clin Pract 2003;61:93–101.
19 Hirata C, Nakano K, Nakamura N, et al: Advanced glycation end products induce expression of vascular endothelial growth factor by retinal Muller cells. Biochem Biophys Res Commun 1997;236:712–715.
20 Yoshida S, Sotozono C, Ikeda T, Kinoshita S: Interleukin-6 (IL-6) production by cytokine-stimulated human Muller cells. Curr Eye Res 2001;22:341–347.
21 Walker RJ, Steinle JJ: Role of beta-adrenergic receptors in inflammatory marker expression in Muller cells. Invest Ophthalmol Vis Sci 2007;48:5276–5281.
22 Cotinet A, Goureau O, Hicks D, Thillaye-Goldenberg B, de Kozak Y: Tumor necrosis factor and nitric oxide production by retinal Muller glial cells from rats exhibiting inherited retinal dystrophy. Glia 1997;20:59–69.
23 Jingjing L, Xue Y, Agarwal N, Roque RS: Human Muller cells express VEGF183, a novel spliced variant of vascular endothelial growth factor. Invest Ophthalmol Vis Sci 1999;40:752–759.
24 Robbins SG, Conaway JR, Ford BL, Roberto KA, Penn JS: Detection of vascular endothelial growth factor (VEGF) protein in vascular and non-vascular cells of the normal and oxygen-injured rat retina. Growth Factors 1997;14:229–241.
25 Hollborn M, Jahn K, Limb GA, Kohen L, Wiedemann P, Bringmann A: Characterization of the basic fibroblast growth factor-evoked proliferation of the human Muller cell line, MIO-M1. Graefes Arch Clin Exp Ophthalmol 2004;242:414–422.
26 Hollborn M, Tenckhoff S, Jahn K, et al: Changes in retinal gene expression in proliferative vitreoretinopathy: glial cell expression of HB-EGF. Mol Vis 2005;11:397–413.
27 Zhang SX, Wang JJ, Gao G, Parke K, Ma JX: Pigment epithelium-derived factor downregulates vascular endothelial growth factor (VEGF) expression and inhibits VEGF-VEGF receptor 2 binding in diabetic retinopathy. J Mol Endocrinol 2006;37:1–12.
28 Casaroli Marano RP, Preissner KT, Vilaro S: Fibronectin, laminin, vitronectin and their receptors at newly-formed capillaries in proliferative diabetic retinopathy. Exp Eye Res 1995;60:5–17.
29 Nagase H, Visse R, Murphy G: Structure and function of matrix metalloproteinases and TIMPs. Cardiovasc Res 2006;69:562–573.
30 Jin M, Kashiwagi K, Iizuka Y, Tanaka Y, Imai M, Tsukahara S: Matrix metalloproteinases in human diabetic and nondiabetic vitreous. Retina 2001;21:28–33.
31 Salzmann J, Limb GA, Khaw PT, et al: Matrix metalloproteinases and their natural inhibitors in fibrovascular membranes of proliferative diabetic retinopathy. Br J Ophthalmol 2000;84:1091–1096.
32 Das A, McGuire PG, Eriqat C, et al: Human diabetic neovascular membranes contain high levels of urokinase and metalloproteinase enzymes. Invest Ophthalmol Vis Sci 1999;40:809–813.
33 Hoffmann S, He S, Ehren M, Ryan SJ, Wiedemann P, Hinton DR: MMP-2 and MMP-9 secretion by rpe is stimulated by angiogenic molecules found in choroidal neovascular membranes. Retina 2006;26:454–461.
34 Limb GA, Daniels JT, Pleass R, Charteris DG, Luthert PJ, Khaw PT: Differential expression of matrix metalloproteinases 2 and 9 by glial Muller cells: response to soluble and extracellular matrix-bound tumor necrosis factor-alpha. Am J Pathol 2002;160:1847–1855.
35 Ahuja S, Ahuja P, Caffe AR, Ekstrom P, Abrahamson M, van Veen T: rd1 mouse retina shows imbalance in cellular distribution and levels of TIMP-1/MMP-9, TIMP-2/MMP-2 and sulfated glycosaminoglycans. Ophthalmic Res 2006;38:125–136.
36 Limb GA, Matter K, Murphy G, et al: Matrix metalloproteinase-1 associates with intracellular organelles and confers resistance to lamin A/C degradation during apoptosis. Am J Pathol 2005;166:1555–1563.
37 Arevalo JC, Wu SH: Neurotrophin signaling: many exciting surprises! Cell Mol Life Sci 2006;63:1523–1537.
38 Landi S, Sale A, Berardi N, Viegi A, Maffei L, Cenni MC: Retinal functional development is sensitive to environmental enrichment: a role for BDNF. FASEB J 2007;21:130–139.
39 Garcia M, Forster V, Hicks D, Vecino E: In vivo expression of neurotrophins and neurotrophin receptors is conserved in adult porcine retina in vitro. Invest Ophthalmol Vis Sci 2003;44:4532–4541.
40 Oku H, Ikeda T, Honma Y, et al: Gene expression of neurotrophins and their high-affinity Trk receptors in cultured human Muller cells. Ophthalmic Res 2002;34:38–42.

41 Taylor S, Srinivasan B, Wordinger RJ, Roque RS: Glutamate stimulates neurotrophin expression in cultured Muller cells. Brain Res Mol Brain Res 2003;111:189–197.
42 Lewis GP, Linberg KA, Geller SF, Guerin CJ, Fisher SK: Effects of the neurotrophin brain-derived neurotrophic factor in an experimental model of retinal detachment. Invest Ophthalmol Vis Sci 1999;40:1530–1544.
43 Mansour-Robaey S, Clarke DB, Wang YC, Bray GM, Aguayo AJ: Effects of ocular injury and administration of brain-derived neurotrophic factor on survival and regrowth of axotomized retinal ganglion cells. Proc Natl Acad Sci USA 1994;91:1632–1636.
44 Pinzon-Duarte G, Arango-Gonzalez B, Guenther E, Kohler K: Effects of brain-derived neurotrophic factor on cell survival, differentiation and patterning of neuronal connections and Muller glia cells in the developing retina. Eur J Neurosci 2004;19:1475–1484.
45 Wahlin KJ, Campochiaro PA, Zack DJ, Adler R: Neurotrophic factors cause activation of intracellular signaling pathways in Muller cells and other cells of the inner retina, but not photoreceptors. Invest Ophthalmol Vis Sci 2000;41:927–936.
46 Dicou E, Nerriere V, Naud MC, de Kozak Y: NGF involvement in ocular inflammation: secretion by rat resident retinal cells. Neuroreport 1994;6:26–28.
47 Hammes HP, Federoff HJ, Brownlee M: Nerve growth factor prevents both neuroretinal programmed cell death and capillary pathology in experimental diabetes. Mol Med 1995;1:527–534.
48 Ghazi-Nouri SM, Ellis JS, Moss S, Limb GA, Charteris DG: Expression and localisation of BDNF, NT4 and TrkB in proliferative vitreoretinopathy. Exp Eye Res 2008;86:819–827.
49 Raymond PA, Hitchcock PF: Retinal regeneration: common principles but a diversity of mechanisms. Adv Neurol 1997;72:171–184.
50 Moshiri A, Close J, Reh TA: Retinal stem cells and regeneration. Int J Dev Biol 2004;48:1003–1014.
51 Tropepe V, Coles BL, Chiasson BJ, et al: Retinal stem cells in the adult mammalian eye. Science 2000;287:2032–2036.
52 Gu P, Harwood LJ, Zhang X, Wylie M, Curry WJ, Cogliati T: Isolation of retinal progenitor and stem cells from the porcine eye. Mol Vis 2007;13:1045–1057.
53 Coles BL, Angenieux B, Inoue T, et al: Facile isolation and the characterization of human retinal stem cells. Proc Natl Acad Sci USA 2004;101:15772–15777.
54 Turner DL, Cepko CL: A common progenitor for neurons and glia persists in rat retina late in development. Nature 1987;328:131–136.
55 Finley MF, Devata S, Huettner JE: BMP-4 inhibits neural differentiation of murine embryonic stem cells. J Neurobiol 1999;40:271–287.
56 Fischer AJ, Reh TA: Muller glia are a potential source of neural regeneration in the postnatal chicken retina. Nat Neurosci 2001;4:247–252.
57 Sugimori M, Nagao M, Bertrand N, Parras CM, Guillemot F, Nakafuku M: Combinatorial actions of patterning and HLH transcription factors in the spatiotemporal control of neurogenesis and gliogenesis in the developing spinal cord. Development 2007;134:1617–1629.
58 Scheer N, Groth A, Hans S, Campos-Ortega JA: An instructive function for Notch in promoting gliogenesis in the zebrafish retina. Development 2001;128:1099–1107.
59 Raymond PA, Barthel LK, Bernardos RL, Perkowski JJ: Molecular characterization of retinal stem cells and their niches in adult zebrafish. BMC Dev Biol 2006;6:36.
60 Singhal S, Lawrence JM, Bhatia B, et al: Chondroitin sulfate proteoglycans and microglia prevent migration and integration of grafted Muller stem cells into degenerating retina. Stem Cells 2008;26:1074–1082.
61 Fawcett JW, Asher RA: The glial scar and central nervous system repair. Brain Res Bull 1999;49:377–391.
62 Fisher EJ, McLennan SV, Yue DK, Turtle JR: Cell-associated proteoglycans of retinal pericytes and endothelial cells: modulation by glucose and ascorbic acid. Microvasc Res 1994;48:179–189.
63 Zeng HY, Green WR, Tso MO: Microglial activation in human diabetic retinopathy. Arch Ophthalmol 2008;126:227–232.
64 Ma N, Streilein JW: Contribution of microglia as passenger leukocytes to the fate of intraocular neuronal retinal grafts. Invest Ophthalmol Vis Sci 1998;39:2384–2393.
65 Close JL, Gumuscu B, Reh TA: Retinal neurons regulate proliferation of postnatal progenitors and Muller glia in the rat retina via TGF beta signaling. Development 2005;132:3015–3026.
66 Wan J, Zheng H, Xiao HL, She ZJ, Zhou GM: Sonic hedgehog promotes stem-cell potential of Muller glia in the mammalian retina. Biochem Biophys Res Commun 2007;363:347–354.
67 Osakada F, Ooto S, Akagi T, Mandai M, Akaike A, Takahashi M: Wnt signaling promotes regeneration in the retina of adult mammals. J Neurosci 2007;27:4210–4219.

Dr. G. Astrid Limb
UCL Institute of Ophthalmology
11–43 Bath Street
London, EC1V 9EL (UK)
Tel. +44 20 7608 6974, Fax +44 20 7608 4034, E-Mail g.limb@ucl.ac.uk

Hammes H-P, Porta M (eds): Experimental Approaches to Diabetic Retinopathy.
Front Diabetes. Basel, Karger, 2010, vol 20, pp 109–123

Growth Factors in the Diabetic Eye

Rafael Simó · Cristina Hernández

CIBERDEM (Carlos III Health Institute) and Diabetes and Metabolism Research Unit, Institut de Recerca Hospital Universitari Vall d'Hebron, Universitat Autònoma de Barcelona, Barcelona, Spain

Abstract

Proliferative diabetic retinopathy (PDR) remains a leading cause of blindness in working age individuals in developed countries. Although tight control of both blood sugar and blood pressure are essential in preventing PDR, laser photocoagulation remains the primary treatment. However, laser photocoagulation is a late, destructive intervention that does not specifically address the underlying etiology of diabetic retinopathy (DR). Therefore, new pharmacological treatments based on the understanding of the pathophysiological mechanisms of DR are required. Growth factors and, in particular, vascular endothelial growth factor (VEGF) play a key role in the development of PDR. Hypoxia, hyperglycemia, advanced glycation end-products, proinflammatory cytokines and several growth factors upregulate VEGF expression. Intraocular delivery of anti-VEGF therapies is now widely used to treat age-related macular degeneration, and is currently undergoing evaluation in clinical trials for the treatment of DR. Other growth factors involved in the pathogenesis of DR are insulin-like growth factor-1, platelet-derived growth factor, basic fibroblast growth factor, hepatocyte growth factor, angiopoietins, connective tissue growth factor and stromal cell-derived factor-1. Increasing the knowledge of the molecular mechanisms involved in their regulation will permit us to develop new therapeutic strategies addressed to ease the burden of this devastating disease.

Proliferative diabetic retinopathy (PDR) remains the leading cause of blindness among working age population, and diabetic macular edema (DME) is one of the primary causes of poor visual acuity in patients with diabetic retinopathy (DR) [1]. Whereas PDR is the commonest sight-threatening lesion in type 1 diabetes, DME is more frequent in type 2 diabetes. Apart from vascular endothelial growth factor (VEGF), which plays an essential role in both DME and RDP, most of growth factors have been involved in the pathogenesis of PDR rather than DME [2].

PDR, the end stage of DR, is characterized by neovascularization, which is easily identified by ophthalmoscopic examination. At this stage, although the metabolic pathways triggered by hyperglycemia such as the polyol and the hexosamine pathways, de novo synthesis of diacylglycerol-protein kinase C, and the production of free radicals and advanced glycosylation end-products (AGEs) continue to operate as pathogenic factors, the production of angiogenic growth factors is a determinant event and, therefore, its blockade is a crucial therapeutic strategy [3].

Acellular capillaries (capillaries without pericytes and endothelial cells), leukostasis (the inappropriate adherence of leukocytes to the retinal capillaries) and platelet aggregation constitute the main structural changes leading to the capillary

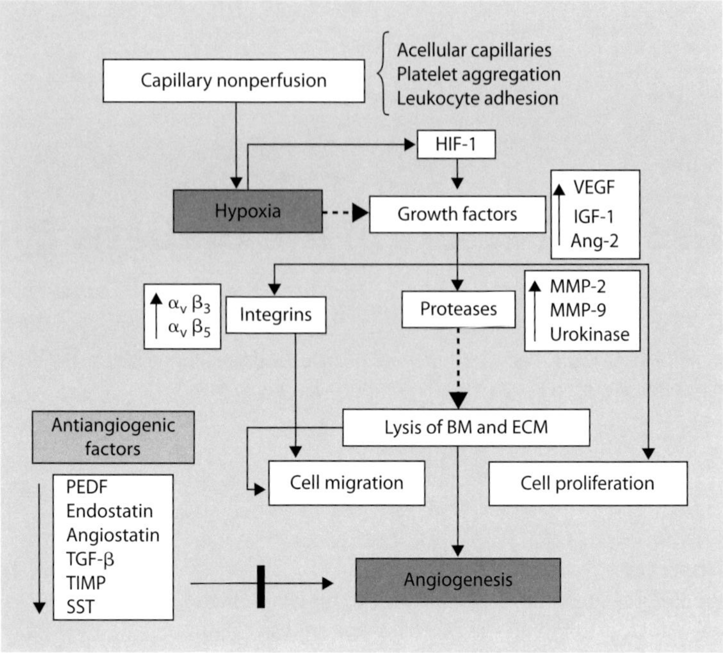

Fig. 1. Main mechanisms involved in PDR development. Capillary occlusion leads to hypoxia which is crucial to stimulate the synthesis of growth factors and, in particular, VEGF. The increase in the synthesis of integrins and proteases mediated by growth factors plays an essential role in angiogenesis. It should be stressed that a downregulation of antiangiogenic factors also exists and promotes neovascularization. MMP = Matrix metalloproteinase; BM = basement membrane; ECM = extracellular matrix; PEDF = pigment epithelium-derived factor.

occlusion. Severe hypoxia due to capillary occlusion is the main condition for the initiation of neovascularization in PDR. The main pathways involved in PDR development due to hypoxia are summarized in figure 1. Hypoxia upregulates the expression of angiogenic factors directly or through hypoxia-inducible factor (HIF-1). Apart from promoting endothelial cell proliferation, angiogenic factors can also cause increased expression of proteinases and integrins, both of which are important for cell migration. Behind the advancing front of proliferating endothelial cells is an area where the endothelial cells stop proliferating and join together to form a lumen that becomes a new capillary tube. Finally, these vessels fuse and generate a network that circulates blood into the newly vascularized region. This new vascular network subsequently matures and undergoes remodeling to form a stable vascular network. However, these new vessels are fragile and prone to bleeding. In addition, they tend to grow towards the vitreous body in which they are eventually anchored by means of fibrovascular tissue. This fibrotic tissue tends to contract and can lead to retinal detachment, which can be accompanied by catastrophic visual loss.

The complex cascade of events involved in the process of neovascularization requires the coordinated action of growth-promoting and growth-inhibiting angiogenic factors. In adult mammalian eyes, the vasculature is quiescent because of a balance between the action of angiogenic factors and antiangiogenic factors. The endogenous inhibitors prevent new vessel growth in the eye, and any alteration in this delicate balance leads to angiogenesis.

The main growth factors involved in the pathogenesis of PDR are VEGF, insulin-like growth factor-1 (IGF-1), platelet-derived growth factor (PDGF), basic fibroblast growth factor (bFGF), hepatocyte growth factor (HGF) and angiopoietins. Recently, other factors such as connective tissue growth factor (CTGF) and stromal cell-derived factor 1 (SDF-1) have been involved in DR development and will also be included herein. Finally, proinflammatory cytokines also play an important role in the pathogenesis of DR but they are beyond the scope of this review.

Vascular Endothelial Growth Factor

VEGF-A is part of a family that includes VEGF-A to VEGF-E and placenta growth factor (PIGF). VEGF-A, which we refer to as VEGF, is the main and most well-studied growth factor. VEGF is a critical component for angiogenesis (sprouting new blood vessels from existing vascular structures) and vasculogenesis (de novo blood vessel formation). VEGF is a potent mitogen for micro- and macrovascular endothelial cells derived from arteries, veins and lymphatics, but it is devoid of consistent and appreciable mitogenic activity for other cell types [4]. VEGF plays an essential role in the development of pathological microvascular complications, and DR in particular. However, it is also a survival factor for endothelial cells, increases microvascular permeability and is a potent vasodilator. Renal glomerular capillary function is under the strict control of VEGF and its role as neurotrophic and neurogenic agent has recently been demonstrated in preclinical work. VEGF also participates in skeletal muscle regeneration, cardiac remodeling and in endochondral bone formation. Finally VEGF plays an important role in the female reproductive cycle.

Apart from physiological actions, VEGF has other effects that although triggered by pathological stimuli are very important. These include the capacity to promote the formation of collateral vessels, which is essential in the recovery from ischemic events, and a substantial role in wound healing. In this regard, it is important to note that VEGF acts as a chemoattractant to mobilize endothelial cells from the bone marrow.

VEGF can be synthesized by numerous retinal cell types including retinal pigment epithelial (RPE) cells, pericytes, endothelial cells, glial cells, choroidal fibroblasts, Müller cells and ganglion cells [2]. RPE is the major source of VEGF in the ocular fundus and RPE-derived VEGF seems to be essential for the maintenance of RPE-choriocapillary complex [5]. There are seminal works indicating the critical participation of VEGF in vascular retinal development and survival, and it has been suggested that VEGF maintains the integrity of endothelial cells via anti-apoptotic signaling. Endogenous VEGF plays a role in the survival of retinal ganglion cells and is critical for the survival of retinal neuronal cells in response to ischemic injury [6]. Furthermore, pericyte support of vessel survival is closely related to VEGF [7].

The human VEGF gene is organized in eight exons, separated by seven introns and is localized in chromosome 6p21.3. By alternative exon splicing, four main VEGF isoforms can be generated having 121, 165, 189, and 206 amino acids, respectively ($VEGF_{121}$, $VEGF_{165}$, $VEGF_{189}$, $VEGF_{206}$). The predominant molecular variant is $VEGF_{165}$, a basic, heparin-binding homodimeric glycoprotein of 45 kDa [4]. The affinity for heparin may profoundly affect the bioavailability of VEGF. $VEGF_{121}$ fails to bind to heparin and, therefore, is a freely soluble protein. In contrast, $VEGF_{189}$ and $VEGF_{206}$ bind to heparin with high affinity and, in consequence, they are almost completely sequestered in the extracellular matrix. $VEGF_{165}$ has intermediate properties because it is secreted and circulates as a diffusible protein, but a significant fraction remains bound to the cell surface and the extracellular matrix. However, the isoforms quenched in the extracellular matrix may be released in a diffusible form by either heparin, heparinase or plasmin. Hence, VEGF molecular variants may become available to endothelial cells by at least two different mechanisms: freely diffusible proteins ($VEGF_{121}$, $VEGF_{165}$) or after protease activation and cleavage of the longer isoforms ($VEGF_{189}$, $VEGF_{206}$). In addition, it should be noted that loss of the heparin-binding domain, whether it is due to alternative splicing of RNA or plasmin cleavage, results in a substantial loss of mitogenic activity for vascular endothelial cells [4].

$VEGF_{165}$ is the most abundantly expressed VEGF-A isoform and has optimal characteristics of bioavailability combined with high biological potency. Ishida et al. [8] showed in a mouse model of ocular neovascularization that during pathological neovascularization, both the absolute and relative expression levels of $VEGF_{164}$ (the equivalent to $VEGF_{165}$ in humans) increased to a greater degree than during physiological neovascularization. Intravitreous injection of pegaptanib (a selective blocker of $VEGF_{164}$) potently suppressed the pathological neovascularization, whereas it had little or no effect in physiological neovascularization. In parallel experiments, genetically altered $VEGF_{164}$-deficient mice exhibited no difference in physiological neovascularization when compared with wild-type (VEGF+/+) controls. In contrast, administration of a VEGFR-1/Fc fusion protein (1 μl), which blocks all VEGF isoforms, led to significant suppression of both pathological and physiological neovascularization. Therefore, at least in experimental retinopathy, $VEGF_{164}$ plays an essential role in pathological but not in physiological neovascularization or, in other words, VEGF isoforms other than $VEGF_{164}$, in combination, may be sufficient to promote normal physiological neovascularization. These findings have led to $VEGF_{164/165}$ being proposed as an optimal target to be blocked in terms of both efficacy and safety.

In recent years, an antiangiogenic family of VEGF isoforms has been discovered, and termed $VEGF(_{xxx})b$, where xxx is the number of amino acids encoded [9]. $VEGF(_{xxx})b$ isoforms arise from an alternative 3′ splice site in exon 8, and differ by a mere six amino acids at the C-terminus. These alternative six amino acids radically change the functional properties of VEGF. The first member of this family to be identified was $VEGF_{165}b$, and it is the only form which has been characterized in terms of its action on endothelial cells [9]. A single injection of $VEGF_{165}b$ can significantly reduce preretinal neovascularization without inhibition of physiological intraretinal angiogenesis in the oxygen-induced retinopathy mouse model of ocular neovascularization [10]. DR is associated with a switch in splicing from anti- to proangiogenic isoforms of VEGF [11]. Therefore, understanding what regulates $VEGF(_{xxx})b$ alternative splicing, and therefore, the balance of pro- and antiangiogenic isoforms is of great importance and may provide a novel therapeutic strategy for DR.

The main mechanisms by which VEGF expression is regulated are displayed in figure 2. Among them, hypoxia is one of the most important. VEGF mRNA expression is rapidly and reversibly induced by exposure to low pO_2 in a variety of pathophysiological circumstances. Transcriptional activation leading to VEGF upregulation in response to hypoxia is mainly mediated by HIF-1, and it has been found that the increased levels of HIF-1α had temporal and spatial correlation with the increased expression of VEGF [12].

VEGF exerts its action through two high-affinity tyrosine kinase receptors, VEGFR-1 (Flt-1) and VEGFR-2 (KDR, human; Flk-1, mouse) which are mainly expressed on the cell surface of vascular endothelium. VEGFR-3 is a member of the same family but binds VEGF-C and -D. VEGF signaling pathway is very complex, and the cross talk between VEGF receptors as well as other molecules that act as modulators, such as heparan sulphate proteoglycans (HSPGs) and the neuropilins, further complicates the picture [4]. The main characteristics of VEGF receptors are displayed in table 1 and figure 3. It is important to note that VEGFR-2 expression becomes increased during DR development [13].

VEGF concentration has been found strikingly higher in the vitreous fluid of PDR patients

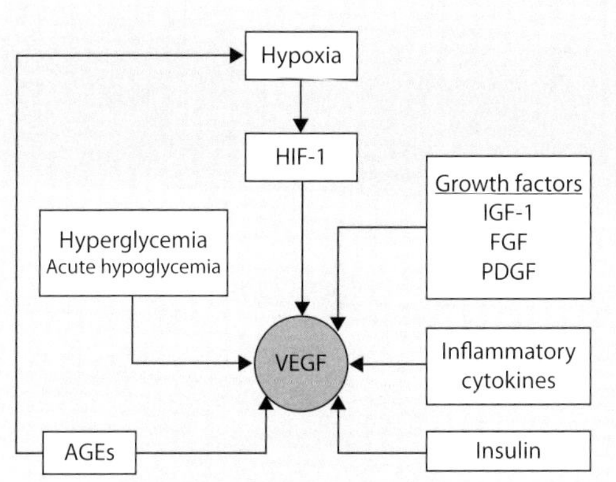

Fig. 2. Apart from hypoxia (see text), changes in glucose levels are another major factor involved in VEGF expression. Long-term high glucose concentration and acute glucose deprivation can upregulate VEGF in cultured bovine RPE cells. AGE production could be one of the mechanisms by which chronic hyperglycemia could stimulate VEGF mRNA expression, and conversely this could also explain the angiogenic properties of AGEs. In addition, activation of HIF-1α by AGEs through an extracellular-regulated kinase-dependent pathway could also be involved in VEGF expression mediated by AGEs. Apart from hypoxia and AGEs, a variety of growth factors including IGF-1, FGF and PDGF, as well as inflammatory cytokines (i.e. IL-1α, IL-6), and several hormones and oncogenes could upregulate VEGF mRNA expression. Finally, a relationship between insulin and VEGF expression has been observed by several researchers. In this regard, it is important to note that acute intensive insulin therapy produces a transient worsening of diabetic BRB breakdown via an HIF-1α-mediated increase in retinal VEGF expression. This observation could contribute to the understanding of the transient worsening of DR that follows the institution of intensive insulin therapy.

than in nondiabetic control subjects, and it was related to retinopathy activity [2]. The excess of nondiffusible VEGF isoforms generated by the retina in diabetes could be quenched by the heparan-sulfate macromolecules contained in the vitreous fluid. Therefore, the vitreous fluid could act as a VEGF reservoir. It should be noted that the vitreal levels of VEGF detected in PDR patients are in the same range that induces neovascularization in vitro and, in consequence, vitreous accumulation of VEGF derived from widespread production of this factor by ischemic retina can contribute significantly to intraocular neovascularization.

The signaling pathways by which VEGF induces neovascularization in PDR are very complex and they are beyond the scope of this review. However, activation of PKC β_2-isoform has been reported to be important for VEGF-dependent retinal neovascularization. Apart from the mitogenic effect, VEGF has other properties that contribute to neovascularization. VEGF induces expression of serine proteases urokinase-type and tissue-type plasminogen activators as well as several metalloproteinases. In addition, VEGF significantly decreases the tissue inhibitors of metalloproteinases TIMP-1 and TIMP-2 in human dermal microvascular endothelial cells. These effects will be crucial in favoring the proteolysis of the basement membrane which, as mentioned above, is the first step in the angiogenic process that leads to PDR [2].

VEGF is known also as vascular permeability factor (VPF) due to its ability to induce vascular leakage. The main mechanism by which VEGF induces vascular leakage in the retina is by lowering the levels and activity of occludin and zonula occludens 1, two critical proteins for the integrity of tight junctions, and/or by increasing vesicular transport [2].

The crucial role of VEGF in retinal neovascularization and vascular permeability has led to the development of VEGF inhibitors in experimental studies for the treatment of PDR and DME. In order to avoid systemic side effects, intravitreous rather than systemic administration of anti-VEGF agents has been used. There are many strategies for blocking VEGF action, but until now only those based on blocking VEGF by means of antibodies or aptamers are used in clinical practice [3, 14]. In this regard, pegaptanib sodium (Macugen Eyetech Pharmaceuticals/

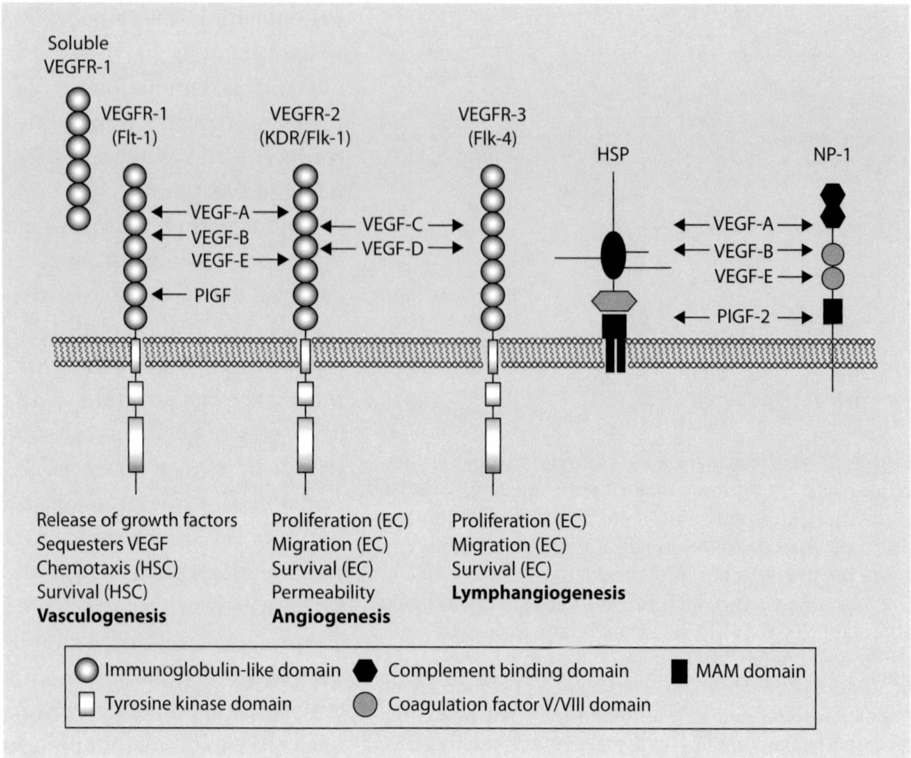

Fig. 3. VEGF isoforms and their interaction with VEGFR. VEGF tyrosine kinase receptors consist of seven extracellular immunoglobulin-like domains, a transmembrane region and an intracellular tyrosine kinase domain interrupted by a kinase insert domain. VEGFR-1 binds VEGF-A, VEGF-B and PIGF. VEGFR-1 has an alternatively spliced soluble form that sequesters VEGF and inhibits its activity. VEGFR-1 may limit cell proliferation induced by activation of VEGFR-2 and, thus, may limit VEGF-induced angiogenesis. There is considerable 'cross-talk' between VEGFR-1 and VEGFR-2, and depending on conditions, VEGFR-1 can act as a pro- or antiangiogenic regulator of VEGFR-2. VEGFR-1 has a role in the recruitment of endothelial progenitors. VEGFR-2 binds VEGF-A, VEGF-C, VEGF-D and VEGF-E, and it is responsible for angiogenesis as well as the permeability effects of VEGF. VEGFR-3 binds VEGF-C and VEGF-D and its expression becomes primarily restricted to the lymphatic endothelium of adult tissues. The interaction of VEGFR with either HSPG or neuropilin-1, a semaphorin receptor, may facilitate the presentation and binding of VEGF to its receptor. MAM = Meprin, A5, m tyrosine phosphatase; EC = endothelial cells; HSC = hematopoietic stem cells.

Pfizer) and ranibizumab (Lucentis, Novartis) have been approved by the US Food and Drug Administration (FDA) for the treatment of choroidal neovascularization in wet age-related macular degeneration (AMD) and are currently in clinical trials for treatment of DR. Bevacizumab (Avastin, Genentech/Roche) was originally developed for systemic treatment of colon cancer and was approved by the FDA for metastatic colorectal cancer. Despite the lack of any randomized trial data, intravitreal injection of bevacizumab is being used 'off-label' for AMD and

Table 1. Type of VEGF receptors, cell type location and pathological consequences associated with their activation

Receptor	Cell type location	Pathological consequences of activation
VEGFR-1 (Flt-1)	Vascular endothelial cells, monocytes, macrophages, neurons and glial cells	Tumor growth, metastases, inflammation, atherosclerosis, rheumatoid arthritis
Soluble VEGFR-1 (sFlt-1)	Not membrane bound Serum and body fluids	Hypertension, pre-eclampsia, proteinuria, and renal dysfunction Prevention of ocular neovascularization
VEGFR-2 (Flk-1/KDR)	Vascular and lymphatic endothelial cells	Pathological angiogenesis (diabetic retinopathy, cancer) and hypertension
VEGFR-3 (Flt-4)	Lymphatic endothelial cells	Lymph node metastasis

DR, as it is thought to behave with similar efficacy and safety as ranibizumab but is less costly. Pegaptanib is a pegylated neutralizing RNA aptamer with an extremely high affinity for human $VEGF_{165}$, whereas ranibizumab and bevacizumab, which are humanized monoclonal antibodies, bind and inhibit the biological activity of all VEGF isoforms ($VEGF_{121,\ 165,\ 189,\ 206}$) [14]. Aflibercept, known as a 'VEGF trap' due its ability to block all six VEGF proteins (VEGF-A to VEGF-E, and PIGF) is currently in clinical trial for both AMD and DME.

The main prospective clinical trials using intravitreal anti-VEGF agents have been conducted in patients with AMD [15]. Several phase III studies with anti-VEGF agents in the diabetic population are currently in various stage of recruitment. However, because the results in AMD have been very impressive and preliminary data in DR are promising, intravitreal anti-VEGF therapy is currently widely used in clinical practice for both PDR and DME [14, 15]. In addition, anti-VEGF therapy is currently used by many ophthalmologists as a pretreatment of vitrectomy for severe PDR and its usefulness as an adjunct to traditional laser treatment is being investigated. Nevertheless, in contrast to the rapid response of retinal neovascularization, the response of DME to anti-VEGF treatment is not prolonged and is subject of significant variability. In this regard, DME without a significant ischemic component may not benefit from anti-VEGF therapy as much as PDR [16].

Although intraocular delivery of VEGF by means of intravitreal injections permits the placement of small amounts of anti-VEGF drugs within the eye, a significant portion of intraocular anti-VEGF can pass into systemic circulation and, therefore, systemic adverse effects can appear. The most frequent systemic adverse effects are hypertension, proteinuria, cardiovascular events (due to the impairment of collateral vessel development) and bleeding associated with impaired wound healing [14]. These systemic adverse effects are particularly worrisome in the diabetic population. Apart from systemic adverse effects, ocular adverse effects such as endophthalmitis, traumatic injury of the lens, retinal detachment and potential loss of neural retinal cells have been reported. While the incidence of serious complications associated with intraocular injections is low, cumulative risk exposure may be significant for patients, such as those with diabetes, who require serial treatments over many years.

Insulin-Like Growth Factor 1

IGF-1, a polypeptide made up of 70 amino acids and with a molecular weight of 7.6 kDa, is a member of the IGF family of growth factors and related molecules. The IGF family is made up of ligands (IGF-I, IGF-II, and insulin), at least six well-characterized binding proteins (IGFBP-1 through -6), and cell surface receptors that mediate the actions of the ligands (IGF-I receptor, the insulin receptor, and the IGF-II mannose-6-phosphate receptor). IGF-1 stimulates growth, differentiation and metabolism in a variety of cell types by acting through the tyrosine kinase receptor IGF-1R, and plays an important role in both embryonic and postnatal growth. In addition, its systemic levels regulate growth hormone (GH) secretion through a negative feedback [17].

IGF-I is mainly synthesized by the liver and has been considered the main mediator of the growth-promoting and metabolic actions of GH. However, IGF-1 has also autocrine and paracrine effects, which are not related to GH levels. In fact, it has been shown in rats that IGF-1 expression is preserved in numerous tissues, including the retina, after hypophysectomy [17]. In addition, GH can itself produce direct effects mediated by GHR and not involving IGF-1. These dual observations suggest that GH has both direct and indirect (via IGF-1) effects on growth and emphasizes local, autocrine/paracrine action by IGF-1.

IGF-1 expression is increased by GH and insulin and decreased by malnutrition. Most IGF-1 circulates bound to IGFBPs and less than 1% circulates as free form. Free IGF-1 represents the active form and, indeed, it is the main factor responsible for inhibiting the pituitary production of GH. The affinity of IGF-1 for each of the six IGFBPs is 5- to 50-fold greater than IGF-I affinity for IGF-IR. Therefore, the in vivo equilibrium favors the binding of IGF-I to the IGFBPs [17]. In serum, most IGF-1 circulates as a ~150-kDa complex (ternary complex) which consists of IGF-I (γ-subunit) bound to IGFBP-3 (β-subunit) and acid-labile subunit (α-subunit). IGFBPs are mainly synthesized in the liver and they have major functions that are essential for coordinating and regulating the biological activities of IGF-1 [17].

Several in vitro studies have shown that IGF-1 is expressed in microvascular endothelial cells, pericytes, Müller cells, and RPE cells. In addition, IGFR-1 expression has been found in cultures of HREC, Müller cells, and RPE cells. Furthermore, IGFBPs are also synthesized by retinal cells [2, 18]. These findings suggest that the IGF-1/IGF-1R/IGFBPs complex participates in the physiological events that occur in the retina. Indeed, IGF-1 as well as IGF-1 analogues prolong the survival of neuroretinal cells in vitro, under conditions of hypoxia or serum starvation. In addition, IGF-I (10 ng/ml) also protects HREC from apoptosis induced by high glucose and serum starvation. Hellström et al. [19] examined retinal vessel morphology by digital image analysis of ocular fundus photographs in patients with genetic defects of the GH/IGF-I axis and low levels of IGF-I and demonstrated that these patients had significantly less retinal vascularization, thus providing evidence that IGF-1 is critical for normal vascularization of the human retina. In this regard, we have found that the contribution of free IGF-1 to total IGF-1 in vitreous fluid was 42% in nondiabetic controls. This percentage greatly exceeds that obtained in serum (<1%), thereby suggesting not only that a significant amount of free IGF-1 is produced intraocularly, but also that it plays a relevant role in retinal homeostasis [20].

Although extensive claims have been made for the stimulating or accelerating the role of serum IGF-1 in the development of DR, the results of clinical studies have been controversial, and this concept has not been supported by clinical intervention trials. More important than circulating IGF-1 is its intraocular production (fig. 4). As mentioned above, several retinal cell types express both IGF-1 and its receptor, and this expression is independent of GH levels. The proliferative effect of IGF-1 on retinal endothelial cells

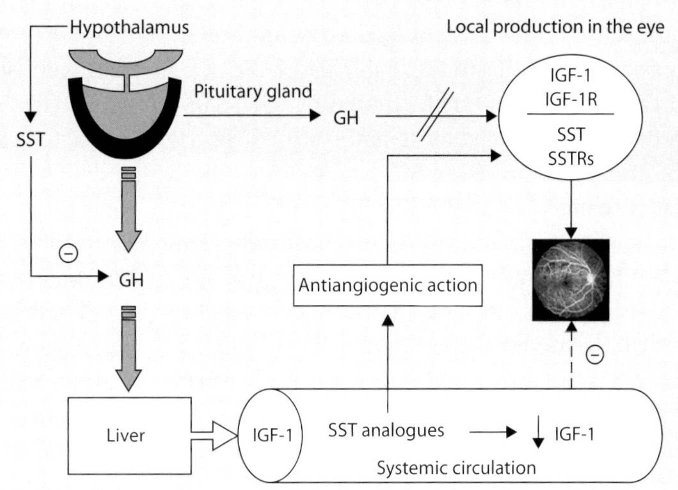

Fig. 4. Production of GH/IGF-1 is inhibited by SST. This inhibitory effect has been the rationale for using SST analogues in the treatment of DR. However, the role of circulating IGF-1 in the pathogenesis of DR is controversial. SST analogues could, by means of their antiangiogenic action, prevent or arrest DR development independent of their ability to lower IGF-1. However, because they have inadequate penetration of the BRB following systemic administration and poor tissue distribution in the retina, novel formulations specifically addressing DR are needed.

has been reported in several in vitro studies, and the essential role of IGF-1 in regulating not only retinal neovascularization, but also VEGF action, has been established in RPE cells and in the oxygen-induced retinopathy (OIR) mouse model. In addition, it has been shown that IGF-1 injected intravitreally induces retinal neovascularization and/or blood-retinal barrier (BRB) breakdown in several experimental models. In this way, transgenic mice overexpressing IGF-1 in the retina developed most of the alterations seen in human diabetic eye disease and neovascularization was consistent with increased IGF-1 induction of VEGF expression in retinal glial cells [21]. However, it should be noted that in all these studies the concentrations of IGF-1 within the eye were supraphysiological and nondiabetic animal models were used. In fact, in another model of transgenic mice with subtle IGF-1 overexpression (2.5-fold elevation of IGF-1 mRNA and 29% increase in IGF-1 protein in the retina) a lack of spontaneous ocular neovascularization was observed [22]. In addition, several authors have failed to detect mitogenic effects when IGF-1 was added in physiological concentrations to cultured retinal endothelial cells. Moreover, it has been demonstrated in rats that either hypoxia or diabetes produces a significant decrease in retinal IGF-1 mRNA levels, and also that both the immunoreactive protein and mRNA for IGF-1 are reduced in HREC of diabetic origin as compared to nondiabetic HREC cultures [2]. Gerhardinger et al. [23] have reported a three-fold decrease in IGF-1 mRNA levels in retinas obtained post-mortem from diabetic human donors with incipient retinal microangiopathy compared with retinas of age-matched nondiabetic donors. Finally, although elevated intravitreous levels of IGF-1 have been found in the vitreous fluid of diabetic patients with PDR [2], we have demonstrated that serum diffusion is the main factor accounting for this enhancement [20]. In fact, we observed a deficit of free IGF-1 in the vitreous fluid of PDR patients in comparison with nondiabetic control subjects, thus suggesting that in patients with PDR there is a lower production of free IGF-1 by the retina [20]. In addition, a relationship between intravitreous free IGF-1 and either PDR activity or intravitreous VEGF was not detected [24]. Taken together, these results suggest that although IGF-1 participates in the pathogenesis of DR it is not the main cause of ocular neovascularization and its precise role remains to be established.

The observation that circulating GH-IGF-1 production is reduced by somatostatin (SST) has been the basis for using SST analogues in both PDR and macular edema [25]. However, as mentioned above, circulating IGF-1 does not seem to be an important factor in the pathogenesis of DR. Supporting this idea, the results obtained in the multicentered clinical trial with a long-acting SST analogue (Sandostatin LAR®, Novartis Pharmaceuticals) given by intramuscular injections every 4 weeks in patients with severe non-PDR and non-high risk PDR have been inconclusive. In recent years, growing evidence has accumulated indicating that SS analogues have an angiostatic effect [2]. In addition, an SST deficit in the vitreous fluid and a lower expression in the retina have been found in diabetic patients [26, 27]. Furthermore, a significantly worsened neovascularization has been detected in a model of transgenic mice lacking the SST receptor type 2 (SSTR-2), whereas a chronic overexpression of SSTR-2 attenuated the hypoxia induced neovascularization by limiting VEGF increase [18]. Therefore, a treatment to target SST receptors can be theoretically effective in reducing neovascularization. However, given that SST analogues have inadequate penetration of the BRB following systemic administration and poor tissue distribution in the retina, novel formulations specifically addressing DR are needed. Alternatively, new SST analogues for intravitreous or intraretinal delivery could be envisaged as a new strategy in DR treatment.

Platelet-Derived Growth Factor

Platelet-derived growth factor (PDGF), a ≈35-kDa protein originally isolated from human platelets, is one of the most ubiquitous growth factors that stimulates cellular proliferation and directs cellular movement. The PDGF family of growth factors is composed of four different polypeptide chains encoded by four different genes. The classical PDGF chains, PDGF-A and PDGF-B, are well characterized, while the novel PDGFs, PDGF-C and PDGF-D, are less well known. PDGF isoforms exert their effects on target cells by activating two structurally related protein tyrosine kinase receptors (α- and β-receptors) [28].

PDGF induces mitogenic, chemoattractant and survival cell responses on fibroblasts and endothelial and vascular smooth muscle cells. In addition, it appears to be an important factor in endothelial/pericyte interactions and in tissue regeneration [29]. PDGF has been implicated in PDR as well as in proliferative vitreoretinopathy (PVR). It has been shown that PDGF acts as a paracrine growth factor for RPE cells in culture stimulating their proliferation and chemotaxis and mediates contraction of the fibrovascular tissue that produces retinal detachment. Moreover, PDGF-B induces the expression of VEGF and endothelin-1 in cultured bovine retinal pericytes. Immunocytochemical studies have shown the presence of PDGF and its receptors in epiretinal membranes in DR. In addition, increased levels of PDGF have been described in vitreous fluid of patients with PVR and PDR [2].

Hypoxia and hyperglycemia increase PDGF production in cultured human vascular endothelial cells and bovine pericytes. PDGF-B is a potent survival factor for the retinal microvasculature in general and pericytes in particular [7]. Inhibition of PDGF in a OIR model promotes pericyte loss and increases VEGF and VEGFR-2 retinal expression. On the other hand, transgenic mice showing overexpression of PDGF-B develop a proliferation of endothelial cells, pericytes and glial cells leading to traction retinal detachment as seen in the end stages of DR. Therefore, it seems that PDGF acts as a survival factor and is necessary for normal retinal vascularization but its overexpression could be deleterious and, in consequence, it is a key mediator in the pathogenesis of PDR. In recent years, several therapeutic approaches aimed at blocking PDGF action have been successfully used in experimental models.

Fibroblast Growth Factor

The fibroblast growth factor family contains over 20 structurally related heparin-binding proteins, and bFGF or FGF-2 is the prototype member. FGF-2 exists in four different molecular weight isoforms owing to differential splicing or initiation from alternative start codons. FGF is a potent angiogenic inducer, and its biological effects are mediated by binding to four distinct high-affinity tyrosine kinase receptors (FGFR1-FGFR4) which in order to be fully activated operate in conjunction with low affinity HSPGs. In addition, the binding of FGF-2 to heparan sulphate serves as a storage of inactive FGF-2 and protects FGF-2 from degradation by heparanases [2].

In the retina, FGF-2 expression has been reported in the ganglion inner and outer nuclear layers, basement membranes of Müller cells, blood vessels and RPE cells. FGF receptors are also widely distributed in the neuroretina, and their expression is most abundant in photoreceptors. In this regard it should be noted that FGF-2 neurotrophic effects protecting against photoreceptor damage and retinal degeneration have been extensively reported [2]. FGF-2 participates in retinal physiological vascularization. However, it seems that FGF-2 itself does not play an essential role in retinal neovascularization.

Hepatocyte Growth Factor

HGF, also named *scatter factor*, is a 90-kDa cytokine mainly synthesized by the liver. HGF regulates cell growth, cell motility, and the morphogenesis of various types of cells. Its name originates from its capacity to induce the mitogenesis in hepatocytes, but it is also a potent angiogenic factor. HGF targets and signals epithelial and endothelial cells in a paracrine manner via its high-affinity c-Met surface receptor, a tyrosine kinase receptor [30].

In the retina, vascular endothelial cells, fibroblasts, glial cells and RPE cells have the ability to produce and release HGF. HGF can act as an anti-apoptotic factor for endothelial cells, and prevents endothelial cell death which is induced by either serum deprivation, high glucose concentrations, hypoxia or glutathione depletion. Furthermore, intravitreous injection of recombinant human HGF is neuroprotective in a rat model of retinal ischemia-reperfusion injury [2]. Therefore, HGF could be considered as a survival growth factor physiologically synthesized by the retina.

Several authors have shown elevated levels of HGF in the vitreous fluid of PDR patients [2]. We have found 25-fold higher levels of HGF in the vitreous fluid than in the serum of diabetic patients with PDR, and no relationship between intravitreous and serum concentrations was detected [31]. These findings strongly suggest that intraocular synthesis is a significant contributing factor to the high intravitreous levels of HGF observed in patients with PDR. It has been recently reported in experimental models that HGF may play an important role in the initial stages of retinal angiogenesis as well as in increasing retinal vascular permeability. However, we have found that HGF levels per mg of intravitreal proteins were lower in diabetic patients than in nondiabetic subjects, and no relationship between intravitreous levels of HGF and either retinopathy activity or intravitreous VEGF was found [32]. In addition, it should be pointed out that, unlike VEGF, both high glucose concentration and hypoxia downregulate HGF expression in endothelial cells. Finally, we have not found any difference in the expression of HGF receptor (c-Met) on the epiretinal membranes from PDR patients in comparison with the idiopathic epiretinal membranes [33]. All this leads us to think that the role of HGF might be more important in the wound healing process and fibrosis than in neovascularization itself. In fact, HGF serves as a chemoattractant for bone marrow-derived stem, which participates in the regeneration of injured RPE. However, it should be noted that the role of HGF in the eye in both health and disease is only just beginning to be appreciated, and future studies are required to determine its precise role in the pathogenesis of DR.

Angiopoietins

The angiopoietins are a class of growth factors that activate the Tie2 receptor and play important roles in the regulation of angiogenesis. Whereas angiopoietin-1 (Ang-1) is a widespread receptor agonist, angiopoietin-2 (Ang-2) represents a natural angiopoietin-1/Tie2 inhibitor and is highly expressed only at sites of vascular remodeling in the adult, in particular in the female reproductive tract. The presence of Ang-2 destabilizes the vessels, a necessary step for the remodeling process that takes place in angiogenesis, whereas the presence of Ang-1 and the activation of Tie2 stabilizes vessels. In contrast to VEGF, which can initiate vessel growth in vitro and in vivo, neither Ang-1 nor Ang-2 alone can promote in vivo neovascularization [34].

Ang-1 promotes the survival of endothelial cells and pericytes in vitro without causing endothelial cell proliferation, stabilizes endothelial interactions with surrounding support cells, and blocks the leak-inducing action of VEGF in vivo [2]. Joussen et al. [35] have shown that angiopoietin-1, when given intravitreally to newly diabetic rats, normalizes VEGF and intercellular adhesion molecule-1 mRNA and protein levels, leading to reductions in leukocyte adhesion, endothelial cell injury, and BRB breakdown. Alternatively, when an adenovirus coding for angiopoietin-1 was given systemically to mice with established diabetes, it similarly inhibited leukocyte adhesion, endothelial cell injury and BRB breakdown.

Ang-2 has been reported as acting differently in the absence and presence of VEGF. In the presence of VEGF, Ang-2 plays a proangiogenic role and also increases the permeability of retinal endothelial cells [36]. By contrast, Ang-2 promotes endothelial cell death and vessel regression in the absence of VEGF [37]. Hammes et al. [38] demonstrated that upregulation of Ang-2 plays a critical role in the loss of pericytes in the diabetic retina.

Takagi et al. [39] demonstrated that inhibition of TIE-2 by soluble TIE-2 fusion protein suppresses the in vitro retinal angiogenesis induced by the hypoxia-conditioned medium as well as retinal angiogenesis in a murine model of retinal ischemia. The inhibition of TIE-2, when combined with inhibition of VEGF, more efficiently suppressed retinal angiogenesis than did inhibition of VEGF alone, thus suggesting that signaling of both TIE-2 and VEGF plays a potential role in ischemia-induced retinal angiogenesis [39]. Similarly, Das et al. [40] reported inhibition of experimentally induced retinal neovascularization in newborn mice using the TIE-2 antagonist muTek delta Fc. Recently, small-molecule Tie2 inhibitors, which blocked Ang-induced Tie2 autophosphorylation and downstream signaling, have been identified, thus constituting a new target in PDR treatment [41].

Connective Tissue Factor

CTGF is a cytokine that stimulates extracellular matrix production and acts as a profibrotic factor in the retina. CTGF immunostaining has been localized in epiretinal membranes obtained from patients with nondiabetic PVR, as well as in epiretinal membranes from PDR patients. Furthermore, it has been demonstrated that vitreous levels of CTGF correlate strongly with the degree of fibrosis in vitreoretinal disorders. It has been shown that recombinant CTGF causes angiogenesis in the cornea and in other in vivo models. However, in CTGF knockout mice, angiogenesis is not impaired in several experimental models of neovascularization. Recently, Kuiper et al. [42] demonstrated that CTGF is primarily a profibrotic factor in the eye and suggest that a shift in the balance between CTGF and VEGF is associated with the switch from angiogenesis to fibrosis in PDR.

CTGF mRNA is expressed at high levels in retinal vascular endothelial cells. Interestingly, it has been demonstrated by immunohistochemistry that in the normal human retina CTGF is mainly expressed in microglia, whereas in diabetic patients without PDR the CTGF staining in microglia was decreased and a predominant pericyte expression was observed.

A variety of cellular mechanisms may be involved in mediating CTGF upregulation in DR. CTGF can be increased by AGEs, TGF-β, hypoxia, cellular stretch, reactive oxygen species and PKC-dependent pathways. In addition, CTGF is upregulated by VEGF in retinal endothelial cells and inhibits VEGF-induced angiogenesis by the formation of VEGF-CTGF complexes.

Stromal Cell-Derived Factor 1

SDF-1, the predominant chemokine that mobilizes hematopoietic stem cells and circulating endothelial progenitor cells, is also involved in DR development. SDF-1 works in conjunction with VEGF to promote the recruitment of endothelial progenitors from remote locations, such as the bone marrow, into the ischemic retina. SDF-1 and its receptor, CXCR4, have hypoxia response elements in the promoter of their genes. In addition, VEGF also increased levels of SDF-1 and CXCR4 mRNA. Recently, it has been found that SDF-1 and CXCR4 are increased in hypoxic retina, with SDF-1 localized in glial cells primarily near the surface of the retina and CXCR4 localized also in glial cells but mainly in bone marrow-derived cells [43]. Butler et al. [44] have shown that intravitreal SDF-1 levels are increased in diabetic patients with either macular edema or PDR, and these levels are able to induce retinopathy in a murine model of proliferative adult retinopathy. In addition, SDF-1 induced HREC to increase expression of VCAM-1 and reduced tight cellular junctions by lowering occludin expression. Moreover, intravitreal injection of blocking antibodies to SDF-1 prevented retinal neovascularization in this murine model, even in the presence of exogenous VEGF. Finally, the same group of investigators has found a dramatic decrease in the intravitreous levels of both SDR-1 and VEGF after intravitreal injection of triamcinolone. Together, these data demonstrate that SDF-1 plays a major role in proliferative retinopathy and may be an ideal target for the prevention of proliferative retinopathy.

Concluding Remarks and Future Clinical Applications

Improvements in diabetes care and management have been crucial in lowering the incidence and severity of DR. Nevertheless, DR remains the leading cause of blindness in working age individuals in developed countries, and retinal neovascularization occurs in up to 20% of patients with diabetes. Therefore, new pharmacological treatments based on the understanding of the pathophysiological mechanisms of DR are needed. The knowledge of the role of growth factors and their signaling pathways is essential to develop new strategies for blocking neovascularization. Among angiogenic factors, VEGF seems to be the most important, and there are ongoing phase III studies evaluating the clinical effectiveness and safety of intravitreal anti-VEGF therapy in both DME and PDR. However, there is now ample evidence to suggest that the development of DR is a multifactorial complex process in which the balance between angiogenic and antiangiogenic factors is crucial. Therefore, a future scenario will involve using a combination of anti-VEGF therapy with not only other antiangiogenic agents aimed at different steps of the angiogenic cascade but with natural antiangiogenic factors. However, it should be emphasized that, at present, the milestones in DR treatment are the optimization of blood glucose control, lowering of blood pressure, and regular fundoscopic screening.

References

1 Congdom N, Friedman DS, Lietman T: Important causes of visual impairment in the world today. JAMA 2003;290:2057–2060.

2 Simó R, Carrasco E, García-Ramírez M, Hernández C: Angiogenic and antiangiogenic factors in proliferative diabetic retinopathy. Curr Diabet Rev 2006;2:71–98.

3 Hernández C, Simó R: Strategies for blocking angiogenesis in diabetic retinopathy: from basic science to clinical practice. Expert Opin Invest Drugs 2007;16:1209–1226.

4 Ferrara N: Vascular endothelial growth factor: basic science and clinical progress. Endocr Rev 2004;24:581–611.

5 Saint-Geniez M, Maldonado AE, D'Amore PA: VEGF expression and receptor activation in the choroid during development and in the adult. Invest Ophthalmol Vis Sci 2006;47:3135–3142.

6 Nishijima K, Ng Y-S, Zhong L, Bradley J, Schubert W, Jo N, Akita J, Samuelsson SJ, Robinson GS, Adamis AP, Shima DT: VEGF-A is a survival factor for retinal neurons and a critical neuroprotectant during the adaptative response to ischemic injury. Am J Pathol 2007;171:53–67.

7 Hammes HP, Lin J, Renner O, Shani M, Lundqvist A, Betsholtz C, Brownlee M, Deutsch U: Pericytes and the pathogenesis of diabetic retinopathy. Diabetes 2002;51:3107–3112.

8 Ishida S, Usui T, Yamashiro K, Kaji Y, Ahmed E, Carrasquillo KG, Amano S, Hida T, Oguchi Y, Adamis AP: $VEGF_{164}$-mediated inflammation is required for pathological, but not physiological, ischemia-induced retinal neovascularization. J Exp Med 2003;198:483–489.

9 Woolard J, Wang WY, Bevan HS, Qiu Y, Morbidelli L, Pritchard-Jones RO, Cui TG, Sugiono M, Waine E, Perrin R, Foster R, Digby-Bell J, Shields JD, Whittles CE, Mushens RE, Gillatt DA, Ziche M, Harper SJ, Bates DO: VEGF165b, an inhibitory vascular endothelial growth factor splice variant: mechanism of action, in vivo effect on angiogenesis and endogenous protein expression. Cancer Res 2004;64:7822–7835.

10 Konopatskaya O, Churchil AJ, Harper SJ, Bates DO, Gardiner TA: VEGF165b an endogenous C-terminal splice variant of VEGF, inhibits retinal neovascularization in mice. Mol Vis 2006;12:626–632.

11 Perrin RM, Konopatskaya O, Qiu Y, Harper S, Bates DO, Churchill AJ: Diabetic retinopathy is associated with a switch in splicing from anti- to proangiogenic isoforms of vascular endothelial growth factor. Diabetologia 2005;48:2422–2427.

12 Ozaki H, Yu AY, Della N, Ozaki K, Luna JD, Yamada H, Hackett SF, Okamoto N, Zack DJ, Semenza GL, Campochiaro PA: Hypoxia inducible factor-1 alpha is increased in ischemic retina: temporal and spatial correlation with VEGF. Invest Ophthalmol Vis Sci 1999;40:182–189.

13 Witmer AN, Vrensen GFJM, Van Noorden CJF, Schlingemann RO: Vascular endothelial growth factors and angiogenesis in eye disease. Prog Retin Eye Res 2003;22:1–29.

14 Simó R, Hernández C: Intravitreous anti-VEGF for diabetic retinopathy: hopes and fears for a new therapeutic strategy. Diabetologia 2008;51:1574–1580.

15 Wong TY, Liew G, Mitchell P: Clinical update: new treatments for age-related macular degeneration. Lancet 2007;370:204–206.

16 Sang DN, D'Amore PA: Is blockade of vascular endothelial growth factor beneficial for all types of diabetic retinopathy? Diabetologia 2008;51:1570–1573.

17 Le Roith D, Bondy C, Yakar S, Liu JL, Butler A: The somatomedin hypothesis: 2001. Endocr Rev 2001;22:53–74.

18 Dal Monte M, Cammalleri M, Martini D, Casini G, Bagnoli P: Antiangiogenic role of somatostatin receptor 2 in a model of hypoxia-induced neovascularization in the retina: results from transgenic mice. Invest Ophthalmol Vis Sci 2007;48:3480–3489.

19 Hellström A, Svensson E, Carlsson B, Niklasson A, Albertsson-Wikland K: Reduced retinal vascularization in children with growth hormone deficiency. J Clin Endocrinol Metab 1999;84:795–798.

20 Simó R, Hernández C, Segura RM, García-Arumí J, Sararols L, Burgos R, Cantón A, Mesa J: Free IGF-I in the vitreous fluid of diabetic patients with proliferative diabetic retinopathy. A case-control study. Clin Sci (Lond) 2003;134:376–382.

21 Ruberte J, Ayuso E, Navarro M, Navarro M, Carretero A, Nacher V, Haurigot V, George M, Llombart C, Casellas A, Costa C, Bosch A, Bosch F: Increased ocular levels of IGF-1 in transgenic mice lead to diabetes-like eye disease. J Clin Invest 2004;113:1149–1157.

22 Hu W, Wang W, Gao H, Zhong J, Yao W, Lee WH, Ye P, Quiao X: Lack of spontaneous ocular neovascularization and attenuated laser-induced choroidal neovascularization in IGF-I overexpression transgenic mice. Vision Res 2007;47:776–782.

23 Gerhardinger C, McClure KD, Romeo G, Podestà F, Lorenzi M: IGF-I mRNA and signaling in the diabetic retina. Diabetes 2001;50:175–183.

24 Simó R, Lecube A, Segura RM, García-Arumí J, Hernández C: Free insulin growth factor-I and vascular endothelial growth factor in the vitreous fluid of patients with proliferative diabetic retinopathy. Am J Ophthalmol 2002;134:376–382.
25 Palii SS, Caballero S Jr, Shapiro G, Grant MB: Medical treatment of diabetic retinopathy with somatostatin analogues. Expert Opin Investig Drugs 2007;16:73–82.
26 Simó R, LecubeA, Sararols L, García-Arumí J, Segura RM, Hernández C: Deficit of somatostatin-like immunoreactivity in the vitreous fluid of diabetic patients. Diabetes Care 2002;25:2282–2286.
27 Carrasco E, Hernández C, Miralles A, Huguet P, Farrés J, Simó R: Lower somatostatin expression is an early event in diabetic retinopathy and is associated with retinal neurodegeneration. Diabetes Care 2007;30:2902–2908.
28 Fredricksson L, Li H, Eriksson U: The PDGF family: four gene products form five dimeric isoforms. Cytokine Growth Factor Rev 2004;15:197–204.
29 Armulik A, Abramsson A, Betsholtz C: Endothelial/pericyte interactions. Circ Res 2005;97:512–523.
30 Grierson I, Heathcote L, Hiscott P, Hogg P, Briggs M, Hagan S: Hepatocyte growth factor/scatter factor in the eye. Prog Retin Eye Res 2000;19:779–802.
31 Cantón A, Burgos R, Hernández C, Mateo C, Segura RM, Mesa J, Simó R: Hepatocyte growth factor in vitreous and serum from patients with proliferative diabetic retinopathy. Br J Ophthalmol 2000;84:732–735.
32 Simo R, Lecube A, Garcia-Arumi J, Carrasco E, Hernandez C: Hepatocyte growth factor in the vitreous fluid of patients with proliferative diabetic retinopathy: its relationship with vascular endothelial growth factor and retinopathy activity. Diabetes Care 2004;27:287–288.
33 Simó R, Vidal MT, García-Arumí J, Carrasco F, García-Ramírez M, Segura RM, Hernández C: Intravitreous hepatocyte growth factor in patients with proliferative diabetic retinopathy: a case-control study. Diabetes Res Clin Pract 2006;71:36–44.
34 Joussen AM: Vascular plasticity-the role of the angiopoietins in modulating ocular angiogenesis. Graefes Arch Clin Exp Ophthalmol 2001;239:972–975.
35 Joussen AM, Poulaki V, Tsujikawa A, Qin W, Qaum T, Xu Q, Moromizato Y, Bursell SE, Wiegand SJ, Rudge J, Ioffe E, Yancopoulos GD, Adamis AP: Suppression of diabetic retinopathy with angiopoietin-1. Am J Pathol 2002;160:1683–1693.
36 Peter S, Cree IA, Alexander R, Turowski P, Pckrim Z, Patel J, Boyd SR, Joussen AM, Ziemessen F, Hykin PG, Moss SE: Angiopoietin modulation of vascular endothelial growth factor: Effect on retinal endothelial cell permeability. Cytokine 2007;40:144–150.
37 Lobov IB, Brooks PC, Lang RA: Angiopoietin-2 displays VEGF dependent modulation of capillary structure and endothelial cell survival in vivo. Proc Natl Acad Sci USA 2002;99:11205–11210.
38 Hammes HP, Lin J, Wagner P, Feng Y, Vom Hagen F, Krzizok T, Renner O, Breier G, Brownlee M, Deutsch U: Angiopoietin-2 causes pericyte dropout in the normal retina: evidence for involvement in diabetic retinopathy. Diabetes 2004;3:1104–1110.
39 Takagi H, Koyama S, Seike H, Oh H, Otani A, Matsumura M, Honda Y: Potential role of the angiopoietin/tie2 system in ischemia-induced retinal neovascularization. Invest Ophthalmol Vis Sci 2003;44:393–402.
40 Das A, Fanslow W, Cerretti D, Warren E, Talarico N, McGuire P: Angiopoietin/Tek interactions regulate MMP-9 expression and retinal neovascularization. Lab Invest 2003;83:1637–1645.
41 Liu J, Lin TH, Cole AG, Wen R, Zhao L, Brescia MR, Jacob B, Hussain Z, Appell KC, Henderson I, Webb ML: Identification and characterization of small-molecule inhibitors of Tie2 kinase. FEBS Lett 2008;582:785–791.
42 Kuiper EJ, Van Nieuwenhoven FA, de Smet MD, van Meurs JC, Tanck MW, Oliver N, Klaassen I, Van Noorden CJF, Goldschmeding R, Schlingemann RO: The angio-fibrotic switch of VEGF and CTGF in proliferative diabetic retinopathy. PLoS ONE 2008;3:e2675.
43 Lima e Silva R, Shen J, Hackett SF, Kachi S, Akiyama H, Kiuchi K, Yokoi K, Hatara MC, Lauer T, Aslam S, Gong YY, Xiao WH, Khu NH, Thut C, Campochiaro PA: The SDF-1/CXCR4 ligand/receptor pair is an important contributor to several types of ocular neovascularization. FASEB J 2007;21:3219–3230.
44 Butler JM, Guthrie SM, Koc M, Afzal A, Caballero S, Brooks HL, Mames RN, Segal MS, Grant MB, Scott EW: SDF-1 is both necessary and sufficient to promote proliferative retinopathy. J Clin Invest 2005;115:86–93.

Dr. Rafael Simó
Diabetes and Metabolism Research Unit
Institut de Recerca Hospital Universitari Vall d'Hebron
Pg. Vall d'Hebron 119–129, ES–08035 Barcelona (Spain)
Tel. +34 93 489 4172, Fax +34 93 489 4032, E-Mail rsimo@ir.vhebron.net

Hammes H-P, Porta M (eds): Experimental Approaches to Diabetic Retinopathy.
Front Diabetes. Basel, Karger, 2010, vol 20, pp 124–141

Balance between Pigment Epithelium-Derived Factor and Vascular Endothelial Growth Factor in Diabetic Retinopathy

Nahoko Ogata[a] · Joyce Tombran-Tink[b]

[a]Department of Ophthalmology, Kansai Medical University, Moriguchi, Osaka, Japan; [b]Department of Neural and Behavioral Sciences and Ophthalmology, Milton S. Hershey Medical Center, College of Medicine, The Pennsylvania State University, Hershey, Pa., USA

Abstract

Formation and maintenance of the normal vasculature is dependent on interactions between several agonists and inhibitors of angiogenesis. There is strong evidence that two key endogenous molecules with opposing effects on angiogenesis are critical in maintaining the structural and functional integrity of blood vessels in the body. These are the well-characterized proteins, vascular endothelial derived growth factor (VEGF) and pigment epithelium-derived factor (PEDF). Overexpression of VEGF, a potent endothelial cell mitogen, is potentiated in response to hypoxia, hyperglycemia, and chronic inflammation to generate pathological angiogenesis. At nonphysiological levels, VEGF transmits increased proangiogenic signals by binding to its receptors on endothelial cells, which, in turn, activates discrete molecular pathways that perturb endothelial cell proliferation, adhesion, migration, tight junction formation, and vascular permeability. PEDF, on the other hand blocks endothelial cell proliferation and migration and in so doing checks the excessive actions of VEGF on blood vessel growth. Both of these molecules are found in a state of equilibrium in the eye, which is essential to maintain healthy retinal vasculature. Disruption in the function or synthesis of these factors by environmental stresses can contribute to vessel abnormalities. In diabetic retinopathy, formation of microvascular lesions is a hallmark event in the development and progression of the disease. Disturbances in the levels of VEGF and PEDF have been noted in this condition in experimental and clinical findings. This chapter highlights recent developments that have widened our understanding of how modulations in expression levels of these opposing angiogenesis factors may exacerbate diabetic retinopathy, the need for better surveillance that would identify early disturbances in their synthesis and secretion in the diabetic retina, and the importance of developing treatments to restore physiological levels of both molecules in the prevention of diabetic retinopathy.

Vascular endothelial growth factor (VEGF), a dimeric glycoprotein of approximately 40 kDa, is a potent endothelial cell mitogen that stimulates proliferation, migration, and tube formation, important processes in the development of new blood vessels. VEGF is essential for angiogenesis during normal embryological development. In mammals, the VEGF family consists of seven members: VEGF-A typically referred to as VEGF, VEGF-B, VEGF-C, VEGF-D, VEGF-E, and VEGF-F. VEGF itself has many variants which are generated from a single gene by alternative splicing [1, 2]. In humans, these include the relatively abundant $VEGF_{121}$, $VEGF_{165}$, $VEGF_{189}$, and $VEGF_{206}$, and several less abundant forms.

The VEGF isoforms are specifically mitogenic for vascular endothelial cells, and are implicated in inducing permeability at blood-tissue barriers [1, 2]. The abnormal expression of VEGF has become a focal point of current research on the pathogenesis of diabetic retinopathy, as well as other retinal and choroidal vascular diseases. Because unchecked production and activity of VEGF can have severe pathological consequences, antiangiogenic factors are quintessential in maintaining physiological levels of this protein or blocking its mitogenic actions on endothelial cells.

One such factor secreted by almost all tissues in the body is pigment epithelium-derived factor (PEDF), a 50-kDa polypeptide first identified in the conditioned-medium of human retinal pigment epithelial cells [3, 4]. This protein was described in initial studies as a potent differentiation factor that induced the formation of neuron-like structures in primitive cultured retinoblastoma cells [4]. Sequence analysis of the human PEDF gene showed that it is a member of the serine protease inhibitor (serpin) gene family, but to date a target substrate has not been identified to validate protease inhibitory activity [5]. However, another important function for PEDF emerged with the studies of Dawson et al. [6] who demonstrated that PEDF can block the migration of endothelial cells in vitro in a dose-dependent manner and was more effective than angiostatin, thrombospondin-1 and endostatin, other potent antagonists of blood vessel growth. The efficacy of PEDF in reducing angiogenesis was also clearly demonstrated in a murine model of ischemia-induced retinopathy [7]. One mechanism proposed for the antiangiogenic actions of PEDF on blood vessel formation is that it counteracts the mitogenic activity of VEGF by inducing apoptosis of activated endothelial cells during neovascularization [7]. These findings placed PEDF among the most potent natural inhibitors of angiogenesis. Since then, many laboratories have focused on determining whether there is a physiological balance in levels of VEGF and PEDF that is critical in coordinating vessel formation.

VEGF and PEDF in the Eye

The expression level of VEGF in the eye is a focal point of research in the pathogenesis of diabetic retinopathy since increased vascularization and vessel permeability are hallmark features of this blinding disease. In normal developmental processes, VEGF expression decreases substantially after birth, but some cells still constitutively secrete picomolar amounts. It is estimated that cells of the neural retina can secrete ~20 pg per milligram of protein, while cells of the choroid and retinal pigment epithelium secrete ~ 50 pg per milligram of protein in the adult [8]. In vitro experiments have shown that VEGF can induce fenestrations in capillary endothelial cells derived from bovine adrenal cortex [9]. Increased endothelial fenestrations are most likely the predominant mechanism for vascular permeability in diabetic retinopathy.

One factor that is a major stimulus for VEGF expression and subsequent retinal neovascularization is hypoxia [10–13]. Reduced retinal blood flow that is associated with hypoxia may be present even before early signs of retinopathy, such as the loss of capillary pericytes and endothelial cells, are detected. These early pathological changes in the diabetic retina are likely to be triggered by an abnormal increase in the synthesis and secretion of VEGF by specific retinal cells that are responding to hypoxic conditions in the eye [14–16]. Immunocytochemical evidence to support this has been reported in studies which show an increase in the levels of the VEGF protein on nonvascular cells in the eyes of patients with diabetes even in the absence of retinopathy. Thus, diabetic retinopathy may actually have its earliest beginnings as a disease of retinal neurons and glia with later involvement of the retinal vasculature [15, 16].

PEDF is also normally synthesized in the eye [17] and other tissues throughout the body. Not surprisingly, this antiangiogenic protein is secreted by cells of the cornea, lens, ciliary body, retina, choroid, and the retinal pigment epithelium, all of which are important structures in the eye that could lose function by the abnormal growth of blood vessels [17].

It is hypothesized that a critical balance in the production and secretion of VEGF and PEDF must be maintained to control the normal structure-function relationship of the retinal and choroidal vasculature and the neural architecture of the retina.

There are numerous experimental studies that support a reciprocal relationship between PEDF and VEGF in the eye. For example, systemic (intraperitoneal) administration of the PEDF protein inhibits VEGF-induced retinal neovascularization in hyperoxygenated neonatal mice, an accepted model of human retinopathy of prematurity [7], and levels of VEGF are known to be increased while those of PEDF are decreased in proliferative diabetic retinopathy (PDR) [18–22]. Both experimental retinal and choroidal neovascularization in the mouse can be inhibited after an intravitreal injection of a replication-deficient adenovirus containing the PEDF gene [23]. This would suggest that gene therapy with this agent in humans might be feasible.

PEDF/VEGF in the Diabetic Retinopathy

Abnormal production or secretion of VEGF and PEDF in retinal tissues may be an underlying cause of some retinal diseases. The vitreous from eyes with PDR contains high levels of VEGF [24–26], which is produced by ischemic retinal cells [27, 28]. In addition, there is upregulation of the VEGF/VEGF receptor system in human diabetic retinas and those from STZ-induced diabetic retinopathy in rats [29, 30].

PEDF, on the other hand, has reduced expression levels in the vitreous of individuals with PDR 6, suggesting that loss of PEDF is involved in the pathogenesis of this condition [18–22]. Evidence to support this was shown in studies by Spranger et al. [19] who reported that PEDF concentrations in the vitreous of patients with PDR or with extensive nondiabetic retinal neovascularization caused by retinal-vein occlusion were significantly lower than those of control patients. We also observed a similar trend in PEDF expression in the vitreous of patients with diabetic retinopathy [20]. Correlations in the expression levels of these molecules were also noted in animal models with the degree of ischemia-induced retinal neovascularization in rats [18]. Retinas with neovascularization had a 5-fold increase in VEGF and a 2-fold decrease in PEDF compared to age-matched controls [18]. A decrease in the level of PEDF and an increase in the level of VEGF have been reported in the vitreous of human eyes with PDR [19–22]. In these studies, the vitreal concentration of PEDF was significantly lower at 1.11 ± 0.14 μg/ml (mean ± SE) in eyes with diabetic retinopathy than in eyes with macular hole at 1.71 ± 0.22 μg/ml ($p = 0.021$, fig. 1a), while the VEGF level was 1,799 ± 478 pg/ml in eyes with diabetic retinopathy and not detectable in eyes with macular hole (fig. 1b). Similarly, PEDF level in eyes with PDR (0.94 ± 0.12 μg/ml) was reduced in nonproliferative diabetic retinopathy (NPDR; 2.25 ± 0.32 μg/ml) and the level in active diabetic retinopathy (0.85 ± 0.14 μg/ml) was lower than that in inactive diabetic retinopathy as well (1.59 ± 0.24 μg/ml; $p = 0.01$; fig. 1a). A comparative study showed that the VEGF level was as high as 2,025 ± 533 pg/ml in eyes with PDR compared to 215 ± 201 pg/ml in eyes with NPDR, and the concentration in active diabetic retinopathy (2,543 ± 673 pg/ml) was significantly higher than that in inactive diabetic retinopathy (395 ± 188 pg/ml; $p = 0.0098$; fig. 1b) [21]. These findings strongly indicate that inverse changes in the intraocular levels of PEDF and VEGF correlate with the degree of retinal neovascularization.

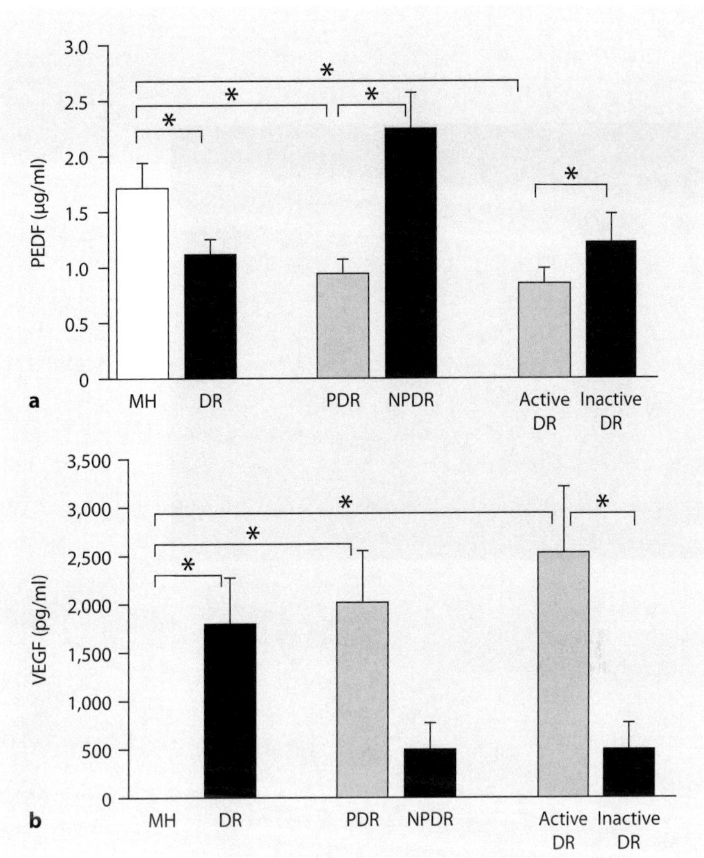

Fig. 1. **a** PEDF levels in the vitreous samples from the eyes with diabetic retinopathy. **b** VEGF levels in the vitreous samples from the eyes with diabetic retinopathy (* $p < 0.05$). Reprinted with permission from [21]. MH = idiopathic macular hole; DR = diabetic retinopathy.

Not only was this relationship noted in the vitreous of patients, but also in retinal cells where a decrease in the expression of PEDF was accompanied by an increase in the expression of VEGF in patients with PDR. Matsuoka et al. [31] observed strong expression of VEGF in the endothelial cells of newly formed vessels in the fibrovascular membranes in eyes with PDR and comparatively weak expression of PEDF in these cells. However, the level of PEDF was prominent in the extracellular matrix and fibrous tissue surrounding the new vessels (fig. 2).

The observations that PEDF blocks VEGF-induced retinal vascular hyperpermeability [32] and downregulates the expression of VEGF [33], and that exogenously administered PEDF inhibits retinal angiogenesis [7, 23] suggest that the decrease in the level of PEDF is mechanistically involved in VEGF overexpression. It is proposed that changes in vitreous constituents including growth factors and cytokines, may exacerbate the diabetic retinopathy condition [21, 26, 34, 35], but changes in the levels of such factors may also be initiating events in the developing pathophysiology at an early stage since VEGF is shown to be increased in vitreous and in nonvascular cells of diabetic eyes without overt retinopathy [15, 16, 36]. Other ocular compartments such as the aqueous humor have similar changes in the levels of VEGF and PEDF in patients with

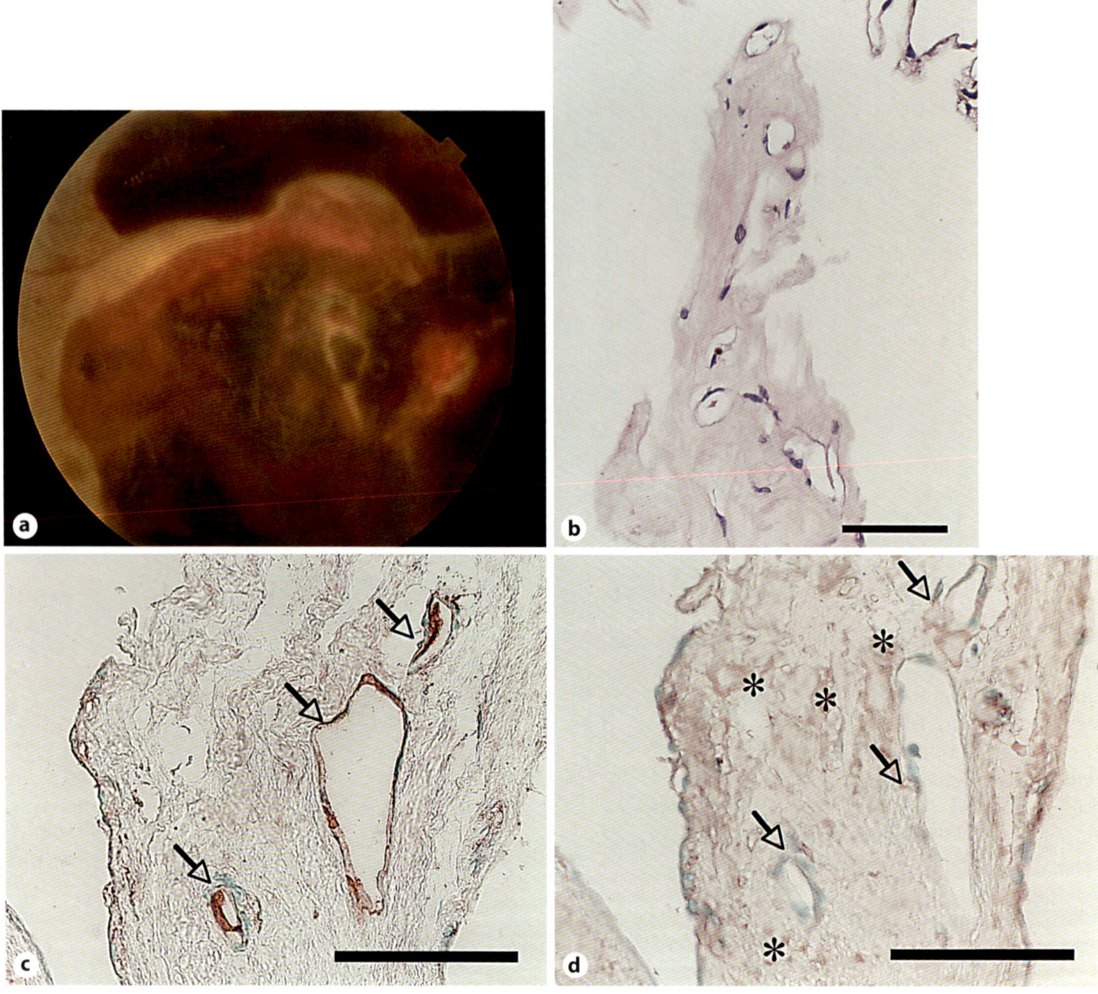

Fig. 2. **a** Preoperative fundus photograph. **b** Section of an excised active fibrovascular membrane showing highly vascularized tissue. New vessels are surrounded by extracellular matrix. HE. Scale bar = 100 μm. **c** Immunohistochemistry for VEGF expression. Strong immunoreactivity for VEGF is observed in endothelial cells (arrows) in the proliferative fibrovascular tissue. Scale bar = 50 μm. **d** Immunohistochemistry for PEDF expression. Immunoreactivity for PEDF is not observed in the endothelial cells (arrows) in the neovascular tissue but it is strongly positive in the extracellular matrix (asterisks) surrounding new vessels. Scale bar = 50 μm. Reprinted with permission from [31].

diabetes including those with no or mild retinopathy [37].

Modulations in the levels of these two angiogenic molecules are evident as well in diabetic macular edema (DME), a major cause of visual loss in patients with diabetes. When their levels in the vitreous were examined by Funatsu et al. [38], they found that VEGF was significantly higher in patients with DME compared to nondiabetic or diabetic individuals without retinopathy (p <

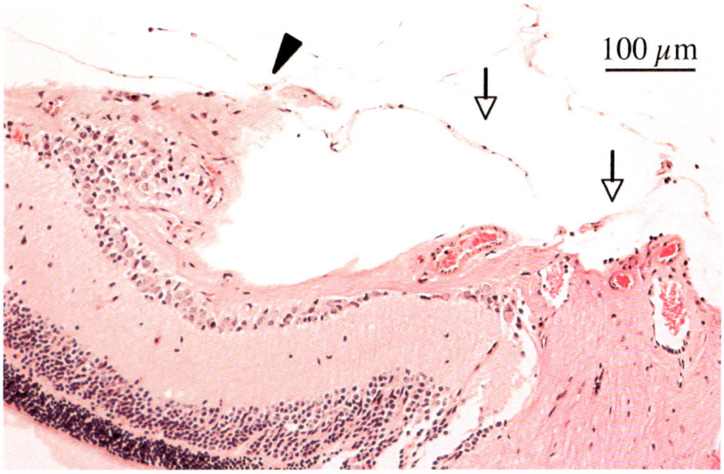

Fig. 3. HE staining of a 56-week-old SDT rat retina. Pathology of the retina with tractional retinal detachment associated with proliferative membranes. Proliferative tissue containing new vessels (arrowhead) and proliferative membranes that extended into the vitreous from the proliferative tissues and optic disc (arrows) are observed. Reprinted with permission from [40].

0.0001 and $p < 0.0001$, respectively). Conversely, vitreous levels of PEDF were decreased in patients with DME compared to nondiabetic or diabetic patients without retinopathy ($p < 0.0001$ and $p < 0.0001$, respectively). They suggested that VEGF and PEDF are independently associated with vascular permeability in the eye [38]. Furthermore, Matsunaga et al. [22] noted that in addition to elevated VEGF levels ($p = 0.003$), the levels of the soluble VEGF receptor sVEGFR-1 were also higher ($p = 0.009$) in the vitreous of patients with PDR and confirmed a reduction in PEDF concentration ($p = 0.041$) compared to normal individuals. Taken together, these studies suggest that the coordinated expression of VEGF and PEDF controls the structural and molecular dynamics of retinal angiogenesis.

VEGF/PEDF in Experimental Studies of Diabetic Retinopathy

Diabetic retinopathy is a major cause of blindness in adults especially when it progresses to the proliferative retinopathy stage. Animal models of diabetes mellitus are few but are important to dissect causes and progression of diabetic retinopathy as well as to test developing drugs that have the potential to reduce the pathology.

A new inbred strain of rats with spontaneous diabetes, Spontaneously Diabetic Torii (SDT) rats, was recently isolated from an outbred colony of Sprague-Dawley (SD) rats and found to be a useful animal model to study diabetic retinopathy [39]. Male SDT rats develop hyperglycemia and glucoseuria spontaneously at about 20 weeks of age with an incidence of 100% at 40 weeks. SDT rats survive for a long time without insulin treatment and more importantly, exhibit severe ocular complications such as tractional retinal detachments, which resemble PDR in humans (fig. 3).

Mature cataracts are found in all SDT rats after 20 weeks of age, and tractional retinal detachment, proliferative tissues from the retina, and proliferative membranes from the retinal surface into the vitreous can be seen at >50 weeks of age in these animals [40]. Neovascularization from retinal vessels is evident in some SDT rats by fluorescein angiography at >40 weeks of age, but the incidence is low, and most interestingly, nonperfused areas that indicate ischemia in the retina are not seen at all ages (fig. 4). The low incidence of neovascular formations and poor development

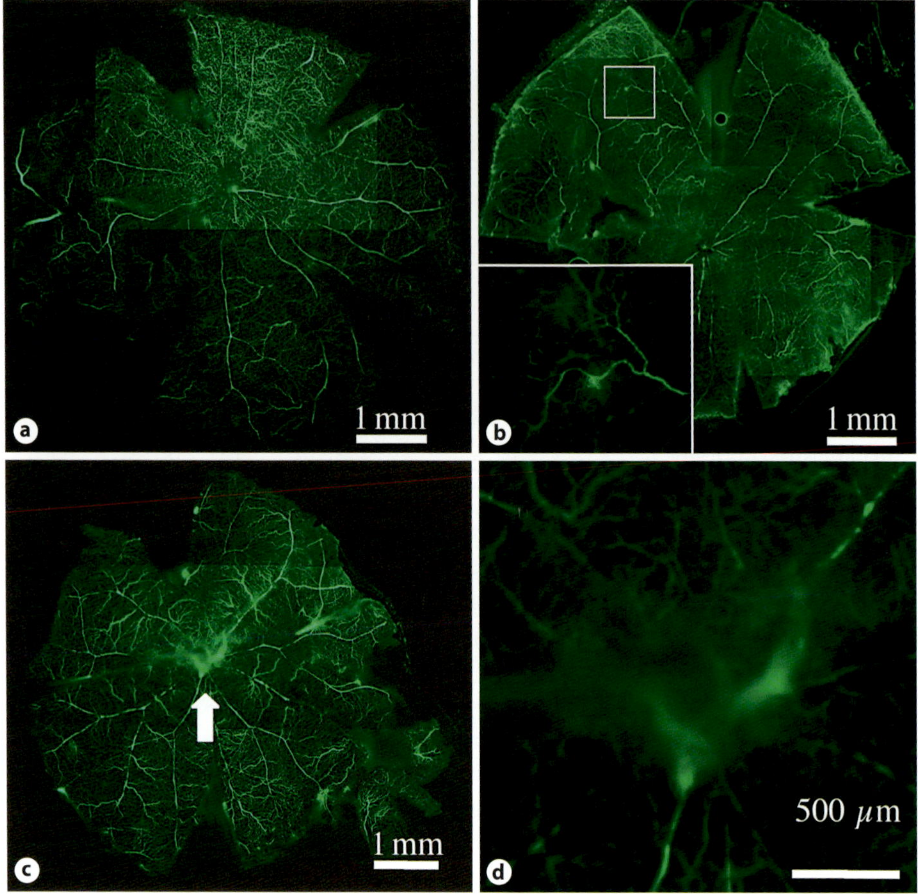

Fig. 4. Retinal angiography with high-molecular-weight fluorescein dextran. **a** 10-week-old SDT rat. **b** 43-week-old SDT rat. Hyperfluorescence that indicates neovascularization is observed but the incidence is low. Nonperfused areas are not detected. The insert is a higher magnification of the square. **c** 56-week-old SDT rat. Hyperfluorescence (arrow) derived from the proliferative membrane around the optic disc can be seen, but nonperfused areas are not observed in the entire retina. **d** Higher magnification of **c**. Reprinted with permission from [40].

of nonperfused areas in the retina of SDT rats are different than in typical PDR in humans. Another interesting feature of this model and one that does not mimic the human condition is that both PEDF and VEGF expressions are upregulated in the SDT rat retinas (fig. 5) [40] as compared to the inverse relationship between these two molecules seen in human eyes with diabetic retinopathy and ischemia-induced retinal neovascularization [6, 7,18–22, 33]. While the SDT model is useful in studying some aspects of diabetic retinopathy, the differences noted between the human and rat condition, especially in the expression of these two key angiogenic molecules, is a concern when studying the role of these factors in controlling retinal vasculature growth and permeability.

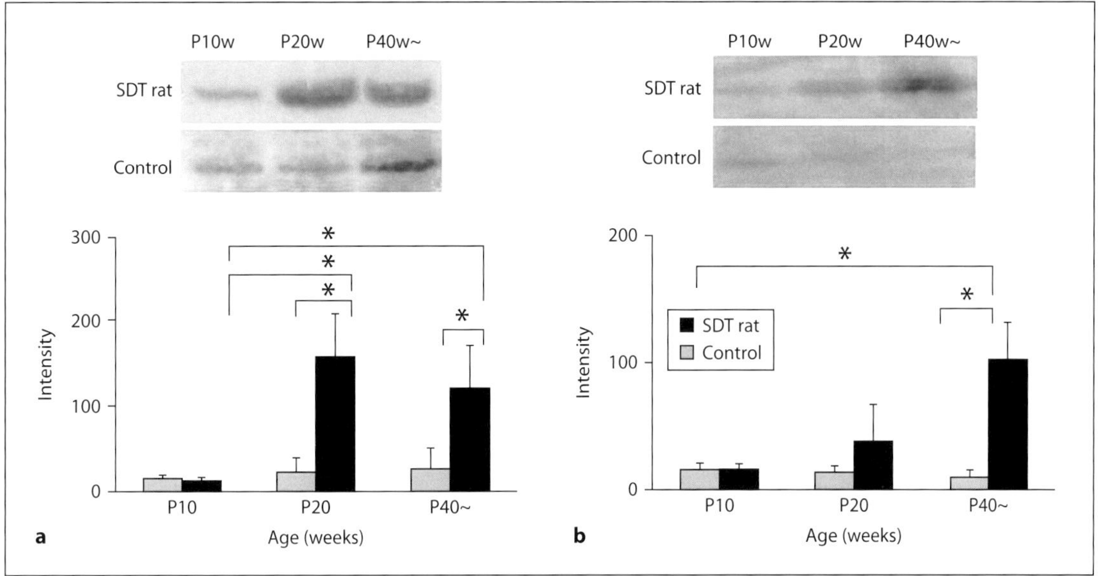

Fig. 5. Western blot analysis for PEDF and VEGF in the retina. **a** Top: PEDF expression. Bottom: The bands of PEDF expression were measured by densitometry with NIH imaging system. The levels of PEDF were dramatically increased in the retinas of 20- and >40-week-old SDT rats compared to those of 10-week-old SDT rats. **b** Top: VEGF expression. Bottom: The VEGF levels in SDT rat retinas were dramatically increased with increasing age. Bars indicate mean ± SEM. * $p < 0.05$. Reprinted with permission from [40].

One explanation for the SDT retinopathy phenotype is the higher expression levels of PEDF in these animals. Recent studies show that hypoxia-treated Brown Norway rats have lower levels of PEDF, more nonperfused areas and increased retinal neovascularization when compared to hypoxia-treated SD rats, which had higher levels of PEDF, fewer nonperfused areas, and less neovascularization [41]. Thus, the levels of PEDF in the retina may alter retinal susceptibility to neovascularization and the progression of diabetic retinopathy.

Some studies have also shown that PEDF can inhibit advanced glycation end-product (AGE)-induced death of pericytes [42] and monocyte chemoattractant protein-1 production in microvascular endothelial cells [43], suggesting that the increased PEDF levels in the SDT rat retina are likely to contribute to reduced AGE functions as well. Studies in support of this concept showed that PEDF or pyridoxal phosphate, an AGE inhibitor, decreased retinal levels of 8-OHdG, an oxidative stress marker, and subsequently suppressed ICAM-1 gene expression and retinal leukostasis in diabetic rats [44]. Furthermore, PEDF was effective in blocking the increased expression of ICAM-1 as well as retinal leukostasis after intravenous administration of AGE to normal rats [44]. An additional affect on leukostasis was observed by Matsuoka et al. [45] who demonstrated that exposure of human umbilical vein endothelial cells (HUVECs) to VEGF increased the number of adhering monocytes, and that PEDF was efficacious in reducing VEGF-induced leukostasis in a dose-dependent manner (fig. 6). Therefore, PEDF may be a useful strategy to prevent retinal leukostasis induced by VEGF, diabetes, or AGE.

The effects of PEDF on blood vessel growth were also clearly demonstrated in a murine model

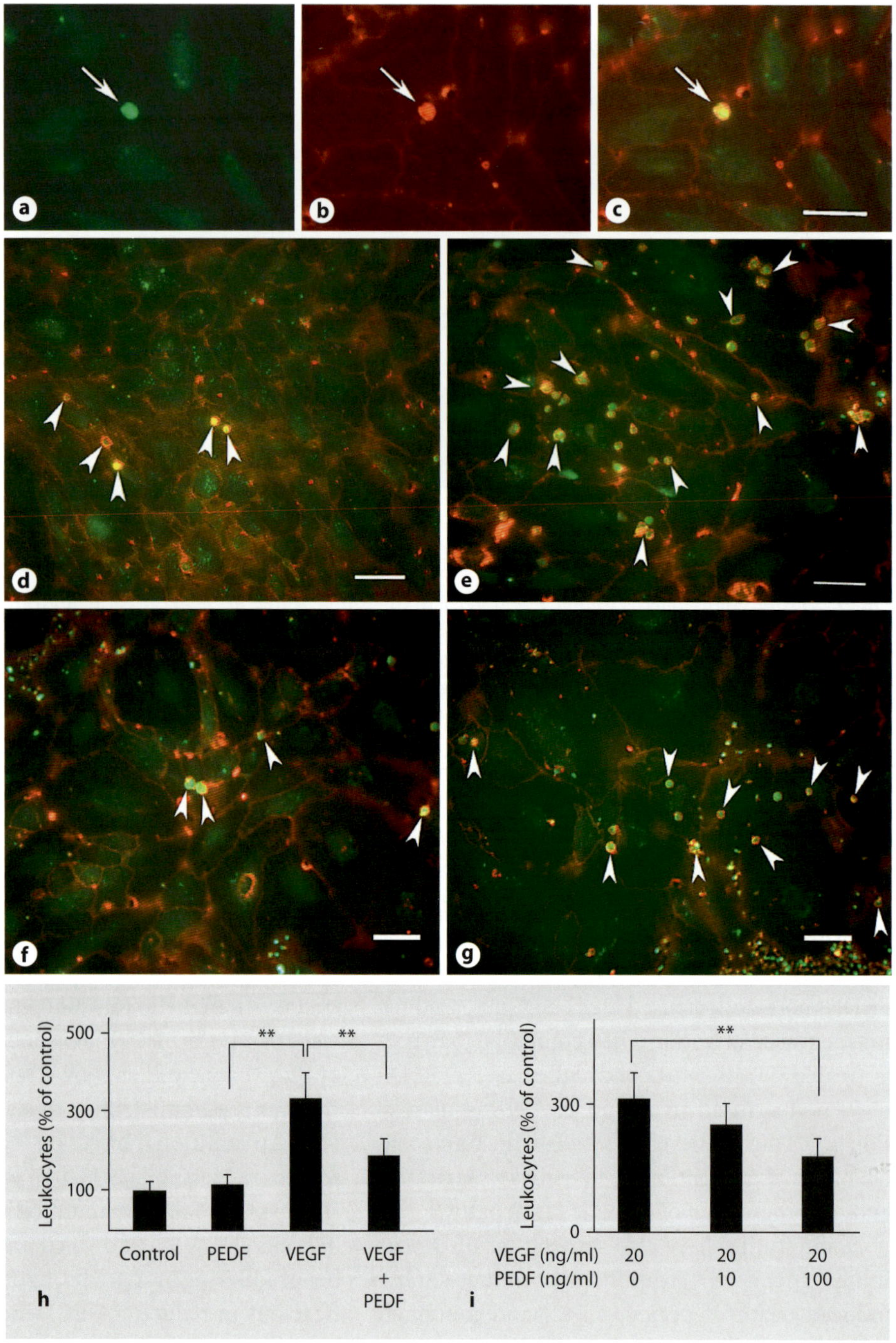
a
b
c
d
e
f
g
Leukocytes (% of control)
500
300
100
**
**
Control
PEDF
VEGF
VEGF + PEDF
h
Leukocytes (% of control)
300
0
**
VEGF (ng/ml) 20 20 20
PEDF (ng/ml) 0 10 100
i

of ischemia-induced retinopathy, where administrated PEDF was shown to inhibit the aberrant growth of blood vessels by causing apoptosis of VEGF-activated endothelial cells [7]. Moreover, PEDF-deficient mice exhibit an increased rate of retinal vascular expansion and are more sensitive to hyperoxia-mediated vessel obliteration [46]. These findings strongly suggest that the increased expression of PEDF could attenuate the progression of diabetic retinopathy by inducing apoptosis of activated endothelial cells, suppressing VEGF functions, and attenuating the deleterious effects of AGE.

One mechanism through which PEDF may counteract VEGF actions is through the regulation of Poly (ADP-ribose) polymerase (PARP). PARP inhibitors are known to decrease angiogenesis by blocking VEGF-induced proliferation, migration, and tube formation of HUVECs, and PARP inhibition has been shown to be associated with the increased expression of PEDF in HUVECs [47].

A second mechanism for PEDF's antiangiogenic actions is that it decreases the expression of VEGF. Studies suggested that PEDF is an endogenous negative regulator of VEGF in retinal capillary endothelial cells (RCECs) and in the retina of rats with oxygen-induced retinopathy [48]. Additional confirmation of this effect by PEDF was seen in Müller cells, where the silencing of the PEDF gene in these cells by siRNA resulted in a significant upregulation of VEGF expression. The effect of PEDF on VEGF expression appears to be at the transcriptional level since PEDF inhibits hypoxia-induced increase in VEGF promoter activity, HIF-1 nuclear translocation and mitogen-activated protein kinase phosphorylation.

A third mechanism of PEDF's effect on VEGFs action may be mediated through the VEGF receptor. There are studies showing that PEDF can effectively inhibit VEGF binding to RCECs, and in vitro receptor-binding assays demonstrate that PEDF competes with VEGF for binding to VEGF receptor 2. On the other hand, VEGF has reciprocal effects on PEDF since it can decrease PEDF gene expression in RCECs, suggesting a VEGF receptor-mediated process for the expression of both genes. These results suggest that there is a reciprocal regulation between VEGF and PEDF that is important in angiogenic control [48].

Plasma PEDF Levels – Diabetes and Nephropathy

PEDF is synthesized by a wide range of human tissues including the lung, brain, kidney, and especially by the liver [49], which may explain the high levels of PEDF in the blood. It has been reported that PEDF is present in the plasma of normal individuals at a concentration of approximately 5 μg/ml, indicating that this is one of the most abundantly circulating proteins in humans

Fig. 6. Confocal fluorescence microscopy for detection of adherent monocytes to HUVECs. **a** Monocytes and nuclei of HUVECs were labeled in green with calcein-AM. **b** Cell surfaces of the monocytes and HUVECs were labeled red with rhodamine-conjugated Con-A lectin. **c** Adherent monocytes appeared yellow in the merged images obtained by combining FITC and rhodamine images. Arrows show monocytes. **d–g** Merge images of the HUVECs and adherent monocytes. HUVECs were treated with PBS as a control (**d**), VEGF (**e**), PEDF (**f**), and both VEGF and PEDF (**g**). **h** Quantification of adherent monocytes. Administration of PEDF did not significantly alter the number of adherent monocytes compared to that of controls. Alternatively, when VEGF was added, the number of adherent monocytes was significantly increased ($p < 0.01$). On the other hand, when PEDF was coadministrated with VEGF, the increase in adherent monocytes induced by VEGF was significantly reduced ($p < 0.01$). **i** Effects of PEDF on adherent monocytes induced by VEGF. PEDF appears to inhibit the increase in adherent monocytes induced by VEGF in a dose-dependent manner. Data were analyzed by ANOVA with Fisher's LSD (** $p < 0.01$). Bars indicate mean ± SEM. Reprinted with permission from [45].

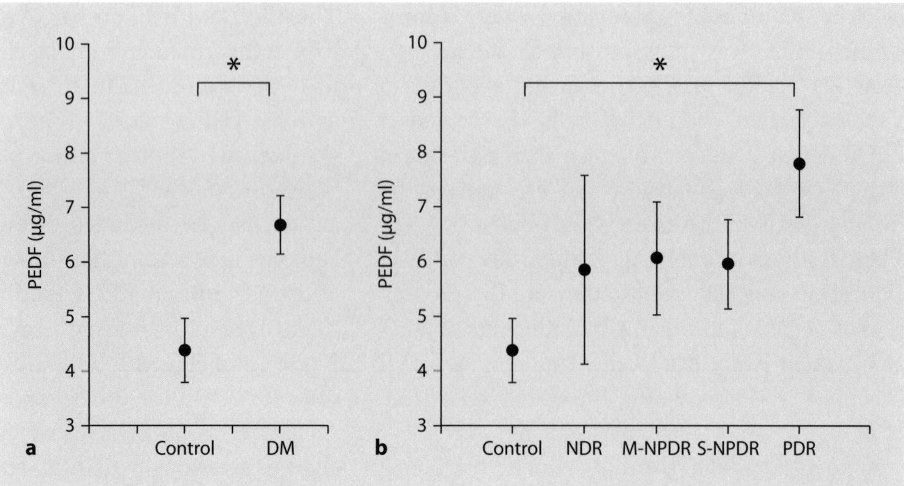

Fig. 7. PEDF levels in diabetic patients and controls. **a** The PEDF level in diabetic patients is significantly higher than that in controls. **b** PEDF levels and the stage of diabetic retinopathy. DM = Diabetes mellitus; NDR = no apparent diabetic retinopathy; M-NPDR = mild to moderate nonproliferative diabetic retinopathy; S-NPDR = severe nonproliferative diabetic retinopathy. * $p < 0.05$. Bars indicate mean ± SEM. Reprinted with permission from [51].

[50]. However, little is known about the regulation of circulating levels of PEDF in patients with diabetes or the importance of PEDF in the plasma of normal individuals.

Although the PEDF levels in the eyes of patients with diabetic retinopathy have been reported to be low [19–22], the plasma level of this polypeptide in patients with diabetes mellitus was found to be elevated [51–53] especially in those with PDR [51]. Quantitative analysis of blood samples from 112 patients with type 2 diabetes and 33 healthy volunteers indicated that the plasma PEDF level in the diabetic patients (6.68 ± 0.54 µg/ml; mean ± SEM) was significantly higher than that in controls (4.38 ± 0.59 µg/ml, p = 0.03). The level of plasma PEDF was found to be 5.84 ± 1.72 µg/ml in individuals with no apparent diabetic retinopathy, 6.05 ± 1.02 µg/ml in those with mild to moderate NPDR, 5.95 ± 0.80 µg/ml in patients with severe NPDR, and 7.79 ± 0.98 µg/ml in the plasma of those with PDR. The PEDF level was especially high in patients with PDR compared to that of controls (p = 0.005; fig. 7) [51].

In addition, PEDF levels in the blood and clinical systemic status of diabetic patients, e.g. gender, age, insulin treatment, the levels of HbA1c, blood urea nitrogen (BUN), and triglycerides, when analyzed showed that plasma PEDF levels increased with aging in controls but not in the diabetic group and that gender (p = 0.03), BUN (p = 0.005), and triglycerides (p = 0.04) were all significant and independent determinants of plasma PEDF levels in diabetic patients (table 1) [51]. Among the diabetic patients studied, PEDF level in men was higher than that in women, but the reason for this difference is still unknown, although it was suggested that the hormonal environment may affect gender-related PEDF levels. The relationship between blood PEDF levels and the systemic status of diabetic patients is still

Table 1. Multiple regression analysis of PEDF levels in diabetic patients (n = 112). Reprinted with permission from [51]

Sex		$p < 0.03$*
Male	54 (48.2%)	
Female	58 (51.8%)	
Age, years	60.9±0.9[1]	$p = 0.84$
Insulin treatment		$p = 0.91$
Yes	40 (35.7%)	
No	72 (64.3%)	
HbA1c, %	7.5±0.2[1]	$p = 0.83$
Serum urea nitrogen, mg/ml	22.3±1.1[1]	$p < 0.001$*
Serum triglycerides, mg/dl	147.0±10.0[1]	$p = 0.04$*

Gender, serum urea nitrogen, and serum triglycerides were significant independent determinants of plasma PEDF levels in diabetic patients. * $p < 0.05$.
[1] Mean ± SEM.

vague and further studies are warranted to understand the role of plasma PEDF in diabetes.

Diabetic nephropathy is also a serious vascular complication of diabetic mellitus [54]. It has been reported that there are high levels of PEDF in the serum of patients with end-stage renal disease [51, 55], that the levels of this protein in the kidney were reduced, but that serum levels were lower in a rat model of diabetic nephropathy [56].

Matsuyama et al. [57] evaluated the relationship between diabetic retinopathy, levels of PEDF, and renal function. They showed that the levels of BUN and creatinine increased significantly as the stage of diabetic retinopathy advanced and that plasma PEDF levels correlated with the levels of BUN and creatinine ($r = 0.54$, $p < 0.0001$; $r = 0.57$, $p < 0.0001$, respectively; fig. 8). Both retinopathy and nephropathy are common microvascular complications associated with diabetes and both are associated with increased plasma PEDF as these conditions progress. Thus, increased levels of PEDF in the blood may indicate microvascular damage in diabetic patients and may be a predictor of the progression of both retinopathy and nephropathy.

In adipose tissue, the synthesis of PEDF is decreased during the differentiation of the cells to mature adipocytes [58]. This expression pattern is in contrast to that of adiponectin, and an association between PEDF plasma levels, obesity and insulin resistance was proposed [59]. Yamagishi et al. [60] reported that PEDF levels were higher in proportion to the number of components of the metabolic syndrome. They suggested that serum PEDF concentrations may increase as a mechanism to counteract coronary risk factors in metabolic syndrome. Together with the results of previous studies, PEDF is most likely associated with the metabolism of patients with diabetes mellitus and may be elevated to counteract vascular cell damage caused by chronic, low-grade inflammation [61, 62].

Although the PEDF receptor has not been cloned, a lipase-linked cell membrane protein (PLA2) that interacts with PEDF has been reported

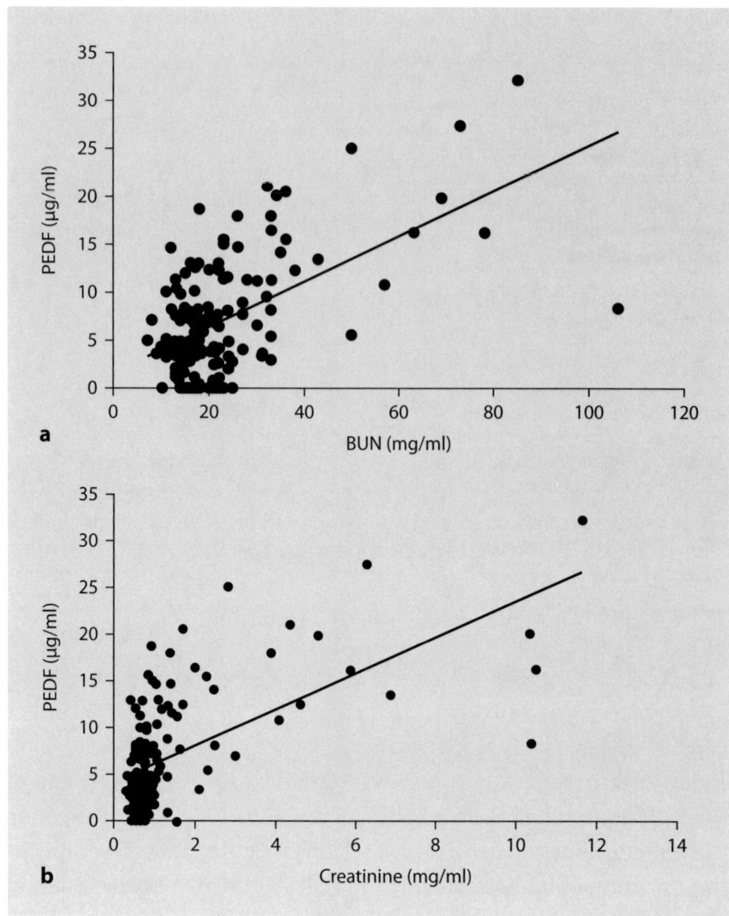

Fig. 8. Relationship between PEDF and renal function. **a** Correlation between PEDF levels and BUN. r = 0.54, p < 0.0001. **b** Correlation between PEDF levels and creatinine. r = 0.57, p < 0.0001. Reprinted with permission from [57].

in the retinal pigment epithelium by Notari et al. [63]. The derived polypeptide has putative transmembrane, intracellular and extracellular regions, and a phospholipase domain. This binding partner of PEDF [TTS-2.2/independent phospholipase A(2) (PLA(2)) zeta and mouse desnutrin/ATGL] has been described in adipose cells as a member of the new calcium-independent PLA(2)/nutrin/patatin-like phospholipase domain-containing 2 (PNPLA2) family that possesses triglyceride lipase and acylglycerol transacylase activities. PLA2 is a regulator of several processes including inflammation, oxidative stress, release of fatty acids, insulin production, angiogenesis, and obesity. This protein has specific and high binding affinity for PEDF, and has potent phospholipase A(2) activity that liberates fatty acids. Thus, it is likely that some of the effects of PEDF in diabetes may be mediated through PLA2 activity.

Recently, the relationship between plasma PEDF levels and anthropometric and metabolic variables in type 2 diabetic patients were examined [64]. The percentage change in serum levels of PEDF during a 1-year observational period showed a positive correlation with the patient's BMI. In addition, the mRNA levels of PEDF in primary cultures of adipocytes, especially omental adipocytes, derived from these individuals were increased in parallel to their BMI values. The level of PEDF was positively associated with metabolic components and TNF-α in patients with type 2 diabetes. These studies suggest that PEDF may be generated from adipose tissues and may play a role in visceral obesity in type 2 diabetic patients possibly through its interaction with PLA2 on adipocytes [64].

The role of PEDF in plasma may be associated with proliferative inflammatory responses since PEDF can prevent endothelial cell migration induced by VEGF and fibroblast growth factor [6, 65], inhibit expression of TNF-α, VEGF, monocyte chemoattractant factor-1, and intercellular adhesion molecule-1 (ICAM-1) [66], and reduce the activity of AGEs in microvascular endothelial cells [43].

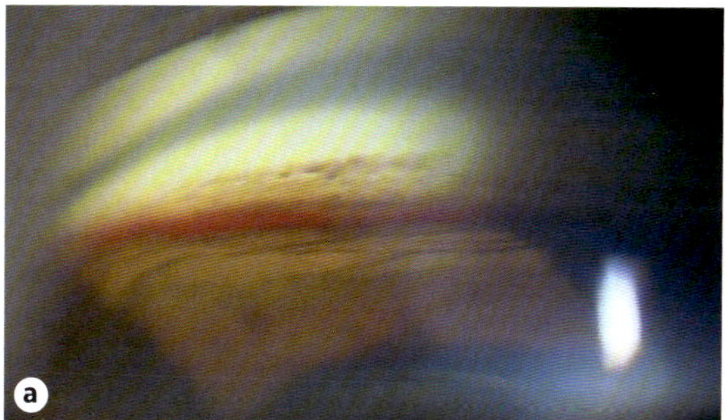

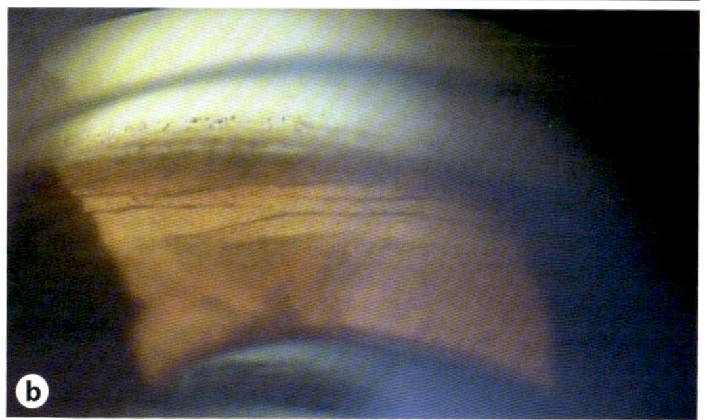

Fig. 9. Angle neovascularization before and after the injection of bevacizumab. **a** Before the injection of bevacizumab, rubeosis of angle structures is marked. **b** Seven days after the injection of bevacizumab, a marked regression of the neovascular vessels can be seen. Reprinted with permission from [81].

Anti-VEGF Therapy for Diabetic Retinopathy

In early anti-angiogenesis studies, it was shown that blocking the activity of VEGF with an anti-VEGF antibody can reduce iris neovascularization and suppress the formation of new retinal vessels in primates [67, 68]. VEGF is thought to be the key candidate gene involved in promoting the pathology seen in diabetic retinopathy. Therefore, reducing its expression or activity in vivo, provides the rationale for anti-VEGF therapy in retinal vascular diseases associated with new vessel formation such as diabetic retinopathy.

One anti-VEGF molecule widely used is bevacizumab (Avastin, Genentech, Inc., San Francisco, Calif., USA), a recombinant human monoclonal IgG1 antibody that inhibits the activity of all isoforms of human VEGF. Bevacizumab has been approved by the United States Food and Drug Administration for intravenous use to control metastatic colorectal cancer. Initial experimental data on primates suggest that the full-length antibody might not penetrate the inner limiting membrane of the retina [69]; however, follow-up studies show that it does penetrate the retinas of rabbits [70] and monkeys [71] within 24 h.

Several case series have been recently published on the off-label use of intravitreal bevacizumab in VEGF-mediated diseases, such as choroidal neovascularization [72], retinal vein occlusion [73], PDR [74–76], cystoid macular edema [77], and neovascular glaucoma [78–80]. In most of these studies, 1.25 mg (0.05 ml) bevacizumab (100 mg/4 ml) was injected into the vitreous of humans and the results were a marked regression of neovascular vessels after 7 days (fig. 9) [81]. When intravitreal injection of bevacizumab was used before vitrectomy for PDR, all patients had less intraoperative bleeding when the neovascular tissues were dissected.

The effect of bevacizumab, however, appears to be transient since most eyes showed signs of a reactivation of the neovascular process 6–8 weeks after injection of the antibody [80]. Bakri et al. [82] measured free bevacizumab after intravitreal injections of 1.25 mg of the compound in rabbits, and reported that the vitreous concentration of bevacizumab declined in a mono-exponential fashion with a half-life of 4.32 days. A concentration >10 μg/ml bevacizumab was maintained in the vitreous humor for 30 days. When the same concentration was injected into the vitreous of eyes with PDR, the levels of VEGF in aqueous humor were significantly reduced at 7 days [81, 83]. We found that VEGF levels were reduced from 676.5 ± 187 pg/ml (mean ± SEM, before injection) to 7.1 ± 7.1 pg/ml ($p < 0.005$) after 7 days, suggesting that bevacizumab is a potent inhibitor of VEGF expression in the eye. The levels of PEDF in the aqueous humor were not altered in PDR after injections with bevacizumab [81, 84]; however, in choroidal neovascularization secondary to age-related macular degeneration or pathologic myopia, intravitreal bevacizumab injections reduced aqueous VEGF and increased PEDF levels [85].

Although further studies with larger samples and longer follow-up times are necessary, these studies strongly suggest that intravitreal bevacizumab may be useful for the treatment of PDR. PEDF gene therapy strategies are currently in phase II clinical trials for age-related macular degeneration where neovascularization and retinal degeneration are predominant features in the pathology of this disease. It would be interesting to develop therapeutic strategies that have greater efficacy in reducing vessel growth and limiting damage to the retina in diseases such as diabetic retinopathy by using a combination of anti-VEGF and pro-PEDF compounds.

References

1 Ferrara N, Davis-Smyth T: The biology of vascular endothelial growth factor. Endocr Rev 1997;18:4–25.

2 Ferrara N: Vascular endothelial growth factor: basic science and clinical progress. Endocr Rev 2004 ;25:581–611.

3 Tombran-Tink J, Johnson LV: Neuronal differentiation of retinoblastoma cells induced by medium conditioned by human RPE cells. Invest Ophthalmol Vis Sci 1989;30:1700–1707.

4 Tombran-Tink J, Chader GJ, Johnson LV: PEDF: A pigment epithelium-derived factor with potent neuronal differentiative activity. Exp Eye Res 1991;53:411–414.

5 Steele FR, Chader GL, Johnson LV, Tombran-Tink J: Pigment epithelium-derived factor: Neurotrophic activity and identification as a member of the serine protease inhibitor gene family. Proc Natl Acad Sci USA 1992;90:1526–1530.

6 Dawson DW, Volpert OV, Gillis P, et al: Pigment epithelium-derived factor: a potent inhibitor of angiogenesis. Science 1999;285:245–248.

7 Stellmach V, Crawford SE, Zhou W, Bouck N: Prevention of ischemia-induced retinopathy by the natural ocular antiangiogenic agent pigment epithelium-derived factor. Proc NatL Acad Soc USA 2001;98:2593–2597.

8 Kim I, Ryan AM, Rohan R, et al: Constitutive expression of VEGF, VEGFR-1, and VEGFR-2 in normal eyes. Invest Ophthalmol Vis Sci 1999;40:2115–2121.

9 Esser S, Wolburg K, Wolburg H, Breier G, Kurzchalia T, Risau W: Vascular endothelial growth factor induces endothelial fenestrations in vitro. J Cell Biol 1998;140:947–959.

10 Shweiki D, Itin A, Soffer D, Keshet E: Vascular endothelial growth factor induced by hypoxia may mediate hypoxia-initiated angiogenesis. Nature 1992;359:843–845.

11 Aiello LP, Northrup JM, Keyt BA, Takagi H, Iwamoto MA: Hypoxic regulation of vascular endothelial growth factor in retinal cells. Arch Ophthalmol 1995;113:1538–1544.

12 Henkind P: Ocular neovascularization. Am J Ophthalmol 1978;85:287–301.

13 Patz A: Clinical and experimental studies on retinal neovascularization. Am J Ophthalmol 1982;94:715–743.

14 Ishii H, Jirousek MR, Koya D, et al: Amelioration of vascular dysfunctions in diabetic rats by an oral PKC beta inhibitor. Science 1996;272:728–731.

15 Amin RH, Frank RN, Kennedy A, Eliott D, Puklin JE, Abrams GW: Vascular endothelial growth factor is present in glial cells of the retina and optic nerve of human subjects with nonproliferative diabetic retinopathy. Invest Ophthalmol Vis Sci 1997;38:36–47.

16 Lutty GA, McLeod DS, Merges C, Diggs A, Plouét J: Localization of vascular endothelial growth factor in human retina and choroid. Arch Ophthalmol 1996;114:971–977.

17 Ogata N, Wada M, Otsuji T, Jo N, Tombran-Tink J, Matsumura M: Expression of pigment epithelium-derived factor in normal adult rat eye and experimental choroidal neovascularization. Invest Ophthalmol Vis Sci 2002;43:1168–1175.

18 Gao G, Li Y, Zhang D, Gee S, Crosson C, Ma J: Unbalanced expression of VEGF and PEDF in ischemia-induced retinopathy. FEBS Lett 2001;489:270–276.

19 Spranger J, Osterhoff M, Reimann M, et al: Loss of antiangiogenic pigment epithelium-derived factor in patients with angiogenic eye diseases. Diabetes 2001;50:2641–2645.

20 Ogata N, Tombran-Tink J, Nishikawa M, et al: Pigment epithelium-derived factor in the vitreous is low in diabetic retinopathy and high in rhegmatogenous retinal detachment. Am J Ophthalmol 2001;132:378–382.

21 Ogata N, Nishikawa M, Nishimura T, Mitsuma Y, Matsumura M: Unbalanced vitreous levels of pigment epithelium-derived factor and vascular endothelial growth factor in diabetic retinopathy. Am J Ophthalmol 2002;134:348–353.

22 Matsunaga N, Chikaraishi Y, Izuta H, Ogata N, Shimazawa M, Matsumura M, Hara H: Role of Soluble Vascular Endothelial Growth Factor Receptor-1 in the Vitreous in Proliferative Diabetic Retinopathy. Ophthalmology 2008;115:1916–1922.

23 Mori K, Duh E, Gehlbach P, et al: Pigment epithelium-derived factor inhibits retinal and choroidal neovascularization. J Cell Physiol 2001;188:253–263.

24 Adamis AP, Miller JW, Bernal MT, et al: Increased vascular endothelial growth factor levels in the vitreous of eyes with proliferative diabetic retinopathy. Am J Ophthalmol 1994;118:445–450.

25 Aiello LP, Avery RL, Arrigg PG, et al: Vascular endothelial growth factor in ocular fluid of patients with proliferative diabetic retinopathy and ocular retinal disorders. N Engl J Med 1994;331:1480–1487.

26 Shinoda K, Isida S, Kawashima S, et al: Comparison of the levels of hepatocyte growth factor and vascular endothelial growth factor in aqueous fluid and serum with grades of retinopathy in patients with diabetes mellitus. Br J Ophthalmol 1999;83:834–837.

27 Pe'er J, Folberg R, Itin A, Gnessin H, Hemo I, Keshet E: Upregulated expression of vascular endothelial growth factor in proliferative diabetic retinopathy. Br J Ophthalmol 1996;80:241–245.

28 Pierce EA, Avery RL, Foley ED, Aiello LP, Smith LE: Vascular endothelial growth factor/vascular permeability factor expression in a mouse model of retinal neovascularization. Proc Natl Acad Sci USA 1995;92:905–909.

29 Ishida S, Shinoda K, Kawashima S, Oguchi Y, Okada Y, Ikeda E: Coexpression of VEGF receptors VEGF-R2 and neuropilin-1 in proliferative diabetic retinopathy. Invest Ophthalmol Vis Sci. 2000;41:1649–1656.

30 Hammes HP, Lin J, Bretzel RG, Brownlee M, Breier G: Upregulation of the vascular endothelial growth factor/vascular endothelial growth factor receptor system in experimental background diabetic retinopathy of the rat. Diabetes 1998;47:401–406.

31 Matsuoka M, Ogata N, Minamino K, Matsumura M: Expression of pigment epithelium-derived factor and vascular endothelial growth factor in fibrovascular membranes from patients with proliferative diabetic retinopathy. Jpn J Ophthalmol 2006;50:116–120.

32 Liu H, Ren J-G, Cooper WL, Hawkins CE, Cowan MR, Tong PY: Identification of the anti-vasopermeability effect of pigment epithelium derived factor and its active site. Proc Natl Acad Sci USA 2004;101:6605–6610.

33 Gao G, Li Y, Gee S, et al: Down-regulation of VEGF and upregulation of PEDF: a possible mechanism for the anti-angiogenic activity of plasminogen kringle 5. J Biol Chem 2002;277:9492–9499.

34 Sebag J, Buckingham B, Charles MA, Reiser K: Biochemical abnormalities in vitreous of humans with proliferative diabetic retinopathy. Arch Ophthalmol 1992;110:1472–1476.

35 Elner SG, Elner VM, Jaffe GJ, Stuart A, Kunkel SL, Strieter RM: Cytokines in proliferative diabetic retinopathy and proliferative vitreoretinopathy. Curr Eye Res 1995;14:1045–1053.

36 Cohen MP, Hud E, Shea E, Shearman CW: Vitreous fluid of db/db mice exhibits alterations in angiogenic and metabolic factors consistent with early diabetic retinopathy. Ophthalmic Res 2008;40:5–9.

37 Boehm BO, Lang G, Volpert O, et al: Low content of the natural ocular anti-angiogenic agent pigment-epithelium derived factor (PEDF) in aqueous humor predicts progression of diabetic retinopathy. Diabetologia 2003;46:394–400.

38 Funatsu H, Yamashita H, Nakamura S, Mimura T, Eguchi S, Noma H, Hori S: Vitreous levels of pigment epithelium-derived factor and vascular endothelial growth factor are related to diabetic macular edema. Ophthalmology 2006;113:294–301.

39 Shinohara M, Masuyama T, Shoda T, et al: A new spontaneously diabetic non-obese Torii rat strain with severe ocular complications. Int J Exp Diabetic Res 2000;1:89–100.

40 Matsuoka M, Ogata N, Minamino K, Higuchi A, Matsumura M: High levels of pigment epithelium-derived factor in the retina of a rat model of type 2 diabetes. Exp Eye Res 2006;82:172–178.

41 Gao G, Li Y, Crosson CE, Becerra SP, Ma J-X: Difference in ischemic regulation of vascular endothelial growth factor and pigment epithelium-derived factor in Brown-Norway and Sprague Dawley rats contributing to different susceptibility to retinal neovascularization. Diabetes 2002;51:1218–1225.

42 Yamagishi S, Inagaki Y, Amano S, Okamoto T, Takeuchi M, Makita Z: Pigment epithelium-derived factor protects cultured retinal pericytes from advanced glycation end product-induced injury through its antioxidative properties. Biochem Biophy Res Comm 2002;296:877–882.

43 Inagaki Y, Yamagishi S, Okamoto T, Takeuchi M, Amano S: Pigment epithelium-derived factor prevents advanced glycation end products-induced monocyte chemoattractant protein-1 production in microvascular endothelial cells by suppressing intracellular reactive oxygen species generation. Diabetologia 2003;46:284–287.

44 Yamagishi S, Matsui T, Nakamura K, Takeuchi M, Imaizumi T: Pigment epithelium-derived factor (PEDF) prevents diabetes- or advanced glycation end products (AGE)-elicited retinal leukostasis. Microvasc Res 2006;72:86–90.

45 Matsuoka N, Ogata N, Minamino M, Matsumura M: Leukostasis and pigment epithelium-derived factor in rat models of diabetic retinopathy. Molecular Vision 2007;13:1058–1065.

46 Huang Q, Wang S, Sorenson CM, Sheibani N: PEDF-deficient mice exhibit an enhanced rate of retinal vascular expansion and are more sensitive to hyperoxia-mediated vessel obliteration. Exp Eye Res 2008;87:226–241.
47 Chen H, Jia W, Xu X, Fan Y, Zhu D, Wu H, Xie Z, Zheng Z: Upregulation of PEDF expression by PARP inhibition contributes to the decrease in hyperglycemia-induced apoptosis in HUVECs. Biochem Biophys Res Commun 2008;369:718–724.
48 Zhang SX, Wang JJ, Gao G, Parke K, Ma JX: Pigment epithelium-derived factor downregulates vascular endothelial growth factor (VEGF) expression and inhibits VEGF-VEGF receptor 2 binding in diabetic retinopathy. J Mol Endocrinol 2006;37:1–12.
49 Tombran-Tink J, Mazuruk K, Rodriguez IR, et al: Organization, evolutionary conservation, expression and unusal Alu density of the human gene for pigment epithelium-derived factor, a unique neurotrophic serpin. Mol Vis 1996;2:11.
50 Petersen SV, Valnickova Z, Enghild JJ: Pigment epithelium-derived factor (PEDF) occurs at a physiologically relevant concentration in human blood: purification and characterization. Biochem J 2003;374:199–206.
51 Ogata N, Matsuoka M, Matsuyama K, Shima C, Tajika A, Nishiyama T, Wada M, Jo N, Higuchi A, Minamino K, Matsunaga H, Takeda T, Matsumura M: Plasma concentration of pigment epithelium-derived factor in patients with diabetic retinopathy. J Clin Endocrin Metab 2007;92:1176–1179.
52 Jenkins A, Zhang SX, Gosmanova A, Aston C, Dashti A, Baker MZ, Lyons T, Ma JX: Increased serum pigment epithelium derived factor levels in type 2 diabetes patients. Diabetes Res Clin Pract 2008;82:5–7.
53 Palmieri D, Watson JM, Rinehart CA: Age-related expression of PEDF/EPC-1 in human endometrial stroma fibroblasts: implications for interactive senescence. Exp Cell Res 1999;247:142–147.
54 Herman WH, Teutsch SM: Kidney disease associated with diabetes; in National Diabetes Data Group. Diabetes in America: Diabetes Data Compiled 1984. Bethesda, US Department of Health and Human Services, chapter XIX, 1985.
55 Motomiya Y, Yamagishi S, Adachi H, Abe A: Increased serum concentration of pigment epithelial derived factor in patients with end-stage renal disease. Clin Chem 2006;52:1970–1971.
56 Wang JJ, Zhang SX, Lu K, et al: Decreased expression of pigment epithelium-derived factor is involved in the pathogenesis of diabetic nephropathy. Diabetes 2005;54:243–250.
57 Matsuyama K, Ogata N, Matsuoka M, Shima S, Wada M, Jo N, Matsumura M: Relationship between pigment epithelium-derived factor (PEDF) and renal function in patients with diabetic retinopathy. Mol Vis 2008;14:992–996.
58 Kratchmarova I, Kalume DE, Blagoev B, Scherer P, Podtelejnikov AV, Molina H, Bickel PE, Andersen JS, Femandez MM, Bunkenborg J, Roepstorff P, Kristiansen K, Lodish HF, Mann M, Pandey A: A proteomic approach for identification of secreted proteins during the differentiation of 3T3-L1 preadipocytes to adipocytes. Mol Cell Proteomics 2002;1:213–222.
59 Matsuzawa Y: Therapy Insight: adipocytokines in metabolic syndrome and related cardiovascular diseases. Nat Clin Pract Cardiovasc Med 2006;3:35–42.
60 Yamagishi S, Adachi H, Abe A, Yashiro T, Enomoto M, Furuki K, Hino A, Jinnouchi Y, Takenaka K, Matsui T, Nakamura K, Imaizumi T: Elevated serum levels of pigment epithelium-derived factor (PEDF) in the metabolic syndrome. J Clin Endocrin Metab 2006;91:2447–2450.
61 Joussen AM, Poulaki V, Le ML, et al: A central role for inflammation in the pathogenesis of diabetic retinopathy. FASEB J 2004;18:1450–1452.
62 Saraheimo M, Teppo AM, Forsblom C, Fagerudd J, Groop PH: Diabetic nephropathy is associated with low-grade inflammation in Type 1 diabetic patients. Diabetologia 2003;46:1402–1407.
63 Notari L, Baladron V, Aroca-Aguilar JD, Balko N, Heredia R, Meyer C, Notario PM, Saravanamuthu S, Nueda ML, Sanchez-Sanchez F, Escribano J, Laborda J, Becerra SP: Identification of a lipase-linked cell membrane receptor for pigment epithelium-derived factor. J Biol Chem 2006;281:38022–38037.
64 Nakamura K, Yamagishi SI, Adachi H, Kurita-Nakamura Y, Matsui T, Inoue H: Serum levels of pigment epithelium-derived factor (PEDF) are positively associated with visceral adiposity in Japanese patients with type 2 diabetes. Diabetes Metab Res Rev 2009;25:52–56.
65 Tombran-Tink J, Barnstable CJ: PEDF: a multifaceted neurotrophic factor. Nat Rev Neurosci 2003;4:628–636.
66 Zhang SX, Wang JJ, Gao G, Shao C, Mott R, Ma JX: Pigment epithelium-derived factor (PEDF) is an endogenous antiinflammatory factor. FASEB J 2006;20:323–325.
67 Adamis AP, Shima DT, Tolentino MJ, et al: Inhibition of vascular endothelial growth factor prevents retinal ischemia associated iris neovascularization in a nonhuman primate. Arch Ophthalmol 1996;114:66–71.
68 Aiello LP, Pierce EA, Foley ED, et al: Suppression of retinal neovascularization in vivo by inhibition of vascular endothelial growth factor (VEGF) using soluble VEGF-receptor chimeric proteins. Proc Natl Acad Sci USA 1995;92:10457–10461.
69 Mordenti J, Thomsen K, Licko V, et al: Intraocular pharmacokinetics and safety of a humanized monoclonal antibody in rabbits after intravitreal administration of a solution or a PLGA microsphere formulation. Toxicol Sci 1999;52:101–106.
70 Shahar J, Avery RL, Heilweil G, Loewenstein A, et al: Electrophysiologic and retinal penetration studies following intravitreal injection of bevacizumab. Retina 2006;26:262–269.
71 Heiduschka P, Fietz H, Hofmeister S, et al., Tubingen Bevacizumab Study Group: Penetration of bevacizumab through the retina after intravitreal injection in the monkey. Invest Ophthalmol Vis Sci 2007;48:2814–2823.
72 Avery RL, Pieramici DJ, Rabena MD, Castellarin AA, Nasir MA, Giust MJ: Intravitreal bevacizumab (Avastin®) for neovascular age-related macular degeneration. Ophthalmology 2006;113:363–372.
73 Rosenfeld PJ, Fung AE, Puliafito CA: Optical coherence tomography findings after an intravitreal injection of bevacizumab (Avastin) for macular edema from central retinal vein occlusion. Ophthalmic Surg Lasers Imaging 2005;36:336–339.

74 Avery RL: Regression of retinal and iris neovascularization after intravitreal bevacizumab (Avastin). Retina 2006;26:352–354.
75 Jorge R, Costa RA, Calucci D, Cintra LP, Scott IU: Intravitreal bevacizumab (Avastin) for persistent new vessels in diabetic retinopathy (IBEPE study). Retina 2006;26:1006–1013.
76 Avery RL, Pearlman J, Pieramici DJ, et al: Intravitreal bevacizumab (Avastin) in the treatment of proliferative diabetic retinopathy. Ophthalmology 2006;113:1695–1705.
77 Haritoglou C, Kook D, Neubauer A, et al: Intravitreal bevacizumab (Avastin) therapy for persistent diffuse diabetic macular edema. Retina 2006;26:999–1005.
78 Kahook MY, Schuman JS, Noecker RJ: Intravitreal bevacizumab in a patient with neovascular glaucoma, Ophthalmic Surg Lasers Imaging 2006;37:144–146.
79 Davidorf FH, Mouser JG, Derick RJ: Rapid improvement of rubeosis iridis from a single bevacizumab (Avastin) injection. Retina 2006;26:354–356.
80 Yazdani S, Hendi K, Pakravan M: Intravitreal bevacizumab (Avastin) injection for neovascular glaucoma. J Glaucoma 2007;16:437–439.
81 Matsuyama K, Ogata N, Jo N, Shima C, Matsuoka M, Matsumura M: Levels of vascular endothelial growth factor and pigment epithelium derived factor in eyes before and after intravitreal injection of bevacizumab. Jpn J Ophthalmol 2009;53:243–248.
82 Bakri SJ, Snyder MR, Reid JM, Pulido JS, Singh RJ: Pharmacokinetics of intravitreal bevacizumab (Avastin). Ophthalmology 2007;114:855–859.
83 Sawada O, Kawamura H, Kakinoki M, Sawada T, Ohji M: Vascular endothelial growth factor in aqueous humor before and after intravitreal injection of bevacizumab in eyes with diabetic retinopathy. Arch Ophthalmol 2007;125:1363–1366.
84 Zhang SX, Wang JJ, Gao G, Parke K, Ma JX: Pigment epithelium-derived factor downregulates vascular endothelial growth factor (VEGF) expression and inhibits VEGF-VEGF receptor 2 binding in diabetic retinopathy. J Mol Endocrinol 2006;37:1–12.
85 Chan WM, Lai TY, Chan KP, Li H, Liu DT, Lam DS, Pang CP: Changes in aqueous vascular endothelial growth factor levels and pigment epithelial-derived factor levels following intravitreal bevacizumab injections for choroidal neovascularization (CNV) secondary to age-related macular degeneration or pathologic myopia. Retina 2008;28:1308–1313.

Nahoko Ogata, MD, PhD
Department of Ophthalmology, Kansai Medical University
Fumizono-cho 10-15, Moriguchi
Osaka 570-8507 (Japan)
Tel. +81 6 6992 1001 (ext. 3324), Fax +81 6 6993 2222, E-Mail ogata@takii.kmu.ac.jp

Hammes H-P, Porta M (eds): Experimental Approaches to Diabetic Retinopathy.
Front Diabetes. Basel, Karger, 2010, vol 20, pp 142–157

The Renin-Angiotensin System in the Eye

Katja Ströder · Thomas Unger · Ulrike Muscha Steckelings

Center for Cardiovascular Research, Institute of Pharmacology, Charité-Universitätsmedizin Berlin, Berlin, Germany

Abstract

The renin-angiotensin system (RAS) is a phylogenetically old hormonal system which serves to control blood pressure, volume and electrolyte homeostasis. Apart from these main systemic effects, the RAS – when overactivated – is further involved in a broad spectrum of cardiovascular diseases ranging from arterial hypertension, atherosclerosis, and cardiac hypertrophy to diabetic or autoimmune nephropathy. Experimental data have provided strong evidence that a local RAS is also expressed in the eye, in particular in the retina and in retinal vessels, and that this ocular RAS is overactivated in diabetes, thus contributing to the pathogenesis of diabetic retinopathy. In this context, the ocular RAS promotes retinal damage by (a) direct effects of angiotensin II via the angiotensin AT1-receptor, and (b) bidirectional interaction with the 'classical' hyperglycemia-induced pathobiochemical pathways (generation of advanced glycation end products, increased polyol pathway flux, activation of protein kinase C, increased hexosamine pathway flux, overproduction of superoxide). The involvement of the RAS in the pathomechanisms underlying diabetic retinopathy suggests pharmacological RAS inhibition as a therapeutic option in this disease. Preclinical data in fact indicate that angiotensin-converting enzyme inhibitors and AT1 receptor blockers are able to confer retinoprotection, and this was further supported by recent clinical trials (EURODIAB, DIRECT).

History of the Renin-Angiotensin System

First data pointing to the existence of a hormonal, blood pressure-regulating system, which we nowadays term the renin-angiotensin system (RAS), were published in 1898 by Robert Tigerstedt and Per Bergmann [1]. They reported the presence of a pressor compound in the renal tissue of rabbits, because upon injection of renal homogenates from one healthy rabbit into another healthy rabbit, they observed an increase in blood pressure in the recipient. Based on its origin, they named the substance 'renin' [1]. Further research on renin was hampered by the lack of a reliable and reproducible animal model of hypertension. Such a model (partial occlusion of renal arteries by a silver clip in dogs) was provided by Harry Goldblatt in 1934 [2]. Five years later, the groups of Eduardo Braun-Menendez in Buenos Aires and of Irvine Page in Indianapolis coincidentally but independently found that renin was not the active vasoconstrictor, but an enzyme acting on a specific substrate thus generating a vasoactive peptide, which they called hypertensin or angiogenin [3, 4]. In 1957 at a symposium to celebrate the 25th anniversary of

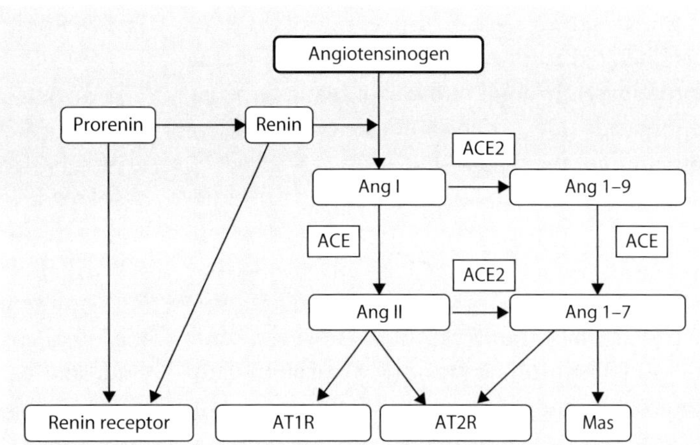

Fig. 1. The RAS.

Goldblatt's first successful experiment, Braun-Menendez and Page agreed on a single nomenclature for the active final compound, which was 'angiotensin', taking half of each original name [5].

Angiotensin-converting enzyme (ACE) and its ability to cleave angiotensin II (Ang II) from angiotensin I (Ang I) was described much later, in 1954, by Leonard T. Skeggs [6]. The discovery of ACE and the realization that ACE and the bradykinin-degrading enzyme kininase II are identical enabled the development of the first RAS-interfering drug, the ACE inhibitor captopril, from the venom of the Brazilian snake *Bothrops jararaca*, which was originally found to prevent inactivation of bradykinin [7].

Other current possibilities of pharmacological RAS interferences comprise the specific and selective blockade of AT1 receptors by AT1 receptor blockers (ARBs) or the inhibition of renin enzymatic activity by renin inhibitors [8, 9]. New developments aim at stimulating the beneficial pathways within the RAS by Ang 1–7 releasing drugs or by nonpeptide AT2 receptor agonists [10, 11].

The Circulating Renin-Angiotensin System

The RAS is an endocrine system primarily known to regulate blood pressure and fluid balance. The first step of the enzymatic cascade eventually leading to the synthesis of the active hormones of the RAS is cleavage of the sole precursor, angiotensinogen, by renin [12] (fig. 1). According to the traditional view of the RAS, angiotensinogen, a glycosylated α_2-plasma protein made up of 452 amino acids, is synthesized in the liver and released into the circulation [12]. Renin is secreted from the juxtaglomerular apparatus of the kidney into the circulation in response to renal sympathetic nerve activation or to a decrease in blood pressure or tubular salt content [12]. In the blood, the major part of the angiotensinogen molecule is cleaved by renin with only the first 10 amino acids remaining to form the inactive decapeptide Ang I. Cleavage of angiotensinogen by renin is the rate-limiting step in the synthesis of angiotensin peptides with the rate of angiotensinogen cleavage set by amount and activity of renin, not by the amount of angiotensinogen which is always available in abundant supply [12].

Ang II is the main effector peptide of the RAS. It is liberated from Ang I by ACE, a zinc-metalloproteinase, through removal of two c-terminal amino acids [13]. A rich source of ACE is the endothelium of the lung [14].

Ang II binds to two main receptor subtypes termed AT1 receptor (AT1R) and AT2 receptor (AT2R) [15]. AT1R and AT2R both belong to the broad family of G-protein-coupled, seven-transmembrane receptors. However, only the AT1R exhibits 'classical' G-protein coupling, while the AT2R only couples to certain G-proteins (Gαi2 and Gαi3) and further signals via distinct binding proteins such as the AT2R-binding protein, SH2 domain-containing phosphatase 1 or PLZF [15–18]. The AT1R is expressed in the vast majority of tissues in the adult organism, and mediates most of the known actions of Ang II, such as vasoconstriction, aldosterone release, sodium retention, fibrosis, hypertrophy and inflammation [15]. The majority of data about the AT2R support the notion that the AT2R in many aspects counteracts AT1R-mediated actions, thus promoting vasodilation, antifibrosis, antihypertrophy and anti-inflammation [15, 19]. As a result of this panel of protective actions, the AT2R is thought (and has been shown experimentally) to be tissue protective and to accelerate tissue repair and regeneration [19, 20].

In addition to the classical RAS components, some new players have been identified in recent years. Ang 1–7, which is cleaved from Ang I and Ang II by the enzyme ACE2, seems to be another active hormone within the RAS [21, 22]. However, Ang 1–7 apparently has actions opposite to Ang II via the AT1R – but similar to Ang II via the AT2R, to which it is also able to bind [22].

Furthermore, a protein has recently been discovered, which binds and activates prorenin and also binds renin in tissues: the (pro)renin receptor (P)PR [16, 23, 24].

Tissue Renin-Angiotensin Systems

The RAS has originally been identified as a circulating hormonal system exerting mainly systemic effects. However, in the early 1990s, the idea developed, that apart from the circulatory system there also exist so called tissue or local RASs [14, 25]. This concept was based on findings of RAS components in 'unorthodox' locations, e.g. the 'renal enzyme' renin in the brain [25], which could not be explained by recruitment from the blood. Tissue-specific differences in the efficiency of RAS inhibition by ACE inhibitors or ARBs also contributed to the concept of a tissue RAS.

Nowadays, it is commonly accepted that the majority of tissues, e.g. heart, liver, brain, reproductive organs, adipose tissue, gut or skin harbor a so called local RAS which generates Ang II independent of circulating factors [14].

The Renin-Angiotensin System in the Eye

Those organs mainly affected by diabetic end organ damage, in particular vessels, kidney, peripheral nerves and the eye, all harbor local RASs [14].

In 1978, Ikemoto and Yamamoto [26] provided first evidence for Ang I-generating activity in the aqueous humor of dogs, rabbits and monkeys by incubating aqueous humor samples with exogenous angiotensinogen and subsequent measurement of Ang I by radioimmunoassay. In 1989/1990 the group of Schalekamp confirmed this finding using human and bovine eyes and, furthermore, found Ang I-generating activity in several other compartments of the eye such as vitreous, bovine retina, pigment epithelium-choroid and anterior uveal tract [27, 28]. In all compartments of the eye, prorenin outweighed renin. Interestingly, prorenin in ocular fluids showed a concentration gradient (posterior vitreous > anterior vitreous > aqueous humor) pointing to local prorenin production within the retina. This assumption is

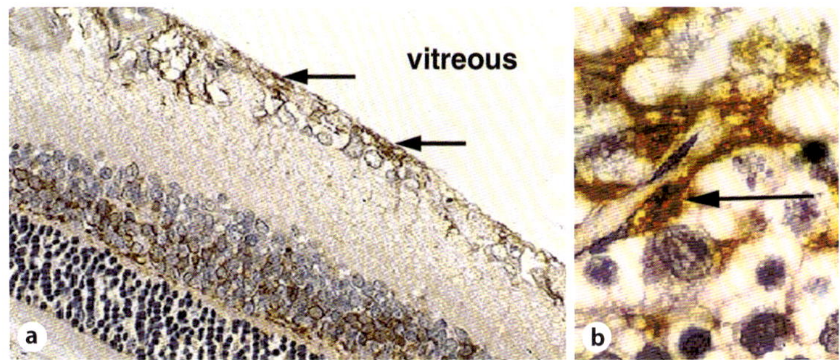

Fig. 2. Three-µm sections of Sprague-Dawley rat retina immunolabeled for renin protein. Hematoxylin was used as the counterstain. **a** Specific labeling for renin protein (arrows) Müller cells distributed from the inner limiting membrane to the outer limiting membrane. ×180. **b** High power of the inner limiting membrane showing renin protein (arrow) immunolabeling in Müller cell end feet abutting a retinal capillary. ×850. With permission from Wilkinson-Berka et al. J Vasc Res 2001;38:527–535.

further supported by the fact that more than 90% of total renin (renin plus prorenin) in ocular fluids and tissues could not be explained by trapped plasma [27, 28]. A similar result was obtained in mice retina [29]. Still, renin production in the retina is modest compared to its main source, the kidney [29]. In later years, concentrations of Ang I and Ang II higher than what could be accounted for by plasma have been measured in the anterior uveal tract, neural retina, retinal pigmented epithelial layer and choroid [30].

In the mid-1990s, with more sensitive laboratory methods available, several groups measured the expression of RAS components in the retina. According to these data, all RAS components (angiotensinogen, prorenin, renin, ACE, chymase, AT1R, AT2R) are present in the retina, either in the neurons and glial cells of the neural retina or in the blood vessels or both [28–33, 35, 37, 38, 40–42] (fig. 2). Recently, the group by Wilkinson-Berka showed that all RAS components are already present in rat retina as early as postnatal day 1 and that this expression pattern persists into adulthood [32]. Furthermore, the presence of a local RAS in the retina has not only been demonstrated in rodents, but also in the human eye [31]. These data, together with other findings demonstrating the presence of RAS components in ocular fluid and tissue, strongly support the existence of an intraocular RAS independent of the circulating RAS.

A more detailed summary of these data can be found in table 1.

The Ocular Renin-Angiotensin System in Diabetes

The status of the systemic RAS in diabetes is rather controversial. On the one hand, it is reported that the circulating RAS is suppressed in diabetes [43], on the other hand several publications agree with the observation that an increase in plasma prorenin is a sensitive marker of the progression from background retinopathy to proliferative retinopathy [44–46].

There is more congruence regarding the tissue RASs in diabetes. In particular, in tissues susceptible to diabetic end organ damage (e.g. in the retina or the kidney), the local or tissue

Table 1. Localization of the RAS in intraocular tissue of different species

RAS component	Localization	Species	References
Prorenin	lens capsule	human	33
	retina	human, bovine, rat	28,32,33
	ciliary body	human	33
	vitreous fluid	human, bovine	27,28
Renin	aqueous humor	dog, rabbit, monkey	26
	retina	human, rat, bovine, murine	28,29,31
	choroid	human	31
	vitreous fluid	human	27
Angiotensinogen	retina	human, rat	31,32
	choroid	human	31,34
	iris	human	34
	vitreous fluid	human	34
	ciliary body	human	31
ACE	retina	human, rabbit, dog, monkey, porcine, rat	31, 35, 38, 40, 41
	ciliary body	human, rabbit, porcine	36, 38, 41
	iris	porcine	41
	cornea	human	38
	tear fluid	human, rabbit	35
	aqueous humor	human, rabbit	35,36
	choroid	human, dog, monkey, porcine	31, 38, 40, 41
	sclera	human, dog, monkey	31, 40
	anterior uveal tract	dog, monkey	40
ACE2	retina	human, rat	37, 42
Chymase	choroid	dog, monkey	40
	vitreous fluid	human	39
	sclera	dog	40
	anterior uveal tract	dog, monkey	40
AT1 receptor	retina	human, rat	32, 38
	choroid	human	37
	cornea	human	38

Table 1. (continued)

RAS component	Localization	Species	References
	ciliary/iris	human	37
	optic nerve	human	37
AT2 receptor	retina	human, rat	32, 37
	choroid	human	37
	optic nerve	human	37
Ang I	anterior uveal tract	porcine	30
	retina	porcine	30
	choroid	porcine	30
	aqueous humor	human	30
	vitreous fluid	human	30
Ang II	retina	human, porcine, rat	30, 32, 37, 38
	choroid	human, porcine, rabbit	30, 38
	cornea	human	38
	aqueous humor	human	30
	ciliary body	human	38
	vitreous fluid	human	30, 37
	anterior uveal tract	porcine	30
Ang 1–7	retina	human	37

RASs have been shown to be activated [47, 48]. An increased prorenin concentration in the vitreous of patients with proliferative retinopathy with retinal detachment when compared to eyes of nondiabetic subjects with spontaneous retinal detachment was already reported by Danser et al. in 1989 [27]. Although renin is the rate-limiting step in Ang II synthesis, elevated levels of angiotensinogen and ACE as demonstrated in the retinas of diabetic rats may further contribute to enhanced retinal Ang II synthesis [48]. Increased levels of Ang II have in fact been measured in the vitreous of diabetic patients, and Ang II levels correlated with the severity of diabetic retinopathy [49].

A novel concept as to how hyperglycemia actually increases RAS activity has been suggested very recently by Toma et al. [50]. They describe a paracrine signaling pathway in the diabetic kidney, in which the hyperglycemia-induced, locally accumulated, citric acid cycle intermediate succinate binds to and activates the G-protein-coupled GPR91 receptor, thus stimulating renin release [50]. Interestingly, the GPR91 receptor seems to be also involved in neovascularization in the hypoxic retina [51].

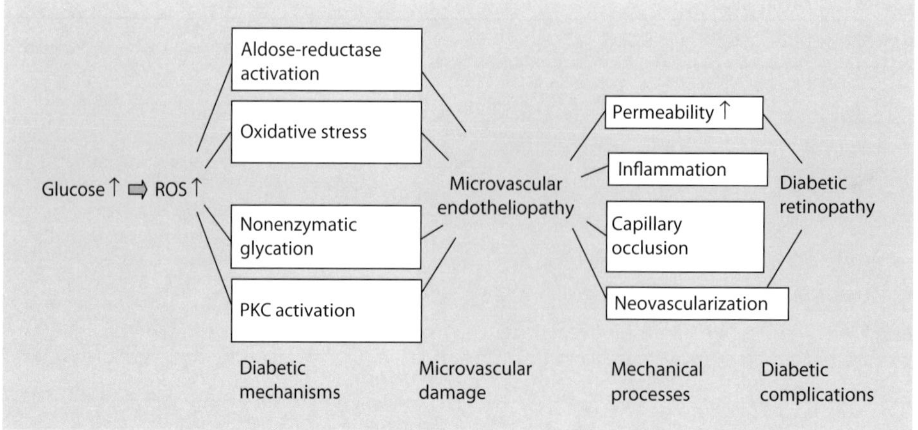

Fig. 3. Pathogenesis of diabetic vasculopathy. Note that the RAS interferes with all steps of this pathological cascade. Adapted from www.diabeticretinopathy.org.uk.

Molecular Mechanisms of Tissue Damage in Diabetes

Hyperglycemia has been established as the primary pathogenic factor of the development of diabetic retinopathy. Knowledge about the biochemical cascades and molecular mechanisms initiated by hyperglycemia and underlying tissue damage in diabetes has grown substantially in recent years. Four major biochemical pathways have been identified to be stimulated by hyperglycemia and to result in disturbed cell homeostasis. These are (1) the intra- and extracellular overproduction of advanced glycation end products (AGEs); (2) increased polyol pathway flux; (3) the activation of protein kinase C, and (4) increased hexosamine pathway flux [for review, see 52, 53] (fig. 3).

1 AGEs are the result of nonenzymatic glycation (Maillard reaction) of proteins in a hyperglycemic environment. The formation of AGEs contributes to hyperglycemic cell damage by three main mechanisms: (a) AGEs bind to specific AGE receptors resulting in the production of reactive oxygen species (ROS) and the activation of NF-κB, which is a key transcription factor for proinflammatory mediators, (b) function of glycated cellular proteins may be disturbed, and (c) AGE precursors interact with and disturb extracellular matrix (ECM) composition [52].
2 The significance of the enhanced polyol pathway flux for diabetic tissue damage is still somewhat controversial, but probably involves a decrease in NADPH, which is required for regenerating reduced gluthation and thereby to control oxidative stress [52].
3 Protein kinase C (PKC), which is activated by increased levels of diacylglycerol, is the initial step of numerous detrimental molecular cascades such as increased synthesis of vascular endothelial growth factor (VEGF), endothelin-1, plasminogen activator inhibitor 1 (PAI-1), or TGF-β (causing increased ECM production), reduced nitric oxide (NO) production, or activation of NF-κB [52].
4 Increased hexosamine pathway activity means that in the hyperglycemic state, part of the intracellular glucose does not undergo glycolysis, but is diverted into another metabolic pathway, the hexosamine pathway,

finally resulting in the synthesis of uridine diphosphate N-acetyl glucosamine. N-acetyl glucosamine then binds to transcription factors like Sp1, which get activated and increase the transcription rate of factors like TGF-β and PA-1 which both contribute to vascular pathology [52].

These pathways interfere with each other in many ways, thus reinforcing one another and exponentiating the detrimental outcome.

Oxidative stress is not only the result of at least two of the above-described pathways, enhanced polyol flux and PKC activation, but the overproduction of ROS may in fact be a first, critical upstream event in hyperglycemic cells which eventually initiates all four biochemical pathways [52, 53]. This so-called 'unifying mechanism', which is excess generation of superoxide by the mitochondrial electron transport chain, is elegantly reviewed in the 2004 Banting Lecture given by Michael Brownlee [53]. An excess ROS production has indeed been demonstrated in a variety of diabetic tissues including the retina [54, 55].

The orchestrated destructive power of the above-described pathways eventually leads to vasculopathy and endothelial dysfunction in macro- and microvessels. In macrovessels, they are a major reason for the susceptibility of these vessels to atherosclerosis. In microvascular disease, they cause pericyte loss, vascular leakage and excess ECM production. More specifically, in the retina they promote exudation of plasma components, vascular occlusion, hypoxia and hypoxia-induced pathological neovascularization, in the kidney they cause proteinuria, mesangial cell expansion and glomerulosclerosis, and in peripheral nerves they contribute to axonal degeneration [52].

The Retinal Renin-Angiotensin System and Diabetic Tissue Damage

The ocular RAS contributes to diabetic tissue damage in two ways:

On the one hand, elevated Ang II levels elicit various detrimental actions by stimulating the AT1R. Such AT1R-mediated actions comprise increased VEGF expression (promoting vascular leakage and disintegration of the blood-retinal barrier) [56], vasoconstriction (adding to impaired blood flow in the diabetic retina) [57], NF-κB activation (acting proinflammatory) [58], increased oxidative stress [55, 59] or ECM accumulation (promoting fibrosis) [60].

On the other hand, the RAS is involved in almost all biochemical events which are initiated by hyperglycemia and eventually lead to cell damage (see the previous section).

1 Ang II has been shown to increase AGE formation and vice versa, thus building up a vicious circle [61].
2 As by diabetes, the polyol pathway flux can also be enhanced by Ang II [62].
3 Retinal PKC is activated in diabetes [63], but also by Ang II [64, 65]. PKC activation elicits a number of unfavorable actions such as increased synthesis of VEGF [63, 66], endothelin-1 [67], PAI-1 [68], or TGF-β (causing increased ECM production) [69], reduced NO production [70], vascular dysfunction [71] or activation of NF-κB [72, 73]. Almost all of these effects can also be obtained by AT1R stimulation in a normoglycaemic environment [56–60]. In particular VEGF, a key factor in the pathogenesis of diabetic retinopathy, which promotes pericyte loss causing vascular leakage, extravasation of plasma components into the retinal tissue, pathological, nonfunctional neovascularization and formation of acellular capillaries and microaneurysms, is not only regulated by hyperglycemia, but also by Ang II [56].
4 Hyperglycemia stimulates angiotensinogen gene expression via the hexosamine pathway, thus contributing to increased Ang II synthesis [74, 75].

Last but not least, the main player within the so-called 'unified mechanism' preceding all four of the above pathways, which is the formation of ROS, is also strongly influenced by Ang II. A myriad of publications has reported increased NADPH oxidase activity or stimulated ROS formation in response to Ang II [54–56]. There is also direct evidence that Ang II-induced oxidative stress plays a role in diabetic retinopathy, e.g. by promoting VEGF expression and leukostasis [56, 76, 77]. Moreover, oxidative stress has been shown to be a direct stimulator of the expression of the AT1R or Ang I-forming cathepsin [78, 79].

Inhibition of the Renin-Angiotensin System in Diabetic Retinopathy

Animal Studies

Animal studies have provided substantial evidence that pharmacological inhibition of the RAS by ACE inhibitors (thus reducing Ang II synthesis) or by AT1R blockers positively influences diabetic retinopathy [80]. In a large number of these studies, RAS blockade has been reported to interfere with the pathogenetic pathways discussed above.

1 The ARB candesartan has been shown to prevent abnormal accumulation of AGEs in diabetic nephropathy and diabetic retinopathy in animal models of type 2 diabetes [81, 82]. In the diabetic kidney, AGE reduction coincided with attenuated oxidative stress [82], in the retina it coincided with reduced VEGF expression [81]. In both studies, ARB treatment led to improved organ function as indicated by decreased albuminuria in diabetic nephropathy and an improved outcome of treated rats in the electroretinogram.

   RAS blockade also has a positive impact on the pathological events induced by AGE accumulation. For example, the ARB telmisartan suppressed retinal inflammation in diabetic retinopathy in mice by inhibition of NF-κB activity [73]. An anti-inflammatory effect in diabetic retinopathy was also observed for the ARB losartan by estimating leukocyte entrapment in the retinal microcirculation [83].

2 There are no data available about an influence of RAS blockade on polyol pathway flux.

3 It has been clearly shown in many models and several species that RAS blockade is able to inhibit PKC activity. In the context of diabetic complications, it is of particular interest that RAS inhibition is also able to inhibit hyperglycemia-induced PKC activation. For example, Malhotra et al. [84] exposed primary rat cardiomyocytes to hyperglycemia in vitro which led to an increase in PKC activity in these cells. Co-treatment of these cells with the ARB losartan completely prevented hyperglycemia-induced (and NOT Ang II-induced) PKC activation [84]. In an in vivo study in a streptozotocin-diabetic rat model, diabetes-related PKC activation in the retina, glomeruli and mesenteric artery was significantly attenuated by ramipril treatment [85]. In terms of organ function, the reduction in PKC activity coincided with ameliorated albuminuria in these animals.

   As stated earlier, PKC activation elicits a number of pathological events such as increased synthesis of VEGF, PAI-1, TGF-β or endothelin-1, reduced NO production, vascular dysfunction or activation of NF-κB. RAS blockade has been demonstrated to have an inhibitory effect on each of these molecular mechanisms.

   The impact of RAS blockade on PAI-1 expression in diabetes has been examined in the vessel wall, albeit not in retinal vessels. In the Otsuka Long-Evans Tokushima Fatty rat, a model of human noninsulin-dependent diabetes mellitus, PAI-1 mRNA and protein levels were increased in the coronary vasculature, and this increase was reversed by candesartan [86]. The same expression pattern and responsiveness to candesartan was found for TGF-β in this study [86].

Retinal hemodynamics are changed in diabetes as a result of a disturbed balance between vasodilatory and vasoconstrictive factors [87, 88]. Expression of two of the main regulators of vascular tone, the vasoconstrictor endothelin-1 and the vasodilator NO, which are both PKC and RAS dependent, is altered in diabetes [87]. Experimental evidence supports the view that impaired hemodynamics in diabetes are due to elevated PKC and RAS activity leading to increased endothelin-1 and decreased NO production, because both, inhibition of PKC and inhibition of the RAS, improve retinal blood flow, decrease endothelin-1 expression and ameliorate reduced NO production in diabetes [89–93]. For example, the ACE inhibitor enalapril significantly lowered plasma endothelin-1 levels in hypertensive patients with type 2 diabetes [91]. Along the same lines, a 1-month treatment of streptozotocin-diabetic rats with losartan significantly reduced endothelin ETB receptor expression in a way comparable to insulin treatment [92]. With regard to NO, oral treatment with candesartan cilexetil or captopril significantly improved acetylcholine-induced vasodilation of retinal vessels in diabetic Sprague-Dawley rats in vivo [90]. A similar effect of ramipril was observed in aortic rings derived from diabetic db/db mice [93].

Regarding VEGF, it has been shown in diabetic normotensive Sprague-Dawley rats, diabetic hypertensive SHR-SP and diabetic hypertensive (mRen-2)27 rats transgenic for the human renin gene that VEGF expression is upregulated by diabetes and can be depressed by ACE inhibition or AT1-receptor blockade [94–96]. Diabetic (mRen-2)27 rats further developed intraocular endothelial hyperproliferation in the retinae and irides, which was also reduced by ACE inhibition, probably through inhibition of VEGF which is regarded to be a key promoter of neovascularization in diabetic retinopathy [96]. VEGF is further thought to play an essential role in the development of vascular malformations in diabetic retinopathy such as acellular capillaries and microaneurysms. RAS inhibition by AT1 receptor blockade reduced the formation of acellular capillaries in diabetic hypertensive (mRen-2)27 rats [97]. Although treatment with valsartan lowered blood pressure in these animals, the inhibitory effect of valsartan on the formation of acellular capillaries was apparently blood pressure independent, because blood pressure reduction by atenolol to the same levels as by valsartan had no such preventive effect [97].

4 No data are available on the impact of RAS blockade on the hexosamine pathway.

Overproduction of superoxide is both the underlying cause and also the result of the pathobiochemical mechanisms implicated in diabetes-induced tissue damage including diabetic retinopathy [52–54]. The overactivated RAS in diabetes further contributes to increased oxidative stress as shown in pericytes in vitro and in a streptozotocin rat model [76, 98]. Chen et al. [76] recently suggested that Ang II-induced superoxide production is causative for retinal leukostasis. In the same experimental setting, Ang II induced retinal leukostasis could be inhibited by AT1-receptor blockade as well as by the general antioxidants tempol and N-acetylcysteine, and by the NAD(P)H oxidase inhibitor apocynin [76]. Other studies support the view that inhibition of the RAS ameliorates diabetic tissue damage at least in part by reduction of oxidative stress, e.g. by an inhibition of NAD(P)H oxidase. For example, a 6-week treatment of diabetic db/db mice with the ACE inhibitor ramipril significantly reduced ROS production resulting in attenuated endothelial dysfunction manifesting in improved acetylcholine-induced vasodilation [93]. A relation between favorable therapeutic effects of RAS inhibition and antioxidant effects has also been shown in diabetic nephropathy in rats [99]. In a small, prospective case-control study conducted among adolescent and young type 1 diabetic patients with early signs of angiopathy (n = 14; 9 of them with retinopathy) or without angiopathy (n = 11), superoxide overproduction was confirmed and attributed to a hyperglycemia-related defective intracellular antioxidant enzyme production and activity in comparison to healthy controls [100]. It was further shown in this study population that a 6-month treatment with the ARB irbesartan significantly improved the production and activity of these enzymes [100]. Interestingly, the established AT1-receptor antagonist candesartan and R-147176, a novel sartan with low affinity for the AT1-receptor, have recently been reported to have direct antioxidant properties independent of AT1 receptor blockade when used in high doses [101, 102]. Both drugs proved to be protective in diabetic nephropathy or retinopathy. The antioxidant features observed for candesartan and R-147176 do not seem to be a class effect but rather restricted to certain sartans, because irbesartan and losartan had no such effect [101]. Still, for some ARBs such antioxidant properties may add to their AT1 blockade-related therapeutic effects in diabetic end organ damage.

Clinical Trials

The effectiveness of RAS inhibition as a therapeutic strategy in diabetic microvascular complications has been extensively tested and substantiated for diabetic nephropathy [103]. The latest 2008 guidelines of the American Diabetes Association recommend ACE inhibitors or ARBs as a first-line treatment in diabetic patients with micro- or macroalbuminuria independent of their blood pressure status [104]. Evidence for RAS blockade as a therapeutic option in diabetic retinopathy is much weaker due to a much lower number of randomized controlled clinical trials enrolling a sufficiently large patient cohort. The United Kingdom Prospective Diabetes Study (UKPDS) first showed the importance of tight control of blood pressure in reducing diabetic retinopathy, and this reduction was achieved by the ACE inhibitor captopril in one of the two treatment groups [105]. While the UKPDS focused more on the effect of blood pressure control, some earlier smaller studies already looked at the effect of RAS inhibition in normotensive diabetic patients and reported encouraging results [106–108]. The EUCLID (EURODIAB controlled trial of lisinopril in insulin-dependent diabetes mellitus) study was a 2-year randomized, double-blind, placebo-controlled study comparing the ACE inhibitor lisinopril with placebo in 530 normotensive, type 1 diabetic patients [109]. However, diabetic retinopathy was only a secondary endpoint in this study, and it was only evaluated in 354 of the 530 originally enrolled patients. Analysis of the EUCLID retinopathy data revealed a significant deceleration of retinopathy progression in the lisinopril-treated group. However, blood pressure and glucose control were slightly better in the lisinopril when compared to the placebo group; small differences but sufficiently robust to may have affected the study outcome [110]. The DIRECT study (DIabetic REtinopathy Candesartan Trials) program reported in September 2008 and represented the first series of clinical trials specifically designed to test the therapeutic efficiency of RAS blockade (by the ARB candesartan) in reducing incidence or progression of diabetic retinopathy in type 1 and type 2 diabetic patients [111, 112]. The DIRECT investigators found that in normotensive type 1 diabetic patients candesartan lowered the incidence of diabetic retinopathy, but had no impact on progression, while in normotensive and hypertensive type 2 diabetic patients progression but not incidence of diabetic retinopathy was reduced. More details of these studies are provided in the chapter by Porta and Hammes [this vol., pp 220–227].

Conclusions

Due to its high incidence among diabetic patients and the danger of vision loss, diabetic retinopathy is one of the mostly feared complications in diabetes. Current measures for the prevention of diabetic retinopathy are restricted to tight blood glucose and blood pressure control, while current treatment only applies to late, progressed stages of retinopathy and consists of quite invasive approaches such as laser photocoagulation or regular intravitreal injections of VEGF inhibitors. In vitro and in vivo preclinical studies have provided strong evidence for an involvement of the RAS in the pathomechanisms underlying diabetic retinopathy. The local, ocular RAS is overactivated in diabetic retinopathy, thus promoting retinal damage in two ways: (a) directly by inducing AT1 receptor-mediated, pathological actions such as increased VEGF expression, vasoconstriction, NF-κB activation, increased oxidative stress or ECM accumulation, and (b) by bidirectional interaction with the 'classical' hyperglycemia-induced pathobiochemical pathways (generation of AGEs, increased polyol pathway flux, activation of protein kinase C, increased hexosamine pathway flux, overproduction of superoxide). Pharmacological interference with the deregulated RAS in diabetic retinopathy by ACE inhibitors or ARBs has proven to be effective in a huge number of preclinical studies and most recently also in the first series of clinical studies specifically designed to test this therapeutic option.

References

1 Tigerstedt R, Bergman PG: Niere und Kreislauf. Skand Arch Physiol 1898;8:223–271.
2 Goldblatt H, Lynch J, Hanzal RF: Studies on experimental hypertension. J Exp Med 1934;59:347–379.
3 Braun-Mendenez E, Fasciolo JC, Leloir LF, Munoz JM: The substance causing renal hypertension. J Physiol 1940;98:283–298.
4 Page IH, Helmer OM: A cristalline pressor substance (angiotonin) resulting from the reaction between renin and renin activator. J Exp Med 1940;71:29–42.
5 Braun-Mendénez E, Page IH: Suggested revision of nomenclature: angiotensin. Science 1958;127:242.
6 Skeggs LT, Jr., Marsh WH, Kahn JR, Shumway NP: The existence of two forms of hypertensin. J Exp Med 1954;99:275–282.
7 Ferreira SH, Bartelt DC, Greene LJ: Isolation of bradykinin-potentiating peptides from Bothrops jararaca venom. Biochemistry 1970;9:2583–2593.
8 Mancia G (ed): Angiotensin II Receptor Antagonists. Abingdon, Informa HealthCare, 2006, pp 1–207.
9 Hershey JC, Steiner B, Fischli W, Feuerstein G: Renin inhibitors: An antihypertensive strategy on the verge of reality. Drug Discov Today Ther Strateg 2005;2:181–185.
10 Hernández Prada JA, Ferreira AJ, Katovich MJ, Shenoy V, Qi Y, Santos RA, Castellano RK, Lampkins AJ, Gubala V, Ostrov DA, Raizada MK: Structure-based identification of small-molecule angiotensin-converting enzyme 2 activators as novel antihypertensive agents. Hypertension 2008;51:1312–1317.
11 Wan Y, Wallinder C, Plouffe B, Beaudry H, Mahalingam AK, Wu X, Johansson B, Holm M, Botoros M, Karlen A, Pettersson A, Nyberg F, Fändriks L, Gallo-Payet N, Hallberg A, Alterman M: Design, synthesis, and biological evaluation of the first selective nonpeptide AT2 receptor agonist. J Med Chem 2004;47:5995–6008.
12 Steckelings, UM, Unger, T: The renin-angiotensin-aldosterone system; in Mancia G, Grassi G, Kjeldsen S (eds): Manual of Hypertension of The European Society of Hypertension. Abingdon, Informa HealthCare, 2008, vol 14, pp 110–116.
13 Jaspard E, Costerousse O, Wei L, Corvol P, Alhenc-Gelas F: The angiotensin I-converting enzyme (kinase II): molecular and regulatory aspects. Agents Actions Suppl 1992;38:349–358.
14 Paul M, Poyan Mehr A, Kreutz R: Physiology of local renin-angiotensin systems. Physiol Rev 2006;86:747–803.
15 de Gasparo M, Catt KJ, Inagami T, Wright JW, Unger T: International union of pharmacology. XXIII. The angiotensin II receptors. Pharmacol Rev 2000;52:415–472.
16 Wruck CJ, Funke-Kaiser H, Pufe T, Kusserow H, Menk M, Schefe JH, Kruse ML, Stoll M, Unger T: Regulation of transport of the angiotensin AT2 receptor by a novel membrane-associated Golgi protein. Arterioscler Thromb Vasc Biol 2005;25:57–64.
17 Nouet S, Amzallag N, Li JM, Louis S, Seitz I, Cui TX, Alleaume AM, Di Benedetto M, Boden C, Masson M, Strosberg AD, Horiuchi M, Couraud PO, Nahmias D: Trans-inactivation of receptor tyrosine kinase by novel angiotensin II AT2 receptor-interacting protein, ATIP. J Biol Chem 2004;279:28989–28997.

18 Senbonmatsu T, Saito T, Landon EJ, Watanabe O, Price E, Roberts RL, Imboden H, Fitzgerald TG, Gaffney FA, Inagami T: A novel angiotensin II type 2 receptor signaling pathway: possible role in cardiac hypertrophy. EMBO J 2003;22:6471–6482.
19 Steckelings UM, Kaschina E, Unger T: The AT2 receptor – a matter of love and hate. Peptides 2005;26:1401–1409.
20 Kaschina E, Grzesiak A, Li J, Foryst-Ludwig A, Timm M, Rompe F, Sommerfeld M, Kemnitz R, Curato C, Namsolleck P, Tschöpe C, Hallberg A, Alterman M, Hucko T, Paetsch I, Dietrich T, Schnackenburg B, Graf C, Dahlöf B, Kintscher U, Unger T, Steckelings UM: AT2-receptor stimulation: a novel option of therapeutic interference with the renin-angiotensin-system in myocardial infarction? Circulation 2008;118:2523–2532.
21 Tipnis SR, Hooper NM, Hyde R, Karran E, Christie G, Turner AJ: A human homolog of angiotensin-converting enzyme. Cloning and functional expression as a captopril-insensitive carboxypeptidase. J Biol Chem 2000;275:33238–33243.
22 Ferrario CM, Trask AJ, Jessup JA: Advances in biochemical and functional roles of angiotensin-converting enzyme 2 and angiotensin-(1–7) in regulation of cardiovascular function. Am J Physiol Heart Circ Physiol 2005;289:H2281–H2290.
23 Burckle C, Bader M: Prorenin and its ancient receptor. Hypertension 2006;48:549–551.
24 Nguyen G, Delarue F, Burckle C, Bouzhir L, Giller T, Sraer JD: Pivotal role of the renin/prorenin receptor in angiotensin II production and cellular responses to renin. J Clin Invest 2002;109:1417–1427.
25 Ganten D, Minnich JL, Granger P, Hayduk K, Brecht HM, Barbeau A, Boucher R, Genest J: Angiotensin-forming enzyme in brain tissue. Science 1971;173:64–65.
26 Ikemoto F, Yamamoto K: Renin-angiotensin system in the aqueous of rabbits, dogs and monkeys. Exp Eye Res 1978;27:723–725.
27 Danser AH, van den Dorpel MA, Deinum J, Derkx FH, Franken AA, Peperkamp E, de Jong PT, Schalekamp MA: Renin, prorenin, and immunoreactive renin in vitreous fluid from eyes with and without diabetic retinopathy. J Clin Endocrinol Metab 1989;68:160–167.
28 Deinum J, Derkx FH, Danser AH, Schalekamp MA: Renin in the bovine eye. J Hypertens Suppl 1989;7:S216–S217.
29 Berka JL, Stubbs AJ, Wang DZ, DiNicolantonio R, Alcorn D, Campbell DJ, Skinner SL: Renin-containing Muller cells of the retina display endocrine features. Invest Ophthalmol Vis Sci 1995;36:1450–1458.
30 Danser AH, Derkx FH, Admiraal PJ, Deinum J, de Jong PT, Schalekamp MA: Angiotensin levels in the eye. Invest Ophthalmol Vis Sci 1994;35:1008–1018.
31 Wagner J, Danser AH, Derkx FH, de Jong TV, Paul M, Mullins JJ, Schalekamp MA, Ganten D: Demonstration of renin mRNA, angiotensinogen mRNA, and angiotensin converting enzyme mRNA expression in the human eye: evidence for an intraocular renin-angiotensin system. Br J Ophthalmol 1996;80:159–163.
32 Sarlos S, Wilkinson-Berka JL. The renin-angiotensin system and the developing retinal vasculature. Invest Ophthalmol Vis Sci 2005;46:1069–1077
33 Sramek SJ, Wallow IH, Day RP, Ehrlich EN: Ocular renin-angiotensin: immunohistochemical evidence for the presence of prorenin in eye tissue. Invest Ophthalmol Vis Sci 1988;29:1749–1752.
34 Sramek SJ, Wallow IH, Tewksbury DA, Brandt CR, Poulsen GL: An ocular renin-angiotensin system. Immunohistochemistry of angiotensinogen. Invest Ophthalmol Vis Sci 1992;33:1627–1632.
35 Vita JB, Anderson JA, Hulem CD, Leopold IH: Angiotensin-converting enzyme activity in ocular fluids. Invest Ophthalmol Vis Sci 1981;20:255–257.
36 Weinreb RN, Sandman R, Ryder MI, Friberg TR: Angiotensin-converting enzyme activity in human aqueous humor. Arch Ophthalmol 1985;103:34–36.
37 Senanayake P, Drazba J, Shadrach K, Milsted A, Rungger-Brandle E, Nishiyama K, Miura S, Karnik S, Sears JE, Hollyfield JG: Angiotensin II and its receptor subtypes in the human retina. Invest Ophthalmol Vis Sci 2007;48:3301–3311.
38 Savaskan E, Loffler KU, Meier F, Muller-Spahn F, Flammer J, Meyer P: Immunohistochemical localization of angiotensin-converting enzyme, angiotensin II and AT1 receptor in human ocular tissues. Ophthalmic Res 2004;36:312–320.
39 Maruichi M, Oku H, Takai S, Muramatsu M, Sugiyama T, Imamura Y, Minami M, Ueki M, Satoh B, Sakaguchi M, Miyazaki M, Ikeda T: Measurement of activities in two different angiotensin II generating systems, chymase and angiotensin-converting enzyme, in the vitreous fluid of vitreoretinal diseases: a possible involvement of chymase in the pathogenesis of macular hole patients. Curr Eye Res 2004;29:321–325.
40 Shiota N, Saegusa Y, Nishimura K, Miyazaki M: Angiotensin II-generating system in dog and monkey ocular tissues. Clin Exp Pharmacol Physiol 1997;24:243–248.
41 Geng L, Persson K, Nilsson SF: Angiotensin converting anzyme (ACE) activity in porcine ocular tissue: effects of diet and ACE inhibitors. J Ocul Pharmacol Ther 2003;19:589–598.
42 Tikellis C, Johnston CI, Forbes JM, Burns WC, Thomas MC, Lew RA, Yarski M, Smith AI, Cooper ME. Identification of angiotensin converting enzyme 2 in the rodent retina. Curr Eye Res 2004;29:419–427
43 Price DA, Porter LE, Gordon M, Fisher NDL, De'Oliviera JMF, Laffel LMB, Passan DR, Williams GH, Hollenberg NK: The paradox of the low-renin state in diabetic nephropathy. J Am Soc Nephrol 1999;10:2382–2391.
44 Franken AA, Derkx FH, Schalekamp MA, Man in t'Veld AJ, Hop WC, van Rens EH, de Jong PT: Association of high plasma prorenin with diabetic retinopathy. J Hypertens Suppl 1988;6:S461–S463.
45 Yokota H, Mori F, Kai K, Nagaoka T, Izumi N, Takahashi A, Nikichi T, Yoshida A, Suzuki F, Ishida Y: Serum prorenin levels and diabetic retinopathy in type 2 diabetes: new method to measure serum level of prorenin using antibody activating direct kinetic assay. Br J Ophthalmol 2005;89:871–873.
46 Wilkinson-Berka JL: Angiotensin and diabetic retinopathy. Int J Biochem Cell Biol 2006;38:752–765.

47 Carey RM, Siragy HM: The intrarenal renin-angiotensin system and diabetic nephropathy. Trends Endocrinol Metab 2003;14:274–281.
48 Ebrahimian TG, Tamarat R, Clergue M, Duriez M, Levy BI, Silvestre JS: Dual effect of angiotensin-converting enzyme inhibition on angiogenesis in type 1 diabetic mice. Arterioscler Thromb Vasc Biol 2005;25:65–70.
49 Funatsu H, Yamashita H, Ikeda T, Nakanishi Y, Kitano S, Hori S: Angiotensin II and vascular endothelial growth factor in the vitreous fluid of patients with diabetic macular edema and other retinal disorders. Am J Ophthalmol 2002;133:537–543.
50 Toma I, Kang JJ, Sipos A, Vargas S, Bansal E, Hanner F, Meer E, Peti-Peterdi J: Succinate receptor GPR91 provides a direct link between high glucose levels and renin release in murine and rabbit kidney. J Clin Invest 2008;118:2526–2534.
51 Sapieha P, Sirinyan M, Hamel D, Zaniolo K, Joyal J-S, Cho J-H, Honoré J-C, Kermorvant-Duchemin E, Varma DR, Tremblay S, Leduc M, Rihakova L, Hardy P, Klein WH, Mu X, Mamer O, Lachapelle P, Di Polo A, Beauséjour C, Andelfinger G, Mitchell G, Sennlaub F, Chemtob S: The succinate receptor GPR91 in neurons has a major role in retinal angiogenesis. Nat Med 2008;14:1067–1076.
52 Brownlee M: Biochemistry and molecular cell biology of diabetic complications. Nature 2001;414:813–820.
53 Brownlee M: Banting lecture 2004. The pathobiology of diabetic complications: a unifying mechanism. Diabetes 2005;54:1615–1625.
54 Ellis EA, Grant MB, Murray FT, Wachowski MB, Guberski DL, Kubilis PS, Lutty GA: Increased NADH oxidase activity in the retina of the BBZ/Wor diabetic rat. Free Rad Biol Med 1998;24:111–201.
55 Förstermann U: Oxidative stress in vascular disease: causes, defense mechanisms and potential therapies. Nat Clin Pract Cardiovasc Med 2008;5:338–349.
56 Yamagishi S, Amano S, Inagaki Y, Okamoto T, Inoue H, Takeuchi M, Choei H, Sasaki N, Kikuchi S: Angiotensin II-type 1 receptor interaction upregulates vascular endothelial growth factor messenger RNA levels in retinal pericytes through intracellular reactive oxygen species generation. Drugs Exp Clin Res 2003;29:75–80.
57 Kawamura H, Kobayashi M, Li Q, Yamanishi S, Katsumura K, Minami M, Wu DM, Puro DG: Effects of angiotensin II on the pericyte-containing microvasculature of the rat retina. J Physiol 2004;561:671–683.
58 Ruiz-Ortega M, Lorenzo O, Egido, J: Angiotensin II increases monocytic chemotactic protein-1 and activates nuclear transcription factor κB and activator protein-1 in cultured mesangial and mononuclear cells. Kidney Int 2000;57:2285–2298.
59 Seshiah PN, Weber DS, Rocic P, Valppu L, Taniyama Y, Griendling KK: Angiotensin II stimulation of NAD(P)H oxidase activity: upstream mediators. Circ Res 2002;91:406–413.
60 Kato H, Suzuki H, Tajima S, Ogata Y, Tominaga T, Sato A, Saruta T: Angiotensin II stimulates collagen synthesis in cultured vascular smooth muscle cells. J Hypertens 1991;9:17–22.
61 Thomas MC, Tikellis C, Burns WM, Bialkowski K, Cao Z, Coughlan MT, Jandeleit-Dahm K, Cooper ME, Forbes JM: Interactions between renin angiotensin system and advanced glycation in the kidney. J Am Soc Nephrol 2005;16:2976–2984.
62 Clements RS Jr, Morrison AD, Winegrad AI: Polyol pathway in aorta: regulation by hormones. Science 1969;166:1007–1008.
63 Xu X, Zhu Q, Xia X, Zhang S, Gu Q, Luo D: Blood-retinal barrier breakdown induced by activation of protein kinase C via vascular endothelial growth factor in streptozotocin-induced diabetic rats. Curr Eye Res 2004;28:251–256.
64 Otani A, Takagi H, Oh H, Koyama S, Honda Y: Angiotensin II induces expression of the Tie2 receptor ligand, angiopoietin-2, in bovine retinal endothelial cells. Diabetes 2001;50:867–875.
65 Policha A, Daneshtalab N, Chen L, Dale LB, Altier C, Khosravani H, Thomas WG, Zamponi GW, Ferguson SSG: Role of angiotensin II type 1A receptor phosphorylation, phospholipase D, and extracellular calcium in isoform-specific protein kinase C membrane translocation responses. J Biol Chem 2006;281:26340–26349.
66 Williams B, Gallacher B, Patel H, Orme D: Glucose-induced protein kinase C activation regulates vascular permeability factor mRNA expression and peptide production by human vascular smooth muscle cells in vitro. Diabetes 1997;46:1497–1503.
67 Yokota T, Ma RC, Park J-Y, Isshiki K, Sotiropoulos KB, Rauniyar RK, Bornfeldt KE, King GL: Role of protein kinase C on the expression of platelet-derived growth factor and endothelin-1 in the retina of diabetic rats and cultured retinal capillary pericytes. Diabetes 2003;52:838–845.
68 Feener EP, Xia P, Inoguchi T, Shiba T, Kunisaki M, King GL: Role of protein kinase C in glucose- and angiotensin II-induced plasminogen activator inhibitor expression. Contrib Nephrol 1996;118:180–187.
69 Koya D, Jirousek MR, Lin YW, Ishii H, Kuboki K, King GL: Characterization of protein kinase C beta isoform activation on the gene expression of transforming growth factor-beta, extracellular matrix components, and prostanoids in the glomeruli of diabetic rats. J Clin Invest 1997;100:115–126.
70 Kuboki K, Jiang ZY, Takahara N, Ha SW, Igarashi M, Yamauchi T, Feener EP, Herbert TP, Rhodes CJ, King GL: Regulation of endothelial constitutive nitric oxide synthase gene expression in endothelial cells and in vivo: a specific vascular action of insulin. Circulation 2000;101:676–681.
71 Ishii H, Jirousek MR, Koya D, Takagi C, Xia P, Clermont A, Bursell SE, Kern TS, Ballas LM, Heath WF, Stramm LE, Feener EP, King GL: Amelioration of vascular dysfunctions in diabetic rats by an oral PKC beta inhibitor. Science 1996;272:728–731.
72 Yerneni KK, Bai W, Khan BV, Medford RM, Natarajan R: Hyperglycemia-induced activation of nuclear transcription factor kappaB in vascular smooth muscle cells. Diabetes 1999;48:855–864.

73 Nagai N, Izumi-Nagai K, Oike Y, Koto T, Satofuka S, Ozawa Y, Yamashiro K, Inoue M, Tsubota K, Umezawa K, Ishida S: Suppression of diabetes-induced retinal inflammation by blocking the angiotensin II type 1 receptor or its downstream nuclear factor-kappaB pathway. Invest Ophthalmol Vis Sci 2007;48:4342–4350.
74 Gabriely I, Yang XM, Cases JA, Ma XH, Rossetti L, Barzilai N: Hyperglycemia modulates angiotensinogen gene expression. Am J Physiol Regul Integr Comp Physiol 2001;281:795–802.
75 Hsieh TJ, Fustier P, Zhang SL, Filep JG, Tang SS, Ingelfinger JR, Fantus IG, Hamet P, Chan JS: High glucose stimulates angiotensinogen gene expression and cell hypertrophy via activation of the hexosamine biosynthesis pathway in rat kidney proximal tubular cells. Endocrinology 2003;144:4338–4349.
76 Chen P, Guo AM, Edwards PA, Trick G, Scicli AG: Role of NADPH oxidase and ANG II in diabetes-induced retinal leukostasis. Am J Physiol Regul Integr Comp Physiol 2007;293:1619–1629.
77 Fukumoto M, Takai S, Ishizaki E, Sugiyama T, Oku H, Jin D, Sakaguchi M, Sakonjo H, Ikeda T, Miyazaki M: Involvement of angiotensin II-dependent vascular endothelial growth factor gene expression via NADPH oxidase in the retina in a type 2 diabetic rat model. Curr Eye Res 2008;33:885–891.
78 Banday AA, Lokhandwala MF: Oxidative stress-induced renal angiotensin AT1 receptor upregulation causes increased stimulation of sodium transporters and hypertension. Am J Physiol Renal Physiol 2008;295:698–706.
79 Cheng XW, Murohara T, Kuzuya M, Izawa H, Sasaki T, Obata K, Nagata K, Nishizawa T, Kobayashi M, Yamada T, Kim W, Sato K, Shi GP, Okumura K, Yokota M: Superoxide-dependent cathepsin activation is associated with hypertensive myocardial remodeling and represents a target for angiotensin II type 1 receptor blocker treatment. Am J Pathol 2008;173:358–369.
80 Clermont A, Bursell SE, Feener EP: Role of the angiotensin II type 1 receptor in the pathogenesis of diabetic retinopathy: effects of blood pressure control and beyond. J Hypertens Suppl 2006;24:73–80.
81 Sugiyama T, Okuno T, Fukuhara M, Oku H, Ikeda T, Obayashi H, Ohta M, Fukui M, Hasegawa G, Nakamura N: Angiotensin II receptor blocker inhibits abnormal accumulation of advanced glycation end products and retinal damage in a rat model of type 2 diabetes. Exp Eye Res 2007;85:406–412.
82 Fan Q, Liao J, Kobayashi M, Yamashita M, Gu L, Gohda T, Suzuki Y, Wang LN, Horikoshi S, Tomino Y: Candesartan reduced advanced glycation end-products accumulation and diminished nitro-oxidative stress in type 2 diabetic KK/Ta mice. Nephrol Dial Transplant 2004;19:3012–3020.
83 Mori F, Hikichi T, Nagaoka T, Takahashi J, Kitaya N, Yoshida A: Inhibitory effect of losartan, an AT1 angiotensin II receptor antagonist, on increased leucocyte entrapment in retinal microcirculation of diabetic rats. Br J Ophthalmol 2002;86:1172–1174.
84 Malhotra A, Kang BPS, Cheung S, Opawumi D, Meggs LG: Angiotensin II promotes glucose-induced activation of cardiac protein kinase C isozymes and phosphorylation of troponin I. Diabetes 2001;50:1918–1926.
85 Osicka TM, Yu Y, Lee V, Panagiotopoulos S, Kemp BE, Jerums G: Aminoguanidine and ramipril prevent diabetes induced increases in protein kinase C activity in glomeruli, retina and mesenteric artery. Clin Sci 2001;100:249–257.
86 Jesmin S, Sakuma I, Hattori Y, Kitabatake A: Role of angiotensin II in altered expression of molecules responsible for coronary matrix remodeling in insulin-resistant diabetic rats. Arterioscler Thromb Vasc Biol 2003;23:2021–2026.
87 Feke GT, Buzney SM, Ogasawara H, Fujio N, Goger DG, Spack NP, Gabbay KH: Retinal circulatory abnormalities in type 1 diabetes. Invest Ophthalmol Vis Sci 1994;35:2968–2975.
88 Das Evcimen N, King GL: The role of protein kinase C activation and the vascular complications of diabetes. Pharmacol Res 2007;55:498–510.
89 Aiello LP, Clermont AC, Arora V, Davis MD, Sheetz MJ, Bursell S-E: Inhibition of PKC beta by oral administration of ruboxistaurin is well tolerated and ameliorates diabetes-induced retinal hemodynamic abnormalities in patients. Invest Ophthalmol Vis Sci 2006;47:86–92.
90 Horio N, Clermont AC, Abiko A, Abiko T, Shoelson BD, Bursell S-E, Feener EP: Angiotensin AT_1 receptor antagonism normalizes retinal blood flow and acetylcholine-induced vasodiliation in normotensive diabetic rats. Diabetologia 2004;47:113–123.
91 Iwase M, Doi Y, Goto D, Ichikawa K, Iino K, Yoshinari M, Fujishima M: Effect of nicardipine versus enalapril on plasma endothelin-1 in hypertensive patients with type 2 diabetes mellitus. Clin Exp Hypertens 2000;22:695–703.
92 Nuwayri-Salti N, Karam CH, Al Jaroudi WA, Usta JA, Maharsy WM, Bitar KM, Bikhazi AB: Effect of type-1 diabetes mellitus on the regulation of insulin and endothelin-1 receptors in rat hearts. Can J Physiol Pharmacol 2007;85:215–224.
93 Liang W, Tan CYR, Ang L, Granville DJ, Wright JM, Laher I: Ramipril improves oxidative stress–related vascular endothelial dysfunction in db/db mice. J Physiol Sci 2008;58:405–411.
94 Gilbert RE, Kelly DJ, Cox AJ, Wilkinson-Berka JL, Rumble JR, Osicka T, Panagiotopoulos S, Lee V, Hendrich EC, Jerums G, Cooper ME: Angiotensin converting enzyme inhibition reduces retinal overexpression of vascular endothelial growth factor and hyperpermeability in experimental diabetes. Diabetologia 2000;43:1360–1387.
95 Nagisa Y, A. Shintani, Nakagawa S: The angiotensin II receptor antagonist candesartan cilexetil (TCV-116) ameliorates retinal disorders in rats Diabetologia. 2001;44:883–888.
96 Moravski CJ, Skinner SL, Stubbs AJ, Sarlos S, Kelly DJ, Cooper ME, Gilbert RE, Wilkinson-Berka JL: The renin-angiotensin system influences ocular endothelial cell proliferation in diabetes: transgenic and interventional studies. Am J Pathol 2003;162:151–160.
97 Wilkinson-Berka JL, Tan G, Jaworski K, Ninkovic S: Valsartan but not atenolol improves vascular pathology in diabetic Ren-2 rat retina. Am J Hypertens 2007;20:423–430.
98 Manea A, Constantinescu E, Popov D, Raicu M: Changes in oxidative balance in rat pericytes exposed to diabetic conditions. J Cell Mol Med 2004;8:117–126.

99 Onozato ML, Tojo A, Goto A, Fujita T, Wilcox CS: Oxidative stress and nitric oxide synthase in rat diabetic nephropathy: effects of ACEI and ARB. Kidney Int 2002;61:186–194.
100 Chiarelli F, Di Marzio D, Santilli F, Mohn A, Blasetti A, Cipollone F, Mezzetti A, Verrotti A: Effects of irbesartan on intracellular antioxidant enzyme expression and activity in adolescents and young adults with early diabetic angiopathy. Diab Care 2005;28:1690–1697.
101 Chen S, Ge Y, Si J, Rifai A, Dworkin LD, Gong R: Candesartan suppresses chronic renal inflammation by a novel antioxidant action independent of AT1R blockade. Kidney Int 2008;74:1128–1138.
102 Izuhara Y, Sada T, Yanagisawa H, Koike H, Ohtomo S, Dan T, Ito S, Nangaku M, van Ypersele de Strihou C, Miyata T: A novel sartan derivative with very low angiotensin II type 1 receptor affinity protects the kidney in type 2 diabetic rats. Arterioscler Thromb Vasc Biol 2008;28:1767–1773.
103 Ruilope LM: Angiotensin receptor blockers: RAAS blockade and renoprotection. Curr Med Res Opin 2008;24:1285–1293.
104 American Diabetes Association. Standards of medical care in diabetes – 2008. Diabetes Care 2008;31(suppl 1): S12–S54.
105 UK Prospective Study Group: Tight blood pressure control and risk of macrovascular and microvascular complications in type 2 diabetes: UKPDS 38, BMJ 1998;317:703–713.
106 Larsen M, Hommel E, Parving HH, Lund-Andersen H: Protective effect of captopril on the blood-retina barrier in normotensive insulin-dependent diabetic patients with nephropathy and background retinopathy, Graefes Arch Clin Exp Ophthalmol 1990;228:505–509.
107 Chase HP, Garg SK, Harris S, Hoops S, Jackson WE, Holmes DL: Angiotensin-converting enzyme inhibitor treatment for young normotensive diabetic subjects: a two-year trial. Ann Ophthalmol 1993;25:284–289.
108 Ravid M, Savin H, Lang R, Jutrin I, Shoshana L, Lishner M: Proteinuria, renal impairment, metabolic control, and blood pressure in type 2 diabetes mellitus. A 14-year follow-up report on 195 patients, Arch Intern Med 1992;152:1225–1229.
109 Chaturvedi N, Sjolie A-K, Stephenson JM, Abrahamian H, Keipes M, Castellarin A, Rogulja-Pepeonik Z, Fuller JH, the EUCLID Study Group: Effect of lisinopril on progression of retinopathy in normotensive people with type 1 diabetes. Lancet 1998;351:28–31.
110 Sjolie AK: Prospects for angiotensin receptor blockers in diabetic retinopathy. Diab Res Clin Prac 2007;76S: S31–S39.
111 Chaturvedi N, Porta M, Klein R, Orchard T, Fuller J, Parving HH, Bilous R, Sjølie AK, for the DIRECT Programme Study Group: Effect of candesartan on prevention (DIRECT-Prevent 1) and progression (DIRECT-Protect 1) of retinopathy in type 1 diabetes: randomised, placebo-controlled trials. Lancet 2008;372:1394–1402.
112 Sjølie AK, Klein R, Porta M, Orchard T, Fuller J, Parving HH, Bilous R, Chaturvedi N, for the DIRECT Programme Study Group: Effect of candesartan on progression and regression of retinopathy in type 2 diabetes (DIRECT-Protect 2): a randomised placebo-controlled trial. Lancet 2008;372:1385–1393.

Dr. Ulrike Muscha Steckelings
Center for Cardiovascular Research, Institute of Pharmacology
Charité-Universitätsmedizin Berlin
Hessische Strasse 3–4, DE–10115 Berlin (Germany)
Tel. +49 30 450 525 024, Fax +49 30 450 525 901, E-Mail ulrike.steckelings@charite.de

Hammes H-P, Porta M (eds): Experimental Approaches to Diabetic Retinopathy.
Front Diabetes. Basel, Karger, 2010, vol 20, pp 158–173

Interactions of Leukocytes with the Endothelium

Triantafyllos Chavakis

Experimental Immunology Branch, NCI, NIH, Bethesda, Md., USA

Abstract

Leukocyte recruitment is integral to both the innate and adaptive immune response. Leukocytes extravasate to sites of inflammation, injury or infection and leukocyte recruitment is crucial to a variety of inflammatory and autoimmune diseases. The process of leukocyte extravasation comprises a complex multistep cascade of adhesive interactions between leukocytes and the endothelium in the vessel wall. These adhesive events are tightly orchestrated by the crosstalk between adhesion receptors on both leukocytes and endothelial cells, as well as by several chemokine receptors, and control how different leukocyte subpopulations are recruited into specific tissues. Targeting leukocyte recruitment is of great therapeutic importance in inflammatory pathologies; specific inhibitors of leukocyte recruitment have already been used successfully in autoimmune diseases. Thus, understanding of the mechanisms regulating the leukocyte adhesion cascade as well as the tissue- and vascular bed-specific leukocyte recruitment will allow for the development of further novel therapeutic approaches with potential application in inflammatory and autoimmune diseases. The present review will (a) focus on the molecular mechanisms of the leukocyte adhesion cascade governing the interactions between leukocytes and endothelial cells and (b) address the potential role of leukocyte-endothelial interactions in the retina, and in particular, the potential role of inflammation in diabetic retinopathy.

Multistep Process of Leukocyte Recruitment

Leukocytes are divided into different subpopulations. Whereas naïve lymphocytes continuously circulate through the secondary lymphoid organs, activated effector lymphocytes as well as neutrophils and macrophages, the latter two representing the first line of defense in innate immunity, respond to inflammatory signals, thereby extravasating from the blood into the site of inflammation, injury or infection. Neutrophils are recruited to the site of acute inflammation within a few hours, and play a major role in tissue destruction by means of their cytotoxic mediators [1–5]. In contrast to the short-lived granulocytes, monocytes arrive to the inflammatory site later and can reside in the tissue for a long time differentiating into macrophages or dendritic cells. Thus, besides being the major phagocytic cells in the defense to pathogens, monocytes also participate in chronic inflammatory diseases, such as atherosclerosis [1, 6].

The present chapter will focus on mechanisms governing the recruitment of leukocytes to the site of inflammation or injury. This process usually takes place at postcapillary venules and comprises a complex multistep cascade of adhesive interactions between the leukocytes and the endothelium as well as migratory events of the leukocytes through the endothelium and beyond. These interactions are mediated by three types of adhesion receptors, the selectins, integrins and the receptors of the immunoglobulin superfamily. These steps are (a) the initial selectin-mediated rolling; (b) the leukocyte activation; (c) the integrin-dependent firm adhesion, and (d) the subsequent transendothelial migration as well as the migration through the subendothelial extracellular matrix [1, 7–13].

Rolling represents the initial tethering of leukocytes along the endothelial cell surface. Rolling adhesions are transient and reversible and function to slow down the flowing leukocytes. They are mediated by weak interactions between selectins, such as the E-, P- or L-selectin with their carbohydrate ligands, such as P-selectin glycoprotein-1 (PSGL-1) [14]. Whereas leukocytes express L-selectin, endothelial cells express P- and E-selectin, which are recognized by leukocyte PSGL-1. The PSGL-1-dependent interactions of leukocytes with P- and E-selectin differ in their temporal regulation, which relies on the different time course of expression/exposure of these selectins on the luminal endothelial cell surface. Whereas P-selectin is stored intracellulary in Weibel-Palade bodies and is rapidly exocytosed to the luminal surface upon endothelial cell activation with several stimuli, E-selectin is constitutively absent from the endothelium, but is newly synthesized after a few hours upon pro-inflammatory stimulation [14, 15]. Besides mediating fast rolling, the interaction between PSGL-1 with P- and E-selectin plays an important role in the slow rolling process. However, slow rolling, which represents the transition between fast rolling and firm adhesion, is a rather complex process. In fact, the classical leukocyte arrest receptors, the leukocyte integrins, and particularly the β_2-integrin lymphocyte function antigen-1 (LFA-1), which are outlined in the next paragraphs, have also been implicated in such slow rolling adhesions promoting firm adhesiveness from rolling [16, 17]. In addition to being the brake for the flowing leukocytes by mediating both fast and slow rolling, selectin-dependent adhesive events between the leukocytes and the endothelium also function to mediate the initial contact of leukocytes with chemokines that are present on luminal endothelial cell surface. This results in the chemokine-induced leukocyte activation, which is required for the integrin activation on leukocytes, thereby priming the subsequent firm adhesion step [18].

The ligation of leukocyte chemokine receptors by chemokine signals present on the luminal surface of the endothelial cells signals the 'inside-out' activation of the leukocyte integrins, thereby promoting strong binding interactions between integrins and their endothelial counter-receptors [13, 18]. Some chemokines, such as CC-chemokine ligand 5 (also known as RANTES) and CXC-chemokine ligand 8 (also known as interleukin-8), are present on the luminal endothelial surface associated with transmembrane heparan sulphate proteoglycans [19, 20], thereby eliciting a rapid integrin activation in rolling leukocytes. Another function of chemoattractants/chemokines and their G-protein-coupled receptors is to guide leukocyte migration within the tissue to the site of inflammation [21].

The firm arrest of leukocytes on the endothelium is mediated by interactions between leukocyte integrins and their endothelial counter-receptors of the immunoglobulin superfamily. The predominant leukocyte integrins involved in firm adhesion are VLA-4 ($\alpha_4\beta_1$), $\alpha_4\beta_7$-integrin, Mac-1 ($\alpha M\beta_2$) and LFA-1 ($\alpha L\beta_2$). The endothelial counter-receptors are the intercellular adhesion molecules (ICAM), the vascular cell adhesion molecule-1 (VCAM-1), the mucosal addressin cell adhesion molecule-1, or the receptor for advanced glycation end products (RAGE), which are constitutively expressed, upregulated or induced on the inflamed endothelium [9, 22–24]. VLA-4 binds to VCAM-1, whereas β_2-integrins (including LFA-1 and Mac-1) bind to ICAM1–5 [9, 22–24]. ICAM-1 and ICAM-2 are the major β_2-integrin ligands on the endothelium; ICAM-3 and ICAM-4 are predominantly expressed on blood cells, and ICAM-5 on brain neurons [24–28]. RAGE serves as a counter-receptor of Mac-1 but not LFA-1 on innate immune cells [23].

Firmly adherent leukocytes move slowly over the endothelial cell surface searching for a near junction. This process is designated crawling or locomotion and requires the integrins Mac-1 and LFA-1 [29, 30]. Leukocytes then migrate through the endothelium. The process of transendothelial migration or diapedesis primarily takes place at the intercellular junctions, i.e. in a paracellular way; however, leukocytes may also extravasate by transcytosis through the endothelial cells [9, 10, 12, 31–36]. Diapedesis involves several heterophilic interactions, such as the binding of integrins Mac-1 and LFA-1 to their counter-receptors ICAM-1, ICAM-2 or to members of the junctional adhesion molecule (JAM) family, as well as several homophilic interactions between platelet endothelial cell adhesion molecule-1 (PECAM-1) or CD99 [31–33]. The process of transendothelial migration will be discussed in detail below.

Regulation of Leukocyte Integrin-Mediated Adhesion

It is clear that integrins are crucial players of the multistep cascade in leukocyte recruitment. Their major importance for leukocyte trafficking and the immune response is suggested by studies utilizing mice deficient in one or more leukocyte β_2-integrins [37–40] and more importantly by the immunodeficiency observed in the leukocyte adhesion deficiency syndrome (LAD) in men lacking β_2-integrins or in men having dysfunctional integrins [41–45]. LAD I in men is due to a complete deficiency in the β_2-integrins $\alpha M\beta_2$, $\alpha L\beta_2$, $\alpha X\beta_2$ and $\alpha D\beta_2$ as a result of mutations in the common β_2-subunit, and these patients exhibit recurrent bacterial infections [22, 41]. In addition, LAD I 'variants' have been reported, in which patients have intact but dysfunctional β_1-, β_2- and β_3-integrins, suggesting a defect in signaling pathways for integrin activation [42–46]. In addition, leukocyte integrins are important therapeutic targets for inflammatory and autoimmune disorders. Inhibitory antibodies against VLA-4 and LFA-1 are effective therapeutic approaches in multiple sclerosis and psoriasis, respectively [47, 48]. Thus, understanding the complex process of the regulation of integrin-mediated leukocyte adhesion is of major importance and will be outlined here.

The activity of leukocyte integrins and thereby the adhesiveness of leukocytes is predominantly regulated by changes in integrin affinity and in integrin valency, whereas integrin expression on leukocytes remains mostly unaffected. The affinity of integrins for their ligands is regulated by conformational changes, whereas integrin valency is modulated by changes in the lateral distribution of the integrins on the plasma membrane [13, 49, 50]. Leukocyte integrins may exist in three different affinity conformations representing the low, intermediate or high affinity [51–54]. The transition into high affinity states of integrins can be induced by 'inside-out' signaling pathways that may result in the separation of the cytoplasmic tails of the α- and β-subunits [55, 56].

Activation of rolling leukocytes by immobilized chemokines or chemokines presented on the apical endothelial cell surface can trigger rapid 'inside-out' activation of integrin affinity [57, 58], in part by signaling that involves phospholipase C [59]. Phospholipase C signaling stimulates the guanidine exchange factor CALDAG-GEFI that activates the small GTPase Rap1. Rap1 belongs to the Ras family of small GTPases and can mediate the chemokine-induced stimulation of LFA-1 and VLA-4-integrin affinity and integrin-dependent leukocyte adhesion [60–62] by utilizing effector proteins such as RAPL and RIAM [63–68].

Whereas the Rap1-RAPL pathway primarily targets the integrin α-chain, the cytoskeletal protein talin can associate with β-integrin subunits, thereby inducing the separation of the cytoplasmic tails and high affinity conformational changes of the integrin. Talin may interact with RIAM, thereby mediating the integrin-activating signals of Rap1 [69–71]. The binding of talin to the integrin β-chain, which is mediated by the NPXY motif of the cytoplasmic tails of β-integrin subunits is enhanced by proteolytic modification of talin by calpain and phosphoinositol phosphate kinase type Iγ-derived signals [72, 73].

The phosphorylation of the cytoplasmic tails of the integrin α- and β-chains is another event during inside-out signaling activation [74–76]. The αL-chain of LFA-1 is constitutively phosphorylated at Ser-1140, and mutation of this residue abrogates the Rap1-induced integrin activation [74], whereas the phosphorylation of T758 of the β-chain of LFA-1 is induced by phorbol ester or downstream of T cell receptor activation [74]. The T758 phosphorylation mediates interactions of the integrin with the multifunctional adaptor proteins of the 14-3-3 family and modulates LFA-1-mediated cell adhesion and spreading [74, 77, 78]. Besides the inside-out signaling pathways regulating integrin activation, lateral associations of the integrins with adaptor molecules on the cell membrane may also regulate leukocyte integrin-mediated adhesion. Tetraspanins, CD47, CD98, RAGE as well as the glycolipid-anchored urokinase receptor and Fc receptors have been indentified as lateral interaction partners of leukocyte integrins that regulate predominantly integrin clustering and valency [79–81].

In contrast to 'inside-out' signaling activation of integrins, which results in increased integrin affinity and leukocyte adhesion, the further stabilization of initial adhesion of leukocytes on the endothelium requires 'outside-in' integrin signaling, i.e. signaling upon integrin ligation, also designated as ligand-induced post-adhesion strengthening [82]. Multiple pathways have been implicated in ligand-induced postadhesion strengthening, including the src-like kinases Hck and Fgr, Vav1 and Vav3, as well as WASP. For example, Vav1/Vav3 double-deficient or WASP-deficient neutrophils displayed normal initial arrest but decreased sustained adhesion associated with reduced resistance to detachment under shear [82–84]. Taken together, integrin-mediated adhesion of leukocytes is regulated by several fine coordinated complex signaling pathways.

Several exogenous and endogenous inhibitors of integrin-mediated leukocyte adhesion have been described. Exogenous microbial-derived inhibitors of the leukocyte adhesion cascade include the canine hookworm *(Ancylostoma caninum)*-derived neutrophil inhibitory factor, the filamentous hemagglutinin of *Bordetella pertussis* and the *Staphylococcus aureus*-derived extracellular adherence protein that block β_2-integrin-dependent inflammatory cell recruitment [85–88]. Less is known about endogenous inhibitors of the leukocyte adhesion cascade. Developmental endothelial locus-1 (Del-1) is a potent inhibitor of leukocyte recruitment. Del-1 is a secreted endothelial-derived protein expressed in embryonic development and in adult immunoprivileged tissues such as the brain and the eye as well as in the lung vessels [89–91]. Del-1 is secreted by endothelial cells and most likely associates with the endothelial surface and matrix [89–92]. Del-1 is a ligand of LFA-1, but it functions to interfere with LFA-1-dependent adhesion to ICAM-1 and the endothelium. Del-$1^{-/-}$ mice displayed increased numbers of leukocytes adhering onto the endothelium of postcapillary venules as compared to wild-type mice, as well as enhanced neutrophil recruitment in LPS-induced lung inflammation. The proinflammatory phenotype of Del-$1^{-/-}$ mice was reversed in Del-1-/LFA-1-double deficient mice, suggesting that Del-1 specifically antagonizes LFA-1-dependent inflammatory cell recruitment [91]. Del-1 acts in an autocrine/paracrine manner as a local inhibitor of leukocyte adhesion. Galectin-1 is another endogenous inhibitor of leukocyte recruitment that inhibits T cell rolling and adhesion to activated endothelial cells. Consistently, effector T cell and neutrophil recruitment was increased in galectin-1-deficient mice [93, 94].

Leukocyte Transendothelial Migration

During transendothelial migration or diapedesis, leukocytes extravasate across the endothelial cell monolayer. Leukocyte transmigration may take place in a paracellular manner between the interendothelial borders or in a transcellular manner through the endothelial cell body [12]. Endothelial cells communicate with each other via interendothelial adhesions or junctions that are crucial in maintaining the endothelial barrier and vascular integrity, thereby also regulating both vascular permeability and the rate of leukocyte transmigration. In contrast to gap junctions that do not constitute a barrier for the transmigrating leukocytes, both tight and adherens junctions regulate the rate of leukocyte transmigration [95, 96]. The hierarchically most important adherens junctions (zonula adherens) are formed by cadherins that promote calcium-dependent, homophilic cell-cell adhesion. VE-cadherin (cadherin-5) is the endothelial-specific cadherin in the interendothelial junctions. Cadherins are linked to the actin cytoskeleton by their interaction with intracellular catenins. VE-cadherin is a major gatekeeper for the passage of leukocytes, since inhibition of VE-cadherin increased the rate of neutrophil extravasation in vivo [97]. Consistently, in vitro studies demonstrated the transient disappearance of VE-cadherin from the junctions during leukocyte transmigration [98]. Tight junctions (zonula occludens) lie apically to adherens junctions, and are formed by adhesive interactions between three different types of transmembrane proteins, occludin, claudins and JAMs [95, 96].

JAMs and the JAM-related endothelial selective adhesion molecule (ESAM) belong to the immunoglobulin superfamily, consisting of two extracellular Ig-like domains [99–102]. At their final carboxy-terminus, JAMs have a class-II PDZ domain-binding motif, which allows them to interact with PDZ-domain-containing molecules, such as the ones found in tight junctions [99–102]. JAM-A is expressed on endothelial and epithelial cells as well as on different circulating blood cells including platelets, monocytes and lymphocytes [103, 104]. JAM-B and JAM-C localize on vascular and lymphatic endothelium [104–106]. JAM-C is also expressed on platelets, activated B-cells and smooth muscle cells [106–108]. JAMs interact homophilically through a conserved motif in their membrane-distal domain [109, 110]. JAMs also function as counter-receptors for leukocyte integrins; in particular, JAM-A binds to LFA-1 [111], JAM-B binds to VLA-4 [112] and JAM-C interacts with Mac-1 [106]. In addition, JAM-C also binds to JAM-B [113, 114]. A role for JAM-A in diapedesis has been shown by experiments with blocking antibodies and genetically modified mice [115–117]. Both the homophilic interaction of JAM-A as well as its heterophilic interaction with β_2-integrin LFA-1 could promote transendothelial migration of leukocytes. The heterophilic binding of JAM-C to Mac-1 was found to mediate a firm platelet-leukocyte interaction [106]. JAM-C overexpression in mice increased neutrophil recruitment, whereas soluble JAM-C reduced neutrophil transmigration in vitro and in vivo [118, 119]. The exact mechanism by which JAMs regulate leukocyte transmigration and recruitment needs further investigation. Interestingly, JAM-C and ESAM can disrupt the interendothelial barrier by regulating the activity of small GTPases such as Rap1 or RhoA and thereby VE-cadherin-mediated adherens junctions [120, 121]. The disruption of the endothelial barrier by JAM-C and ESAM may also contribute to their function in leukocyte diapedesis.

PECAM-1 is a member of the Ig gene superfamily with six Ig-like domains and is expressed on platelets, neutrophils and monocytes as well as at the interendothelial borders [31]. The homophilic interaction mediated by Ig domains 1 and 2 of PECAM-1 is established as a player in transendothelial migration in vitro and in vivo [122–124]. PECAM blockade inhibits transmigration and leukocytes stay adherent on the apical endothelial cell surface [31]. Endothelial PECAM-1 recycles in vesicular structures between the junctions and the subjunctional plasma membrane. This recycling mechanism allows the targeted concentrated localisation of PECAM-1 to the area where leukocyte transmigration takes place [125]. The membrane-proximal Ig domains 5 and 6 of PECAM-1 are involved in heterophilic interactions and the neutrophil-specific antigen CD177 has been identified as an interaction partner of PECAM-1. This heterophilic interaction may also mediate transmigration [126]. Besides its direct participation in transmigration, PECAM-1 homophilic ligation signals to upregulate $\alpha_6\beta_1$-integrin on transmigrating leukocytes, thereby enhancing their subsequent penetration across the basement membrane [127].

CD99 is a molecule expressed on both leukocytes and at the interendothelial cell-cell contacts and functions in a homophilic fashion during transmigration. CD99 controls a distal step in diapedesis through the junctions, as CD99 blockade resulted in monocytes being stopped halfway across the endothelial junction [31, 128].

In addition to the crucial role of ICAM-1 and ICAM-2 in mediating β_2-integrin-dependent leukocyte adhesion to the endothelium, these molecules are also important for transendothelial migration. During transmigration, LFA-1 redistributes and forms a ring-like cluster at the site of contact between the neutrophil and the endothelial junctional surface, where transmigration takes place. The endothelial LFA-1 ligand ICAM-1 colocalizes with the LFA-1 ring [36]. In addition, a 'cuplike' structure that has microvilli-like projections highly enriched in ICAM-1 has been demonstrated to accompany transmigrating leukocytes during transcellular diapedesis through the endothelial cell body [35]. Intravital microscopy studies with ICAM-2-deficient mice and studies engaging ICAM-2-blocking antibodies suggested a role of ICAM-2 in leukocyte transmigration in vivo [129].

Taken together, the recent advances in the understanding of the leukocyte adhesion and transmigration cascade have opened new venues for therapeutic strategies to prevent or modulate leukocyte recruitment in inflammatory and autoimmune pathologies [130].

Leukocyte-Endothelial Interactions in the Diabetic Retina

Multiple studies have established that leukocyte recruitment could be increased under pathophysiological conditions, such as in atherosclerosis, hypercholesterolemia and in diabetes [131]. Animal models of ischemia/reperfusion have shown that the presence of diabetes mellitus further upregulates leukocyte recruitment [132, 133]. These events are dependent on interactions between leukocyte integrins and their endothelial counter-receptors. Elevated expression of ICAM-1 has been demonstrated in blood vessels of diabetic patients and diabetic animals [134, 135] and elevated levels of soluble ICAM-1 and soluble VCAM-1 have been detected in serum of patients with insulin-dependent diabetes [136, 137], a phenomenon that could be linked to the hyperglycemia.

Hyperglycemia can promote leukocyte-endothelial interactions. Glucose can stimulate NF-κB- and protein kinase C-dependent pathways in endothelial cells resulting in the upregulation of endothelial adhesion molecules, such as

ICAM-1 or E-selectin [138–140]. Another pathway by which glucose could stimulate leukocyte-endothelial adhesion is through upregulation of the enzyme activity of 6-N-acetyl glucosaminyl-transferase (core 2 GlcNac-T) in leukocytes. Higher core 2 GlcNac-T activity results in stronger posttranslational modification of glycans on the leukocyte surface, i.e. in increased O-linked glycosylation of PSGL-1, thereby promoting leukocyte rolling interactions to endothelial selectins [141–143].

In addition, chronic diabetes is characterized by the generation and accumulation of advanced glycation end products (AGEs), which are the products of nonenzymatic glycation and oxidation of proteins and lipids. AGEs interact with their cellular receptor, RAGE [144, 145]. In diabetes, AGEs include carboxymethyllysine protein adducts, pentosidine adducts, pyrallines, imidazolones, and methylglyoxal derived AGE adducts [144–146]. RAGE engagement with AGEs triggers intracellular signal transduction involving the activation of NF-κB in endothelial cells [144–146], which promotes the upregulation of the expression of endothelial adhesion molecules such as VCAM-1 or ICAM-1. Thus, increased leukocyte-endothelial interactions in the diabetic vasculature may be attributable to the proinflammatory actions of the interaction between AGEs and RAGE [144]. Furthermore, RAGE could also directly act as an adhesion receptor promoting inflammatory cell recruitment. RAGE was identified as a binding partner for the β_2-integrin Mac-1 and was shown to mediate neutrophil adhesion to the endothelium [23]. In vivo, RAGE-mediated leukocyte recruitment was important in diabetic mice: While RAGE only marginally contributed to leukocyte recruitment in vivo in control mice, in diabetic mice, a higher percentage of leukocyte recruitment could be attributed to RAGE, as evidenced by studies using soluble RAGE as an inhibitor or RAGE-deficient mice. These results support the conclusion that RAGE-mediated leukocyte recruitment is operative in diabetes, when RAGE expression is upregulated [23].

Experimental evidence from animal and clinical studies has suggested a role of leukocyte-endothelial interactions in diabetic retinopathy. During diabetic retinopathy, the pathology of the vascular dysfunction in the retina consists of endothelial cell injury and endothelial cell death, disruption of the blood-retinal barrier, increased leukocyte adhesion to the vascular endothelium and capillary ischemia/nonperfusion [147–150]. Interestingly, increases in leukocytes coincide and correlate with the onset of vascular dysfunction in the diabetic retina. Adhesion of leukocytes to the diabetic vasculature in the retina is an event that is observed early in experimental animal diabetes and is thought to participate in the pathogenesis of diabetic retinopathy [149]. In experimental diabetic retinopathy of the rat, capillary occlusion in the retina correlated with the presence of leukocytes, predominantly neutrophils and monocytes [148, 151, 152]. In men, increased entrapment of neutrophils in the choroid and retina of diabetic individuals was shown [153]. Similar findings were observed in diabetic monkeys that develop retinopathy, which very much resembles human diabetic retinopathy. The number of neutrophils was significantly increased in the retinas of diabetic than of nondiabetic monkeys. Interestingly, neutrophil accumulation was spatially associated with regions with capillary nonperfusion [154]. In summary, these findings have led to the hypothesis that in diabetes, leukocytes may contribute to the capillary occlusion of the retinal microvasculature [149, 150, 155, 156].

Patients with severe nonproliferative diabetic retinopathy had in their serum significantly higher concentrations of chemokines that promote inflammatory cell recruitment, such as SDF-1 and RANTES, as compared with patients who had less severe retinopathy [157]. In particular, higher levels of RANTES were associated with more ischemic forms of diabetic retinopathy. The source of RANTES can be inflammatory cells but also the retinal endothelial and pigment epithelial cells [158]. The increased expression of stromal derived factor-1 (SDF-1) in diabetic retinopathy is an interesting observation, since SDF-1 expression can be regulated by hypoxia, a key component of diabetic retinopathy and because SDF-1 has been shown to act as a proangiogenic factor in vivo and in vitro [159, 160].

In a patient with severe intraretinal diabetic retinopathy, the expression of monocyte chemoattractant protein-1 (MCP-1) was found to be higher than in the normal retina [161]. Moreover, increased MCP-1 has been found in the vitreous of patients with proliferative diabetic retinopathy [162]. The expression of MCP-1 message and protein was upregulated in the mouse model of hypoxia-induced neovascularization in the eye. The localization of MCP-1 was found predominantly in the inner retina in the mouse retinopathy model. Interestingly, antibody blockade of MCP-1 decreased the hypoxia-induced neovascularization in this model [163].

Leukocyte adhesion to the diabetic endothelium is a central process in the scenario of diabetic capillary occlusion due to leukocyte entrapment in the diabetic retinal vasculature. Increased glucose levels can stimulate leukocyte adhesion to the endothelium by several mechanisms as delineated above [138–140]. In models of experimental diabetic retinopathy, leukocytes adhere to and accumulate within the vasculature of the retina [148, 164]. Several studies have indicated that the major receptor/ligand pair mediating adhesive interactions between leukocytes and the retinal endothelial cells is the β_2-integrin-ICAM-1 system. ICAM-1 expression in the diabetic retinal vasculature was increased as assessed by immunohistochemistry analysis [134]. In addition, the expression of leukocyte β_2-integrins was elevated on leukocytes from diabetic patients as well as on leukocytes from diabetic animals [165, 166]. In particular, the levels of the α-integrin chains CD11a and CD11b as well as of the β_2-integrin chain CD18 were higher on the surface of neutrophils from diabetic rats, thereby mediating stronger adhesion to rat endothelial cell monolayers [165]. In experimental diabetes in the rat, the number of leukocytes adhering to the endothelial cells in the retinal vasculature was increased [148]. Increased leukocyte adhesion and leukostasis in the diabetic retina correlated with capillary occlusion and the disruption of the blood-retinal barrier resulting in increased retinal leakiness. Blockade of either CD18 or ICAM-1 in experimental diabetic retinopathy decreased both leukocyte adhesion to the diabetic retinal vasculature and the breakdown of the blood-retinal barrier [148, 164, 165]. Furthermore, inhibition of the β_2-integrin-ICAM-1 interaction could reduce endothelial cell injury and death [151].

The role of the β_2-integrin-ICAM-1 system in diabetic retinopathy was strengthened by findings with mice deficient in either ICAM-1 or CD18. In particular, the formation of acellular capillaries was reduced in ICAM-$1^{-/-}$ and CD$18^{-/-}$ mice in diabetic mouse retinopathy [164], which led to the hypothesis that leukocyte adhesion to the endothelium in the retina is involved in mediating the vascular injury. In addition, ICAM-1- or CD18-deficient mice displayed reduced blood-retinal barrier breakdown in diabetic retinopathy [164].

However, diabetic retinopathy in mice does not result in the development of proliferative pathologic lesions. An alternative model is the model of retinopathy of prematurity, which is also designated as oxygen-induced retinopathy. In this model, 7-day old pups are incubated in high oxygen (75% O_2) for 5 days, which promotes the obliteration of the developing retina vasculature. When pups return to room air on postnatal day 12, this results in dramatic retinal ischemia and hypoxia and in exuberant proangiogenic response and pathological neovascularization [167]. In this model, depletion of myeloid cells by injection of clodronate liposomes into the vitreous cavity resulted in reduced pathological neovascularization in hypoxia-induced retinopathy [168], thus supporting a role for leukocytes in pathological retina angiogenesis.

How can adherent leukocytes mediate the endothelial cell injury and death? One possible mechanism could be Fas-FasL interactions. The surface expression of FasL on leukocytes and particularly on lymphocytes is increased in diabetes, and this phenomenon could induce Fas-mediated endothelial cell injury, apoptosis and death, and blood-retinal barrier breakdown. Blockade of the Fas-FasL system reduced retinal endothelial cell apoptosis without altering leukocyte adhesiveness to the retinal vascular endothelium [169, 170]. However, Fas-deficient mice and FasL-deficient mice did not display any abnormalities in retinal vascular development or the obliteration stage in oxygen-induced retinopathy, whereas the overall neovascularization response in oxygen-induced retinopathy was even increased in FasL-deficient mice [171, 172]. Thus, further detailed studies addressing the underlying mechanisms of the participation of leukocyte-endothelial interactions in retinopathy are required in order to understand whether leukocyte-endothelial interactions play a causative role in the capillary destruction in diabetic retinopathy.

Vascular endothelial growth factor (VEGF) may also play a role in promoting inflammation in the context of diabetic retinopathy. The disruption of the blood-retinal barrier in diabetes correlates with retinal VEGF expression [173, 174]. In addition, VEGF may act in a proinflammatory fashion itself, as it is able to stimulate retinal endothelial ICAM-1 expression and thereby leukocyte adhesion [175–178]. Injection of $VEGF_{164}$ into the vitreous cavity in mice induced ICAM-1 expression in the retinal vasculature [177]. Interestingly, $VEGF_{164}$ was more potent than $VEGF_{120}$ in inducing retinal ICAM-1 expression, leukocyte adhesion and disruption of the blood-retinal barrier [178]. The breakdown of the blood-retinal barrier due to VEGF was abolished by blocking ICAM-1, thereby indicating that ICAM-1 may mediate some of the VEGF-dependent effects in the retina [176]. Moreover, VEGF could stimulate an increase in retinal endothelial NO synthase in the diabetic retina, and this pathway could be involved in the VEGF-induced ICAM-1 upregulation [179]. However, in models of ischemia-reperfusion, ICAM-1 expression was shown to be downregulated by NO [180, 181]. Furthermore, VEGF can also act as a chemoattractant for monocytes [182], which implies that VEGF could directly attract leukocytes to the retinal vasculature.

Taken together, there are several lines suggesting a role for inflammation and inflammatory cell adhesion to endothelial cells in the process of diabetic retinopathy. These findings have prompted several investigators to address the potential of anti-inflammatory therapies as a therapeutic approach in diabetic retinopathy. Anti-inflammatory glucocorticoids could be used to enhance the integrity of the blood-retinal barrier [183]. In diabetic rats, aspirin, a cyclo-oxygenase-2 inhibitor and an inhibitor of tumor necrosis factor-α were effective in suppressing retinal ICAM-1 expression, leukocyte adhesion and blood-retinal barrier disruption [184]. In a dog model of diabetic retinopathy, aspirin was tested and was shown to prevent the formation of acellular capillaries and retinal hemorrhages and thereby the progression of retinopathy [185], whereas no effect of aspirin was found in the Early Treatment Diabetic Retinopathy Study [186]. Whether anti-inflammatory treatments or specifically targeting leukocyte adhesion could prove effective as therapeutic approaches in diabetic retinopathy requires careful evaluation in future studies.

References

1 Luster AD, Alon R, von Andrian UH: Immune cell migration in inflammation: present and future therapeutic targets. Nat Immunol 2005;6:1182–1190.
2 von Andrian UH, Mackay CR: T cell function and migration: two sides of the same coin. N Engl J Med 2000;343:1020–1034.
3 Kunkel EJ, Butcher EC: Plasma cell homing. Nat Rev Immunol 2003;3: 822–829.
4 Nathan C: Neutrophils and immunity: challenges and opportunities. Nat Rev Immunol 2006;6:173–182.
5 Zarbock A, Ley K: Mechanisms and consequences of neutrophil interaction with the endothelium. Am J Pathol 2008;172:1–7.
6 Gleissner CA, Galkina E, Nadler JL, Ley K: Mechanisms by which diabetes increases cardiovascular disease. Drug Discov Today Dis Mech 2007;4:131–140.
7 Springer TA: Traffic signals for lymphocyte recirculation and leukocyte emigration: the multistep paradigm. Cell 1994;76:301–314.
8 Butcher EC: Leukocyte-endothelial cell recognition: three (or more) steps to specificity and diversity. Cell 1991;67:1033–1036.
9 Ley K, Laudanna C, Cybulsky MI, Nourshargh S: Getting to the site of inflammation: the leukocyte adhesion cascade updated. Nat Rev Immunol 2007;7:678–689.
10 Rao RM, Yang L, Garcia-Cardena G, Luscinskas FW: Endothelial-dependent mechanisms of leukocyte recruitment to the vascular wall. Circ Res 2007;101:234–247.
11 Carlos TM, Harlan JM: Leukocyte-endothelial adhesion molecules. Blood 1994;84:2068–2101.
12 Vestweber D: Adhesion and signaling molecules controlling the transmigration of leukocytes through endothelium. Immunol Rev 2007;218:178–196.
13 Kinashi T: Intracellular signalling controlling integrin activation in leukocytes. Nat Rev Immunol 2005;5:546–559.
14 McEver RP: Selectins: lectins that initiate cell adhesion under flow. Curr Opin Cell Biol 2002;14:581–586.
15 Smith ML, Olson TS, Ley K: CXCR2- and E-selectin-induced neutrophil arrest during inflammation in vivo. J Exp Med 2004;200:935–939.
16 Salas A, Shimaoka M, Kogan AN, Harwood C, von Andrian UH, Springer TA: Rolling adhesion through an extended conformation of integrin alphaLbeta2 and relation to alpha I and beta I-like domain interaction. Immunity 2004;20:393–406.
17 Zarbock A, Lowell CA, Ley K: Spleen tyrosine kinase Syk is necessary for E-selectin-induced alpha(L)beta(2) integrin-mediated rolling on intercellular adhesion molecule-1. Immunity 2007;26:773–783.
18 Rot A, von Andrian UH: Chemokines in innate and adaptive host defense: basic chemokinese grammar for immune cells. Annu Rev Immunol 2004;22:891–928.
19 Tanaka Y, Adams DH, Hubscher S, Hirano H, Siebenlist U, Shaw S: T-cell adhesion induced by proteoglycan immobilized cytokine MIP-1β. Nature 1993;361:79–82.
20 Proudfoot AE, Power CA, Wells TN: The strategy of blocking the chemokine system to combat disease. Immunol Rev 2000;177:246–256.
21 Imhof BA, Aurrand-Lions M: Adhesion mechanisms regulating the migration of monocytes. Nar Rev Immunol 2004;4:432–444.
22 Yonekawa K, Harlan JM: Targeting leukocyte integrins in human disease. J Leukoc Biol 2005;77:129–140.
23 Chavakis T, Bierhaus A, Al-Fakhri N, Schneider D, Witte S, Linn T, Nagashima M, Morser J, Arnold B, Preissner KT, Nawroth PP: The pattern recognition receptor (RAGE) is a counterreceptor for leukocyte integrins: a novel pathway for inflammatory cell recruitment, J Exp Med 2003;198:1507–1515.
24 Gahmberg CG, Valmu L, Fagerholm S, Kotovuori P, Ihanus E, Tian L, Pessa-Morikawa T: Leukocyte integrins and inflammation. Cell Mol Life Sci 1998;54:549–555.
25 Staunton DE, Dustin ML, Springer TA: Functional cloning of ICAM-2, a cell adhesion ligand for LFA-1 homologous to ICAM-1. Nature 1989;339:61–64.
26 Fawcett J, Holness CL, Needham LA, Turley H, Gatter KC, Mason DY, Simmons DL: Molecular cloning of ICAM-3, a third ligand for LFA-1, constitutively expressed on resting leukocytes. Nature 1992;360:481–484.
27 Bailly P, Tontti E, Hermand P, Cartron JP, Gahmberg CG: The red cell LW blood group protein is an intercellular adhesion molecule which binds to CD11/CD18 leukocyte integrins. Eur J Immunol 1995;25:3316–3320.
28 Gahmberg CG, Tian L, Ning L, Nyman-Huttunen H: ICAM-5–a novel two-facetted adhesion molecule in the mammalian brain. Immunol Lett 2008;117:131–135.
29 Schenkel AR, Mamdouh Z, Muller WA: Locomotion of monocytes on endothelium is a critical step during extravasation. Nat Immunol 2004;5:393–400.
30 Phillipson M, Heit B, Colarusso P, Liu L, Ballantyne CM, Kubes P: Intraluminal crawling of neutrophils to emigration sites: a molecularly distinct process from adhesion in the recruitment cascade. J Exp Med 2006;203:2569–2575.
31 Muller WA: Leukocyte-endothelial interactions in transmigration and the inflammatory response. Trends Immunol 2003;24:326–333.
32 Chavakis T, Preissner KT, Santoso S: Leukocyte trans-endothelial migration: JAMs add new pieces to the puzzle. Thromb Haemost 2003;89:13–17.
33 Nourshargh S, Marelli-Berg FM: Transmigration through venular walls: a key regulator of leukocyte phenotype and function. Trens Immunol 2005;26:157–165.
34 Millan J, Hewlett L, Glyn M, Toomre D, Clark P, Ridley AJ: Lymphocyte transcellular migration occurs through recruitment of endothelial ICAM-1 to caveola and F-actin rich domains. Nat Cell Biol 2006;8:113–123.
35 Carman CV, Springer TA: A transmigratory cup in leukocyte diapedesis both through individual vascular endothelial cells and between them. J Cell Biol 2004;167:377–388.

36 Shaw SK, Ma S, Kim MB, Rao RM, Hartman CU, Froio RM, Yang L, Jones T, Liu Y, Nusrat A, Parkos CA, Luscinskas FW: Coordinated redistribution of leukocyte LFA-1 and endothelial cell ICAM-1 accompany neutrophil transmigration. J Exp Med 2004;200:1571–1580.

37 Lu H, Smith CW, Perrard J, Bullard D, Tang L, Shappell SB, Entman ML, Beaudet AL, Ballantyne CM: LFA-1 is sufficient in mediating neutrophil emigration in Mac-1-deficient mice. J Clin Invest 1997;99:1340–1350.

38 Ding ZM, Babensee JE, SimonI SI, Lu H, Perrard JL, Bullard DC, Dai XY, Bromley SK, Dustin MK, Entman ML, Smith CW, Ballantyne CM: Relative contribution of LFA-1 and Mac-1 to neutrophil adhesion and migration. J Immunol 1999;163:5029–5038.

39 Berlin-Rufenach C, Otto F, Mathies M, Westermann J, Owen MJ, Hamann A, Hogg N: Lymphocyte migration in lymphocyte function-associated antigen (LFA)-1-deficient mice. J Exp Med 1999;189:1467–1478.

40 Mizgerd JP, Kubo H, Kutkoski GJ, Bhagwan SD, Scharffetter-Kochanek K, Beaudet AL, Doerschuk CM: Neutrophil emigration in the skin, lungs, and peritoneum: different requirements for CD11/CD18 revealed by CD18-deficient mice. J Exp Med 1997;186:1357–1364.

41 Springer TA, Thompson WS, Miller LJ, Schmalstieg FC, Anderson DC: Inherited deficiency of the Mac-1, LFA-1, p150,95 glycoprotein family and its molecular basis. J Exp Med 1984;160:1901–1918.

42 Kuijpers TW, Van Lier RA, Hamann D, de Boer M, Thung LY, Weening RS, Verhoeven, AJ, Roos D: Leukocyte adhesion deficiency type 1 (LAD-1)/variant. A novel immunodeficiency syndrome characterized by dysfunctional β2 integrins. J Clin Invest 1997;100:1725–1733.

43 Harris ES, Shigeoka AO, Li W, Adams RH, Prescott SM, McIntyre TM, Zimmerman GA, Lorant DE: A novel syndrome of variant leukocyte adhesion deficiency involving defects in adhesion mediated by β1 and β2 integrins. Blood 2001;97:767–776.

44 McDowall A, Inwald D, Leitinger B, Jones A, Liesner R, Klein N, Hogg N: A novel form of integrin dysfunction involving β1, β2, and β3 integrins. J Clin Invest 2003;111:51–60.

45 Alon R, Aker M, Feigelson S, Sokolovsky-Eisenberg M, Staunton DE, Cinamon G, Grabovsky V, Shamri R, Etzioni A: A novel genetic leukocyte adhesion deficiency in subsecond triggering of integrin avidity by endothelial chemokines results in impaired leukocyte arrest on vascular endothelium under shear flow. Blood 2003;101:4437–4445.

46 Pasvolsky R, Feigelson SW, Kilic SS, Simon AJ, Tal-Lapidot G, Grabovsky V, Crittenden JR, Amariglio N, Safran M, Graybiel AM, Rechavi G, Ben-Dor S, Etzioni A, Alon R: A LAD-III syndrome is associated with defective expression of the Rap-1 activator CalDAG-GEFI in lymphocytes, neutrophils, and platelets. J Exp Med 2007;204:1571–1582.

47 Steinman L: Blocking adhesion molecules as therapy for multiple sclerosis: natalizumab. Nat Rev Drug Discov 2005;4:510–518.

48 Lebwohl M, Tyring SK, Hamilton TK, Toth D, Glazer S, Tawfik NH, Walicke P, Dummer W, Wang X, Garovoy MR, Pariser D: A novel targeted T-cell modulator, efalizumab, for plaque psoriasis. N Engl J Med 2003;349:2004–2013.

49 Carman CV, Springer TA: Integrin avidity regulation: are changes in affinity and conformation underemphasized? Curr Opin Cell Biol 2003;15:547–556.

50 Dustin ML, Bivona TG, Philips MR: Membranes as messengers in T cell adhesion signaling. Nat Immunol 2004;5:363–372.

51 Shimaoka M, Xiao T, Liu JH, Yang Y, Dong Y, Jun CD, McCormack A, Zhang R, Joachimiak A, Takagi J, Wang JH, Springer TA: Structures of the alpha L I domain and its complex with ICAM-1 reveal a shape-shifting pathway for integrin regulation. Cell 2003;112:99–111.

52 Takagi J, Petre BM, Walz T, Springer TA: Global conformational rearrangements in integrin extracellular domains in outside-in and inside-out signaling. Cell 2002;110:599–511.

53 Takagi J, Springer TA: Integrin activation and structural rearrangement. Immunol Rev 2002;186:141–163.

54 Luo BH, Carman CV, Springer TA: Structural basis of integrin regulation and signaling. Annu Rev Immunol 2007;25:619–647.

55 Nishida N, Xie C, Shimaoka M, Cheng Y, Walz T, Springer TA: Activation of leukocyte beta2 integrins by conversion from bent to extended conformations. Immunity 2006;25:583–594.

56 Kim M, Carman CV, Springer TA: Bidirectional transmembrane signaling by cytoplasmic domain separation in integrins. Science 2003;301:1720–1725.

57 Grabovsky V, Feigelson S, Chen C, Bleijs DA, Peled A, Cinamon G, Baleux F, Arenzana-Seisdedos F, Lapidot T, van Kooyk Y, Lobb RR, Alon R: Subsecond induction of alpha4 integrin clustering by immobilized chemokines stimulates leukocyte tethering and rolling on endothelial vascular cell adhesion molecule 1 under flow conditions. J Exp Med 2000;192:495–506.

58 Shamri R, Grabovsky V, Gauguet JM, Feigelson S, Manevich E, Kolanus W, Robinson MK, Staunton DE, von Andrian UH, Alon R: Lymphocyte arrest requires instantaneous induction of an extended LFA-1 conformation mediated by endothelium-bound chemokines. Nat Immunol 2005;6:497–506.

59 Hyduk SJ, Chan JR, Duffy ST, Chen M, Peterson MD, Waddell TK, Digby GC, Szaszi K, Kapus A, Cybulsky MI: Phospholipase C, calcium, and calmodulin are critical for alpha4beta1 integrin affinity up-regulation and monocyte arrest triggered by chemoattractants. Blood 2007;109:176–184.

60 Katagiri K, Hattori M, Minato N, Irie S, Takatsu K, Kinashi T: Rap1 is a potent activation signal for leukocyte function-associated antigen 1 distinct from protein kinase C and phosphatidylinositol-3-OH kinase. Mol Cell Biol 2000;20:1956–1969.

61 Shimonaka M, Katagiri K, Nakayama T, Fujita N, Tsuruo T, Yoshie O, Kinashi T: Rap1 translates chemokine signals to integrin activation, cell polarization, and motility across vascular endothelium under flow. J Cell Biol 2003;161:417–427.

62 Tohyama Y, Katagiri K, Pardi R, Lu C, Springer TA, Kinashi T: The critical cytoplasmic regions of the αLβ2 integrin in Rap1-induced adhesion and migration. Mol Biol Cell 2003;14:2570–2582.

63 Katagiri K, Maeda A, Shimonaka M, Kinashi T: RAPL, a Rap1-binding molecule that mediates Rap1-induced adhesion through spatial regulation of LFA-1. Nature Immunol 2003;4:741–748.

64 Ghandour H, Cullere X, Alvarez A, Luscinskas FW, Mayadas TN: Essential role for Rap1 GTPase and its guanine exchange factor CalDAG-GEFI in LFA-1 but not VLA-4 integrin mediated human T-cell adhesion. Blood 2007;110:3682–3690.

65 Lafuente E, Boussiotis VA: Rap1 regulation of RIAM and cell adhesion. Methods Enzymol 2005;407:345–358.

66 Kinashi T, Katagiri K: Regulation of immune cell adhesion and migration by regulator of adhesion and cell polarization enriched in lymphoid tissues. Immunology 2005;116:164–171.

67 Bos JL: Linking Rap to cell adhesion. Curr Opin Cell Biol 2005;17:123–128.

68 Lafuente EM, van Puijenbroek AA, Krause M, Carman CV, Freeman GJ, Berezovskaya A, Constantine E, Springer TA, Gertler FB, Boussiotis VA: RIAM, an Ena/VASP and Profilin ligand, interacts with Rap1-GTP and mediates Rap1-induced adhesion. Dev Cell 2004;7:585–595.

69 Han J, Lim CJ, Watanabe N, Soriani A, Ratnikov B, Calderwood DA, Puzon-McLaughlin W, Lafuente EM, Boussiotis VA, Shattil SJ, Ginsberg MH: Reconstructing and deconstructing agonist-induced activation of integrin alphaIIbbeta3. Curr Biol 2006;16:1796–1806.

70 Lee HS, Lim CJ, Puzon-McLaughlin W, Shattil SJ, Ginsberg MH: RIAM activates integrins by linking talin to Ras GTPase membrane-targeting sequences. J Biol Chem 2009;284:5119–5127.

71 Tadokoro S, Shattil SJ, Eto K, Tai V, Liddington RC, de Pereda JM, Ginsberg MH, Calderwood DA: Talin binding to integrin beta tails: a final common step in integrin activation. Science 2003;302:103–106.

72 Calderwood DA: Integrin activation. J Cell Sci 2004;117:657–666.

73 Di Paolo G, Pellegrini L, Letinic K, Cestra G, Zoncu R, Voronov S, Chang S, Guo J, Wenk MR, De Camilli P: Recruitment and regulation of phosphatidylinositol phosphate kinase type 1γ by the FERM domain of talin. Nature 2002;420:85–89.

74 Fagerholm SC, Hilden TJ, Nurmi SM, Gahmberg CG: Specific integrin alpha and beta chain phosphorylations regulate LFA-1 activation through affinity-dependent and -independent mechanisms. J Cell Biol 2005;171:705–715.

75 Fagerholm SC, Hilden TJ, Gahmberg CG: P marks the spot: site-specific integrin phosphorylation regulates molecular interactions. Trends Biochem Sci 2004;29:504–512.

76 Fagerholm S, Morrice N, Gahmberg CG, Cohen P: Phosphorylation of the cytoplasmic domain of the integrin CD18 chain by protein kinase C isoforms in leukocytes. J Biol Chem 2002;277:1728–1738.

77 Hibbs ML, Jakes S, Stacker SA, Wallace RW, Springer TA: The cytoplasmic domain of the integrin lymphocyte function-associated antigen 1 beta subunit: sites required for binding to intercellular adhesion molecule 1 and the phorbol ester-stimulated phosphorylation site. J Exp Med 1991;174:1227–1238.

78 Choi EY, Orlova VV, Fagerholm SC, Nurmi SM, Zhang L, Ballantyne CM, Gahmberg CG, Chavakis T: Regulation of LFA-1-dependent inflammatory cell recruitment by Cbl-b and 14-3-3 proteins. Blood 2008;111:3607–3614.

79 Petty HR, Worth RG, Todd RF 3rd: Interactions of integrins with their partner proteins in leukocyte membranes. Immunol Res 2002;25:75–95.

80 Chavakis T, Kanse SM, May AE, Preissner KT: Haemostatic factors occupy new territory: the role of the urokinase receptor system and kininogen in inflammation. Biochem Soc Trans 2002;30:168–173.

81 Orlova VV, Choi EY, Xie C, Chavakis E, Bierhaus A, Ihanus E, Ballantyne CM, Gahmberg CG, Bianchi ME, Nawroth PP, Chavakis T: A novel pathway of HMGB1-mediated inflammatory cell recruitment that requires Mac-1-integrin. EMBO J 2007;26:1129–1139.

82 Giagulli C, Ottoboni L, Caveggion E, Rossi B, Lowell C, Constantin G, Laudanna C, Berton G: The Src family kinases Hck and Fgr are dispensable for inside-out, chemoattractant-induced signaling regulating beta 2 integrin affinity and valency in neutrophils, but are required for beta 2 integrin-mediated outside-in signaling involved in sustained adhesion. J Immunol 2006;177:604–611.

83 Gakidis MA, Cullere X, Olson T, Wilsbacher JL, Zhang B, Moores SL, Ley K, Swat W, Mayadas T, Brugge JS: Vav GEFs are required for beta2 integrin-dependent functions of neutrophils. J Cell Biol 2004;166:273–282.

84 Zhang H, Schaff UY, Green CE, Chen H, Sarantos MR, Hu Y, Wara D, Simon SI, Lowell CA: Impaired integrin-dependent function in Wiskott-Aldrich syndrome protein-deficient murine and human neutrophils. Immunity 2006;25:285–295.

85 Zhou MY, Lo SK, Bergenfeldt M, Tiruppathi C, Jaffe A, Xu N, Malik AB: In vivo expression of neutrophil inhibitory factor via gene transfer prevents lipopolysaccharide-induced lung neutrophil infiltration and injury by a beta2 integrin-dependent mechanism. J Clin Invest 1998;101:2427–2437.

86 Rozdzinski E, Sandros J, van der Flier M, Young A, Spellerberg B, Bhattacharyya C, Straub J, Musso G, Putney S, Starzyk R, et al: Inhibition of leukocyte-endothelial cell interactions and inflammation by peptides from a bacterial adhesin which mimic coagulation factor X. J Clin Invest 1995;95:1078–1085.

87 Chavakis T, Preissner KT, Herrmann M: The anti-inflammatory activities of Staphylococcus aureus. Trends Immunol 2007;28:408–418.

88 Chavakis T, Hussain M, Kanse SM, Peters G, Bretzel RG, Flock JI, Herrmann M, Preissner KT: Staphylococcus aureus extracellular adherence protein serves as anti-inflammatory factor by inhibiting the recruitment of host leukocytes. Nat Med 2002;8:687–693.

89 Hidai C, Zupancic T, Penta K, Mikhail A, Kawana M, Quertermous EE, Aoka Y, Fukagawa M, Matsui Y, Platika D, Auerbach R, Hogan BL, Snodgrass R, Quertermous T: Cloning and characterization of developmental endothelial locus-1:an embryonic endothelial cell protein that binds the alphavbeta3 integrin receptor. Genes Dev 1998;12:21–33.

90 Ho, H.K., J.J. Jang, S. Kaji, Spektor G, Fong A, Yang P, Hu BS, Schatzman R, Quertermous T, Cooke JP: Developmental endothelial locus-1 (Del-1), a novel angiogenic protein: its role in ischemia. Circulation 2004;109:1314–1319.

91 Choi EY, Chavakis E, Czabanka MA, Langer HF, Fraemohs L, Economopoulou M, Kundu RK, Orlandi A, Zheng YY, Prieto DA, Ballantyne CM, Constant SL, Aird WC, Papayannopoulou T, Gahmberg CG, Udey MC, Vajkoczy P, Quertermous T, Dimmeler S, Weber C, Chavakis T: Del-1, an endogenous leukocyte-endothelial adhesion inhibitor, limits inflammatory cell recruitment. Science 2008;322:1101–1104.
92 Hidai C, Kawana M, Kitano H, Kokubun S: Discoidin domain of Del1 protein contributes to its deposition in the extracellular matrix. Cell Tissue Res 2007;330:83–95.
93 Norling LV, Sampaio AL, Cooper D, Perretti M: Inhibitory control of endothelial galectin-1 on in vitro and in vivo lymphocyte trafficking. FASEB J 2008;22:682–690.
94 Cooper D, Norling LV, Perretti M: Novel insights into the inhibitory effects of Galectin-1 on neutrophil recruitment under flow. J Leukoc Biol 2008;83:1459–1466.
95 Bazzoni G, Dejana E: Endothelial cell-to-cell junctions: molecular organization and role in vascular homeostasis. Physiol Rev 2004;84:869–901.
96 Orlova VV, Chavakis T: Regulation of vascular endothelial permeability by junctional adhesion molecules (JAM). Thromb Haemost 2007;98:327–332.
97 Gotsch U, Borges E, Bosse R, Boggemeyer E, Simon M, Mossmann H, Vestweber D: VE-cadherin antibody accelerates neutrophil recruitment in vivo. J Cell Sci 1997;110:583–588.
98 Shaw SK, Bamba PS, Perkins BN, Luscinskas FW: Real-time imaging of vascular endothelial-cadherin during leukocyte transmigration across endothelium. J Immunol 2001;167:2323–2330.
99 Ebnet K, Suzuki A, Ohno A, Vestweber D: Junctional adhesion molecules (JAMs): more molecules with dual functions? J Cell Sci 2004;117:19–29.
100 Keiper T, Santoso S, Nawroth PP, Orlova V, Chavakis T: The role of junctional adhesion molecules in cell-cell interactions. Histol Histopathol 2005;20:197–203.
101 Bradfield PF, Nourshargh S, Aurrand-Lions M, Imhof BA: JAM family and related proteins in leukocyte migration. Arterioscler Thromb Vasc Biol 2007;27:2104–2112.
102 Weber C, Fraemohs L, Dejana E: The role of junctional adhesion molecules in vascular inflammation. Nat Rev Immunol 2007;7:467–477.
103 Sobocka MB, Sobocki T, Banerjee P, Weiss C, Rushbrook JI, Norin AJ, Hartwig J, Salifu M, Markell MS, Babinska A, Ehrlich YH, Kornecki E: Cloning of the human platelet F11-receptor: a cell adhesion molecule member of the immunoglobulin superfamily involved in platelet aggregation. Blood 2000;95:2600–2609.
104 Palmeri D, van Zante A, Huang CC, Hemmerich S, Rosen SD: Vascular endothelial junction-associated molecule, a novel member of the immunoglobulin superfamily, is localized to intercellular boundaries of endothelial cells. J Biol Chem 2000;275:19319–19345.
105 Aurrand-Lions MA, Johnson-Leger C, Wong C, DuPasquier L, Imhof BA: Heterogeneity of endothelial junctions is reflected by differential and specific subcellular localization of three JAM family members. Blood 2001;98:3699–3707.
106 Santoso S, Sachs UJH, Kroll H, Linder M, Ruf A, Preissner KT, Chavakis T: The junctional adhesion molecule 3 (JAM-3) on human platelets is a counterreceptor for the leukocyte integrin Mac-1. J Exp Med 2002;196:679–691.
107 Ody C, Jungblut-Ruault S, Cossali D, Barnet M, Aurrand-Lions M, Imhof BA, Matthes T: Junctional adhesion molecule C (JAM-C) distinguishes CD27+ germinal center B lymphocytes from non-germinal center cells and constitutes a new diagnostic tool for B-cell malignancies. Leukemia 2007;21:1285–1293.
108 Keiper T, Al-Fakhri N, Chavakis E, Athanasopoulos AN, Isermann B, Herzog S, Saffrich R, Hersemeyer K, Bohle RM, Haendeler J, Preissner KT, Santoso S, Chavakis T: The role of junctional adhesion molecule-C (JAM-C) in oxidized LDL-mediated leukocyte recruitment. FASEB J 2005;19:2078–2080.
109 Kostrewa D, Brockhaus M, D'Arcy A, Dale GE, Nelboeck P, Schmid G, Mueller F, Bazzoni G, Dejana E, Bartfai T, Winkler FK, Hennig M: X-ray structure of junctional adhesion molecule: structural basis for homophilic adhesion via a novel dimerization motif. EMBO J 2001;20:4391–4398.
110 Santoso S, Orlova V, Song K, Sachs UJ, Andrei-Selmer C, Chavakis T: The homophilic binding of junctional adhesion molecule-C mediates tumor cell-endothelial cell interactions. J Biol Chem 2005;280:36326–36333.
111 Ostermann G, Weber KS, Zernecke A, Schroeder A, Weber C: JAM-1 is a ligand of the beta(2) integrin LFA-1 involved in transendothelial migration of leukocytes. Nat Immunol 2002;3:151–158.
112 Cunningham SA, Rodriguez JM, Arrate PM, Tran TM, Brock TA: JAM2 interacts with alpha4beta1. Facilitation by JAM3. J Biol Chem 2002;277:27589–27592.
113 Arrate MP, Rodriguez JM, Tran TM, Brock TA, Cunningham SA: Cloning of human junctional adhesion molecule 3 (JAM3) and its identification as the JAM2 counter-receptor. J Biol Chem 2001;276:45826–45832.
114 Lamagna C, Meda P, Mandicourt G, Brown J, Gilbert RJ, Jones EY, Kiefer F, Ruga P, Imhof BA, Aurrand-Lions M: Dual interaction of JAM-C with JAM-B and alpha(M)beta2 integrin: function in junctional complexes and leukocyte adhesion. Mol Biol Cell 2005;16:4992–5003.
115 Del Maschio A, De Luigi A, Martin-Padura I, Brockhaus M, Bartfai T, Fruscella P, Adorini L, Martino G, Furlan R, De Simoni MG, Dejana E: Leukocyte recruitment in the cerebrospinal fluid of mice with experimental meningitis is inhibited by an antibody to junctional adhesion molecule (JAM). J Exp Med 1999;190:1351–1356.
116 Corada M, Chimenti S, Cera MR, Vinci M, Salio M, Fiordaliso F, De Angelis N, Villa A, Bossi M, Staszewsky LI, Vecchi A, Parazzoli D, Motoike T, Latini R, Dejana E: Junctional adhesion molecule-A-deficient polymorphonuclear cells show reduced diapedesis in peritonitis and heart ischemia-reperfusion injury. Proc Natl Acad Sci USA 2005;102:10634–10639.
117 Khandoga A, Kessler JS, Meissner H, Hanschen M, Corada M, Motoike T, Enders G, Dejana E, Krombach F: Junctional adhesion molecule-A deficiency increases hepatic ischemia-reperfusion injury despite reduction of neutrophil transendothelial migration. Blood 2005;106:725–733.

118 Chavakis T, Keiper T, Matz-Westphal R, Hersemeyer K, Sachs UJ, Nawroth PP, Preissner KT, Santoso S: The junctional adhesion molecule-C promotes neutrophil transendothelial migration in vitro and in vivo. J Biol Chem 2004;279:55602–55608.
119 Aurrand-Lions M, Lamagna C, Dangerfield JP, Wang S, Herrera P, Nourshargh S, Imhof BA: Junctional adhesion molecule-C regulates the early influx of leukocytes into tissues during inflammation. J Immunol 2005;174:6406–6415.
120 Orlova, VV. Economopoulou M, Lupu F, Santoso S, Chavakis T: Junctional adhesion molecule-C regulates vascular endothelial permeability by modulating VE-cadherin-mediated cell-cell contacts. J Exp Med 2006;203:2703–2714.
121 Wegmann F, Petri B, Khandoga AG, Moser C, Khandoga A, Volkery S, Li H, Nasdala I, Brandau O, Fässler R, Butz S, Krombach F, Vestweber D: ESAM supports neutrophil extravasation, activation of Rho, and VEGF-induced vascular permeability. J Exp Med 2006;203:1671–1677.
122 Muller WA, Weigl SA, Deng X, Phillips DM: PECAM-1 is required for transendothelial migration of leukocytes. J Exp Med 1993;178:449–460.
123 Bogen S, Pak J, Garifallou M, Deng X, Muller WA: Monoclonal antibody to murine PECAM-1 (CD31) blocks acute inflammation in vivo. J Exp Med 1994;179:1059–1064.
124 Liao F, Ali J, Greene T, Muller WA: Soluble domain 1 of platelet-endothelial cell adhesion molecule (PECAM) is sufficient to block transendothelial migration in vitro and in vivo. J Exp Med 1997;185:1349–1357.
125 Mamdouh Z, Chen X, Pierini LM, Maxfield FR, Muller WA: Targeted recycling of PECAM from endothelial surface-connected compartments during diapedesis. Nature 2003;421:748–753.
126 Sachs UJ, Andrei-Selmer CL, Maniar A, Weiss T, Paddock C, Orlova VV, Choi EY, Newman PJ, Preissner KT, Chavakis T, Santoso S: The neutrophil-specific antigen CD177 is a counter-receptor for platelet endothelial cell adhesion molecule-1 (CD31). J Biol Chem 2007;282:23603–23612.
127 Dangerfield J, Larbi KY, Huang MT, Dewar A, Nourshargh S: PECAM-1 (CD31) homophilic interaction up-regulates a6b1 on transmigrated neutrophils in vivo and plays a junctional role in the ability of a6 integrins to mediate leukocyte migration through the perivascular basementmembrane. J Exp Med 2002;196:1201–1211.
128 Schenkel AR, Mamdouh Z, Chen X, Liebman RM, Muller WA: CD99 plays a major role in the migration of monocytes through endothelial junctions. Nat Immunol 2002;3:143–150.
129 Huang MT, Larbi KY, Scheiermann C, Woodfin A, Gerwin N, Haskard DO, Nourshargh S: ICAM-2 mediates neutrophil transmigration in vivo: evidence for stimulus specificity and a role in PECAM-1-independent transmigration. Blood 2006;107:4721–4727.
130 Kaneider NC, Leger AJ, Kuliopulos A: Therapeutic targeting of molecules involved in leukocyte-endothelial cell interactions. FEBS J 2006;273:4416–4424.
131 Krieglstein CF, Granger DN: Adhesion molecules and their role in vascular disease. Am J Hyperten 2001;14:44S–54S.
132 Panes J, Kurose I, Rodriguez-Vaca MD, Anderson DC, Miyasaka M, Tso P, Granger DN: Diabetes exacerbates the inflammatory responses to ischemia-reperfusion. Circulation 1996;93:161–167.
133 Salas A, Panes J, Elizalde JI, Casadevall M, Anderson DC, Granger DN, Pique JM: Mechanisms responsible for enhanced inflammatory response to ischemia-reperfusion in diabetes. Am J Physiol 1998;275:H1773–H1781.
134 McLeod DS, Lefer DJ, Merges C, Lutty GA: Enhanced expression of intracellular adhesion molecule-1 and P-selectin in the diabetic human retina and choroid. Am J Pathol 1995;147:642–653.
135 Salas A, Panes J, Rosenbloom CL, Elizalde JI, Anderson DC, Granger DN, Pique JM: Differential effects of a nitric oxide donor on reperfusion-induced microvascular dysfunction in diabetic and non-diabetic rats. Diabetologia 1999;42:1350–1358.
136 Cominacini L, Fratta Pasini A, Garbin U, Campagnola M, Davoli A, Rigoni A, Zenti MG, Pastorino AM, Lo Cascio V: E-selectin plasma concentration is influenced by glycaemic control in NIDDM patients: possible role of oxidative stress. Diabetologia 1997;40:584–589.
137 Ceriello A, Falleti E, Motz E, Taboga C, Tonutti L, Ezsol Z, Gonano F, Bartoli E: Hyperglycemia-induced circulating ICAM-1 increase in diabetes mellitus: the possible role of oxidative stress. Horm Metab Res 1998;30:146–149.
138 Omi H, Okayama N, Shimizu M, Okouchi M, Ito S, Fukutomi T, Itoh M: Participation of high glucose concentrations in neutrophil adhesion and surface expression of adhesion molecules on cultured human endothelial cells: effect of antidiabetic medicines. J Diabetes Complications 2002;16:201–208.
139 Booth G, Stalker TJ, Lefer AM, Scalia R: Mechanisms of amelioration of glucose-induced endothelial dysfunction following inhibition of protein kinase C in vivo. Diabetes 2002;51:1556–1564.
140 Morigi M, Angioletti S, Imberti B, Donadelli R, Micheletti G, Figliuzzi M, Remuzzi A, Zoja C, Remuzzi G: Leukocyte-endothelial interaction is augmented by high glucose concentrations and hyperglycemia in a NF-kB-dependent fashion. J Clin Invest 1998;101:1905–1915.
141 Chibber R, Ben-Mahmud BM, Chibber S, Kohner EM: Leukocytes in diabetic retinopathy. Curr Diabetes Rev 2007;3:3–14.
142 Chibber R, Ben-Mahmud BM, Coppini D, Christ E, Kohner EM: Activity of the glycosylating enzyme, core 2 GlcNAc (beta1,6) transferase, is higher in polymorphonuclear leukocytes from diabetic patients compared with age-matched control subjects: relevance to capillary occlusion in diabetic retinopathy. Diabetes 2000;49:1724–1730.
143 Chibber R, Ben-Mahmud BM, Mann GE, Zhang JJ, Kohner EM: Protein kinase C beta2-dependent phosphorylation of core 2 GlcNAc-T promotes leukocyte-endothelial cell adhesion: a mechanism underlying capillary occlusion in diabetic retinopathy. Diabetes 2003;52:1519–1527.
144 Chavakis T, Bierhaus A, Nawroth PP: RAGE (receptor for advanced glycation endproducts): a central player in the inflammatory response. Microbes Infect 2004;6:1219–1225.
145 Schmidt AM, Yan SD, Yan SF, Stern DM: The multiligand receptor RAGE as a progression factor amplifying immune and inflammatory responses. J Clin Invest 2001;108:949–955.

146 Yan SF, Ramasamy R, Naka Y, Schmidt AM: Glycation, inflammation and RAGE. A scaffold for the macrovascular complications of diabetes and beyond. Circ Res 2003;93:1159–1169.
147 Adamis AP: Is diabetic retinopathy an inflammatory disease? Br J Ophthalmol 2002;86:363–365.
148 Miyamoto K, Khosrof S, Bursell SE, Rohan R, Murata T, Clermont AC, Aiello LP, Ogura Y, Adamis AP: Prevention of leukostasis and vascular leakage in streptozotocin-induced diabetic retinopathy via intercellular adhesion molecule-1 inhibition. Proc Natl Acad Sci USA 1999;96:10836–10841.
149 Adamis AP, Berman AJ: Immunological mechanism in the pathogenesis of diabetic retinopathy. Semin Immunopathol 2008;30:65–84.
150 Kern TS: Contributions of inflammatory processes to the development of the early stages of diabetic retinopathy. Exp Diabetes Res 2007;95103.
151 Joussen AM, Murata T, Tsujikawa A, Kirchhof B, Bursell SE, Adamis AP: Leukocyte-mediated endothelial cell injury and death in the diabetic retina. Am J Pathol 2001;158:147–152.
152 Schroder S, Palinski W, Schmid-Schonbein GW: Activated monocytes and granulocytes, capillary nonperfusion, and neovascularization in diabetic retinopathy. Am J Pathol 1991;139:81–100.
153 Miyamoto K, Hiroshiba N, Tsujikawa A, Ogura Y: In vivo demonstration of increased leukocyte entrapment in retinal microcirculation of diabetic rats. Invest Ophthalmol Vis Sci 1998;39:2190–2194.
154 Kim SY, Johnson MA, McLeod DS, Alexander T, Hansen BC, Lutty GA: Neutrophils are associated with capillary closure in spontaneously diabetic monkey retinas. Diabetes 2005;54:1534–1542.
155 Paques M, Boval M, Richard S, Tadayoni R, Massin P, Mundler O, Gaudric A, Vicaut E: Evaluation of fluorescein-labeled autologous leukocytes for examination of retinal circulation in humans. Curr Eye Res 2000;21:560–565.
156 Cao J, McLeod S, Merges CA, Lutty GA: Choriocapillaris degeneration and related pathologic changes in human diabetic eyes. Arch Ophthalmol 1998;116:589–597.
157 Meleth AD, Agron E, Chan CC, Reed GF, Arora K, Byrnes G, Csaky KG, Ferris FL III, Chew EY: Serum Inflammatory Markers in Diabetic Retinopathy. Invest Ophthalmol Vis Sci 2005;46:4295–4301.
158 Crane IJ, Wallace CA, McKillop Smith S, Forrester JV: Control of chemokine production at the blood-retina barrier. Immunology 2000;101:426–433.
159 Mirshahi F, Pourtau J, Li H, Muraine M, Trochon V, Legrand E, Vannier J, Soria J, Vasse M, Soria C: SDF-1 activity on microvascular endothelial cells: consequences on angiogenesis in in vitro and in vivo models. Thromb Res 2000;99:587–594.
160 Salcedo R Oppenheim JJ: Role of chemokines in angiogenesis: CXCL12/SDF-1 and CXCR4 interaction, a key regulator of endothelial cell responses. Microcirculation 2003;10:359–370.
161 Mitamura Y, Takeuchi S, Yamamoto S, Yamamoto T, Tsukahara I, Matsuda A, Tagawa Y, Mizue Y, Nishihira J: Monocyte chemotactic protein-1 levels in the vitreous of patients with proliferative vitreoretinopathy. Jpn J Ophthalmol 2002;46:218–221.
162 Abu el-Asrar AM, Van Damme J, Put W, Veckeneer M, Dralands L, Billiau A, Missotten L: Monocyte chemotactic protein-1 in proliferative vitreoretinal disorders. Am J Ophthalmol 1997;123:599–606.
163 Yoshida S, Yoshida A, Ishibashi T, Elner SG, Elner VM: Role of MCP-1 and MIP-1alpha in retinal neovascularization during postischemic inflammation in a mouse model of retinal neovascularization. J Leukoc Biol 2003;73:137–144.
164 Joussen AM, Poulaki V, Le ML, Koizumi K, Esser C, Janicki H, Schraermeyer U, Kociok N, Fauser S, Kirchhof B, Kern TS, Adamis AP: A central role for inflammation in diabetic retinopathy. FASEB J 2004;18:1450–1452.
165 Canas-Barouch F, Miyamoto K, Allport JR, Fujita K, Bursell SE, Aiello LP, Luscinskas FW, Adamis AP: Integrin-mediated neutrophil adhesion and retinal leukostasis in diabetes. Invest Ophthalmol Vis Sci 2000;41:1153–1158.
166 Song H, Wang L, Hui Y: Expression of CD18 on the neutrophils of patients with diabetic retinopathy. Graefes Arch Clin Exp Ophthalmol 2007;245:24–31.
167 Smith LE, Wesolowski E, McLellan A, Kostyk SK, D'Amato R, Sullivan R, D'Amore PA: Oxygen-induced retinopathy in the mouse. Invest Ophthalmol Vis Sci 1994;35:101–111.
168 Ishida S, Usui T, Yamashiro K, Kaji Y, Amano S, Ogura Y, Hida T, Oguchi Y, Ambati J, Miller JW, Gragoudas ES, Ng YS, D'Amore PA, Shima DT, Adamis AP: VEGF164-mediated inflammation is required for pathological, but not physiological, ischemia-induced retinal neovascularization. J Exp Med 2003;198:483–489.
169 Joussen AM, Poulaki V, Mitsiades N, Cai WY, Suzuma I, Pak J, Ju ST, Rook SL, Esser P, Mitsiades CS, Kirchhof B, Adamis AP, Aiello LP: Suppression of Fas-FasL-induced endothelial cell apoptosis prevents diabetic blood-retinal barrier breakdown in a model of streptozotocin-induced diabetes FASEB J 2003;17:76–78.
170 Ishida S, Yamashiro K, Usui T, Kaji Y, Ogura Y, Hida T, Honda Y, Oguchi Y, Adamis AP: Leukocytes mediate retinal vascular remodeling during development and vaso-obliteration in disease. Nat Med 2003;9:781–788.
171 Barreiro R, Schadlu R, Herndon J, Kaplan HJ, Ferguson TA: The role of Fas-FasL in the development and treatment of ischemic retinopathy. Invest Ophthalmol Vis Sci 2003;44:1282–1286.
172 Davies MH, Eubanks JP, Powers MR: Increased retinal neovascularization in Fas ligand-deficient mice. Invest Ophthalmol Vis Sci 2003;44:3202–3210.
173 Murata T, Ishibashi T, Khalil A, Hata Y, Yoshikawa H, Inomata H: Vascular endothelial growth factor plays a role in hyperpermeability of diabetic retinal vessels. Ophthalmic Res 1995;27:48–52.
174 Qaum T, Xu Q, Joussen AM, Clemens MW, Qin W, Miyamoto K, Hassessian H, Wiegand SJ, Rudge J, Yancopoulos GD, Adamis AP: VEGF-initiated blood-retinal barrier breakdown in early diabetes. Invest Ophthalmol Vis Sci 2002;42:2408–2413.
175 Melder RJ, Koenig GC, Witwer BP, Safabakhsh N, Munn LL, Jain RK: During angiogenesis, vascular endothelial growth factor and basic fibroblast growth factor regulate natural killer cell adhesion to tumor endothelium. Nat Med 1996;2:992–997.

176 Miyamoto K, Khosrof S, Bursell S-E, Moromizato Y, Aiello LP, Ogura Y, Adamis AP: Vascular endothelial growth factor-induced retinal vascular permeability is mediated by intercellular adhesion molecule-1 (ICAM-1). Am J Pathol 2000;156:1733–1739.

177 Lu M, Perez V, Ma N, Miyamoto K, Peng HB, Liao JK, Adamis AP: VEGF increases retinal vascular ICAM-1 expression in vivo. Invest Ophthalmol Vis Sci 1999;40:1808–1812.

178 Ishida S, Usui T, Yamashiro K, Kaji Y, Ahmed E, Carrasquillo KG, Amano S, Hida T, Oguchi Y, Adamis AP: VEGF is proinflammatory in the diabetic retina. Invest Ophthalmol Vis Sci 2003;44:2155–2162.

179 Joussen AM, Poulaki V, Qin W, Kirchhof B, Mitsiades N, Wiegand SJ, Rudge J, Yancopoulos GD, Adamis AP: Retinal vascular endothelial growth factor induces intercellular adhesion molecule-1 and endothelial nitric oxide synthase expression and initiates early diabetic retinal leukocyte adhesion in vivo. Am J Pathol 2002;160:501–509.

180 Lindemann S, Sharafi M, Spieker M, Buerke M, Fisch A, Grosser T, Veit K, Gierer C, Ibe W, Meyer J, Darius H: NO reduces PMN adhesion to human vascular endothelial cells due to downregulation of ICAM-1 mRNA and surface expression. Thromb Res 2000;97:113–123.

181 Liu P, Xu B, Hock CE, Nagele R, Sun FF, Wong PY: NO modulates P-selectin and ICAM-1 mRNA and hemodynamic alterations in hepatic I/R. Am J Physiol 1998;275:H2191–H2198.

182 Clauss M, Gerlach M, Gerlach H, Brett J, Wang F, Familletti PC, Pan YC, Olander JV, Connolly DT, Stern D: Vascular permeability factor: a tumor-derived polypeptide that induces endothelial cell and monocyte procoagulant activity, and promotes monocyte migration. J Exp Med 1990;172:1535–1545.

183 Felinski EA, Antonetti DA: Glucocorticoid regulation of endothelial cell tight junction gene expression: novel treatments for diabetic retinopathy. Curr Eye Res 2005;30:949–957.

184 Joussen AM, Poulaki V, Mitsiades N, Kirchhof B, Koizumi K, Dohmen S, Adamis AP: Non-steroidal anti-inflammatory drugs prevent early diabetic retinopathy via TNF-alpha suppression. FASEB J 2002;16:438–440.

185 Kern TS, Engerman RL: Pharmacological inhibition of diabetic retinopathy: aminoguanidine and aspirin. Diabetes 2001;50:1636–1642.

186 Early Treatment Diabetic Retinopathy Study: Effects of aspirin treatment on diabetic retinopathy. ETDRS report number 8. Ophthalmology 1991;98:757–765.

Dr. Triantafyllos Chavakis
Experimental Immunology Branch, NCI, NIH
10 Center Drive, Rm 5B17
Bethesda, MD 20892 (USA)
Tel. +1 301 451 2104, Fax +1 301 496 0887, E-Mail chavakist@mail.nih.gov

Hammes H-P, Porta M (eds): Experimental Approaches to Diabetic Retinopathy.
Front Diabetes. Basel, Karger, 2010, vol 20, pp 174–193

Stem and Progenitor Cells in the Retina

Nilanjana Sengupta[a] · Sergio Caballero[a] · Nicanor Moldovan[b] · Maria B. Grant[a]

[a]Department of Pharmacology and Therapeutics, University of Florida, Gainesville, Fla., and [b]Departments of Internal Medicine/Cardiology and Biomedical Engineering, Davis Heart and Lung Research Institute, Columbus, Ohio, USA

Abstract

Regardless of the debate regarding moral issues of using stem cells in research, they are unequivocally useful for understanding pathological angiogenesis, particularly so in the retina. Some important stem cell concepts include a *niche*, as well as the ideas of *self-renewal* and *plasticity*. Self-renewal is the maintenance of a stem cell population, through production of both undifferentiated and further differentiated cells (precursors), while plasticity is the differentiation of a stem cell into various cell types. However, questions regarding plasticity exist, since cell fusion was shown to be the underlying cause for some plasticity observations. Well-studied types of stem cells include neural stem cells, mesenchymal stem cells, hematopoietic stem cells or progenitors such as endothelial precursor cells. Different cell surface markers help classify these cells types. Hematopoietic stem cells and endothelial precursor cells are involved in angiogenesis. Numerous hypoxia-regulated factors have been implicated in angiogenesis, including vascular endothelial growth factor, stromal derived factor-1, insulin-like growth factor, and monocyte chemoattractant protein-1. Progenitor cells, found amongst both early (CD34+) or late (CD14+) blood mononuclear cells, are impaired in diabetes. Studying these types of cells, along with others, can dissect the precise molecular mechanisms underlying stem/progenitor cell activity in the retina.

Despite the ongoing debate about the ethical considerations regarding stem cell use, there is no denying that they are an extremely useful scientific tool for understanding disease and repair processes [1]. Normally, stem cells restore function when there is cell loss due to turnover or damage. The lineage specification of a particular stem cell depends largely on its environment.

There are three mammalian pluripotent embryonic stem (ES) cell lines that have been isolated; they are the embryonal carcinoma, ES and embryonic germ cells [2]. In the adult, the bone marrow (BM) contains the greatest number of stem cells. There are several types of stem cells present, including hematopoietic stem cells (HSCs), mesenchymal stem cells (MSCs) and additional nonhematopoietic cells [3]. The use and manipulation of BM stem cells, such as for therapeutic purposes, requires a better understanding of work characterizing the cell populations and their functions [3].

Niches

A niche is regarded as tissue or extracellular matrix (ECM) that can support the existence of at least one stem cell. In stem cell biology, continuous debate exists on whether or not niches exist and are necessary for stem cells to maintain their characteristics. The most compelling evidence for their existence comes from studies on spermatogenesis, in which germ cells are maintained by specialized stem cells and when the germ cells begin to divide, detach from the basement membrane [4, 5]. The niche also functions to control self-renewal and daughter cell production rates. Often niches function to keep pace with growth from youth to adulthood. In a lineage niche, the number of cells does not change over time. The stem cell divides in such a way that only one daughter cell is preserved in the niche as a stem cell. In the population niche, the fate of cells is somewhat less certain. Both daughter cells may continue to be stem cells or both may differentiate [6].

Characteristics of a Stem Cell

Although the exact definition of a stem cell is difficult to determine, it is generally agreed that stem cells must be capable of self-renewal and plasticity. Stem cells are usually depicted in a hierarchy of differentiation capacity; the totipotent fertilized egg is the ultimate stem cell, resulting in every differentiated cell by way of pluripotent ES cells. ES cells then lead to multipotent adult stem cells, which then give rise to non-self-renewing oligopotent progenitor and or precursor cells (fig. 1). In the hematopoietic lineage, for example, the adult stem cell gives rise to a common myeloid and a common lymphoid progenitor.

Self-Renewal

Self-renewal is the maintenance of a stem cell population, usually through asymmetric division of a cell that produces one cell that is more differentiated than the parent and one that retains the undifferentiated stem cell qualities. This definition can also include the continuance of a stem cell pool, not only the same type of stem cell.

Plasticity

There has been intense debate regarding the extent of plasticity of stem cells. Plasticity is a property that includes the differentiation of a stem cell or a stem cell pool into a wide array of cell types. It also includes *trans*differentiation from a cell that has become somewhat committed to a particular fate into a cell type that has an entirely different fate. Even more radical is the idea of dedifferentiation, where a cell can become *less* committed along a particular lineage and display more primitive characteristics [7]. Some evidence suggests that stem cells are quite flexible and can transdifferentiate extensively. For example, it has been shown that adult stem cells can differentiate into cell types that are quite different from the original cell, even crossing over germ layer distinctions [8, 9]. Cells from the BM have been shown to differentiate into an enormous variety of tissue, including muscle [10, 11], neural cells [12–14], hepatocytes [15–19], kidney [20, 21], lungs [22], GI tract [22], skin [22], myocardium [23–25] and blood [26].

On the other hand, some reports question the degree of plasticity in stem cells, even going so far as to question the existence of cell transdifferentiation. One report shows that stem cells from the central nervous system rarely differentiate into blood [27]. Wagers et al. [28] reported that HSCs did not contribute significantly to nonhematopoietic tissues such as muscle, kidney, gut, liver, or brain. This study showed considerable hematopoietic contribution to blood, but rarely outside of the blood compartment. Only one other cell type studied, a Purkinje cerebellar neuron, was identified as having derived from the HSC. This cell type was also the only identified cell type in two other similar studies [29–31].

Fusion

Cell fusion events have been shown to be at least partially responsible for some cell plasticity observations. When neurosphere-derived cells were cocultured with ES cells, the cells fused [32].

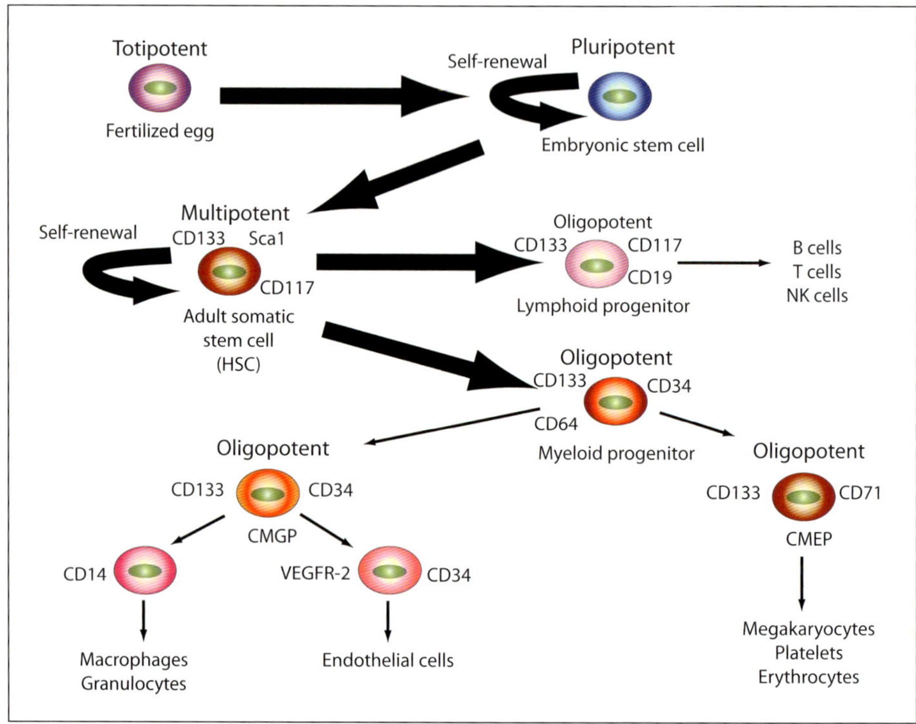

Fig. 1. Stem cells may be categorized by their plasticity. The cell with the greatest potential for differentiation is the totipotent fertilized egg, where a single cell ultimately differentiates into every single tissue of the adult individual. During development, embryonic cells arise that are pluripotent and capable of self-renewal. These cells can then differentiate into multipotent, self-renewing cells such as an HSCs. The HSCs can then differentiate into oligopotent precursor cells such as the lymphoid progenitor or myeloid progenitor. The lymphoid progenitor is then capable of differentiating into B cells, T cells and natural killer (NK) cells, while the myeloid progenitor can differentiate into other precursor cells which, in turn, give rise to macrophages, granulocytes, endothelial cells, megakaryocytes, platelets, or erythrocytes. The cell types are at least partially characterized by the presence or absence of cell surface markers. CMGP = Common macrophage/granulocyte precursor; CMEP = common megakaryocyte/erythrocyte precursor.

Fused cells were also reported by Terada et al. [33] using ES and BM cells. These cells were tetraploid, had the properties of ES and displayed markers of both of the parent cell types. These fused cells were found in the liver, intestine, kidney and heart [33]. Fusion events were also reported in a study involving heat-shocked small airway epithelial cells and human MSCs [34].

Although these fused cells have been seen in more than one study, it is unlikely that they are responsible for the results in all 'transdifferentiation' studies. Fusion is still seen as a relatively rare event. To conclude that fusion has indeed occurred, a study must show evidence of increased chromosome number, as well as the presence of both cell types. It is also important to remember that cell processes that occur in normal animals can be quite different and occur at a different rate from those that occur in injured animals.

Types of Stem and Precursor Cells

Neural Stem Cells

Neural stem cells (NSCs) are progenitor cells that can be isolated from the central nervous system, peripheral nervous system and the embryonic nervous system that can give rise to neurons and glia [35–40]. Based on these findings, it is possible that what was considered an inflexible tissue could have regenerative ability [41]. Cell surface markers that define NSCs have not yet been compiled; rather NSCs are classified based on the cell types they produce. Cultured pluripotent embryonic stem cell can produce a type of NSC, but only approximately 0.2% of embryonic stem cells produce neurospheres [42]. Stem cells have even been found in the ciliary margin of the adult mammalian retina [43].

Mesenchymal Stem Cells

MSCs, also called stromal or skeletal stem cells, are found in the BM and have been thought to differentiate into several cell types, including bone, cartilage, fat, muscle, marrow stroma and tendon [10, 44–49]. When isolated from an adult human, the cells could be stimulated to produce adipocytic, chondrogenic, or osteogenic cells [50]. Compiling the cell surface markers to identify MSCs has proven difficult, partially due to cross-reactivity of markers with other cell types [51, 52]. A distinguishable characteristic of MSCs is their adherence to tissue culture plastic [8].

Work presented by Verfaillie et al. [53] suggests MSCs differentiate into endothelium, liver and neural cells and may be able to differentiate into all cell types [31]. A type of BM-derived cell termed the multipotent adult progenitor cell was shown to co-purify with MSC. These cells were shown to be CD34–, VE-cadherin–, AC133+ and Flk1+, signifying that they were nonendothelial in nature. However, when these cells were cultured in the presence of vascular endothelial growth factor (VEGF), the cells differentiated into cells that express known endothelial markers. In addition, the cells played a role in tumor angiogenesis as well as wound healing. These cells may provide a novel source of endothelial cells for future therapies [53]. The same authors have shown that these multipotent adult progenitor cells differentiate into cells that have mesodermal, neuroectodermal and endodermal characteristics in vitro, and differentiated into cells of the hematopoietic and epithelial lineages in vivo [54].

Hematopoietic Stem Cell

HSCs are believed to be the cells that, besides assisting hematopoiesis, also would drive adult vasculogenesis. They are defined by the ability to differentiate into all cells of the vascular system. The close location of endothelial cells and hematopoietic cells in the early embryonic blood islands has indicated a common ancestor cell, the hemangioblasts [55]. Further evidence for this common ancestor cell is that both lineages display common cell surface markers, such as Flk-1, Tie 2, CD34 and SCL/TAL [56–60]. HSCs home rapidly through the blood to the BM [61]. In vitro studies have shown that when HSCs are in contact with stromal cells, their proliferation rate increases [62, 63]. HSCs may vary in their capacity to self-renew. Krause et al. [22] have shown that one HSC could differentiate into cells of endodermal and ectodermal organs. Multipotent progenitors comprise approximately 0.05% of mouse BM cells. Within this cell population, three groups exist, the long-term and the short-term self-renewing HSCs and the multipotent progenitors that do not have measurable self-renewing capacity [64].

Several studies have shown that recruitment and subsequent differentiation of HSCs to sites of mechanical injury in the retina contribute to retinal neovascularization in a murine model [26, 65–68].

It is still relatively unknown exactly which genes are responsible for HSCs to retain their differentiation characteristics. Early on, it was widely believed that the stem cell leukemia/*tal-1* gene was required for HSCs. However, this notion was placed into question by Mikkola et al. [69] when it was concluded that this gene was seemingly required for the initial *generation* of HSCs, but not for the *retention* of HSC characteristics.

Endothelial Precursor Cells

During development, HSCs are found in the center of blood islands, whereas the endothelial precursor cells (EPCs) are found along the periphery. In 1991, George et al. [70] unequivocally demonstrated the presence of circulating endothelial cells (CECs) in whole blood using an endothelial cell-specific antibody. Since that time, a number of different laboratories have identified CECs in whole blood by the use of endothelial cell-specific monoclonal antibodies and cell culture in a variety of pathologic conditions. In normal individuals, there are approximately 0–20 CEC per milliliter of blood. CECs may be derived from two sources: shed from the vasculature or, more interestingly, released from the BM. Cells derived from the vasculature would be mature endothelial cells and express phenotypic endothelial cell markers such as von Willebrand factor, VE-cadherin, CD146, or TE-7. These mature endothelial cells may detach due to mechanical disruption [71, 72]. If CECs originate from the BM, they are derived from EPCs and can fully differentiate to endothelial cells, expressing mature endothelial cell markers. Unfortunately, few studies have addressed these hypotheses to determine the true origin of CECs [73, 74].

Although it is not clear what markers precisely define an EPC, it is clear that cells derived from the BM will populate an area of neoangiogenesis. In a neovascular mouse model, 8–11% of the endothelial cells were of EPC origin, whereas hematopoietic progenitors populate about 2% of the vasculature in stable adult tissue [75]. Similar results are seen in the neovascularization that occurs in the endometrium during ovulation and wound healing in mice [76]. There are both circulating HSCs and EPCs that have the capacity to populate both the BM and neovasculature [61]. Although HSCs are generally thought to be the ancestor of the EPCs, it has been shown that MSCs can also differentiate into EPCs [22].

Several studies have indirectly addressed the issue of the presence of EPCs in the circulation and their role in postnatal vasculogenesis. The progenitor cell markers CD133 or CD34 are seen on the EPCs. After 7 days of culture on fibronectin, CD34+ mononuclear cells display an endothelial cell phenotype, are able to incorporate acetylated low-density lipoprotein, produce nitric oxide when stimulated with VEGF and express platelet/endothelial cell adhesion molecule-1 and Tie-2 receptor [77]. It is also believed that a unique subset of cells expressing CD133, CD34 and VEGFR-2 may be an additional source of EPC [78, 79]. Cells that express both CD133 and CD34 are believed to be more primitive EPCs, whereas CD133– but CD34+, VEGFR-2+ cells may represent a more mature, differentiated population of EPCs [78, 79]. In support of this, CD34+ cells enriched for CD133+ cells do not express VE-cadherin or von Willebrand factor and only 3% of these cells express VEGFR-2. However, after 3 weeks of culture and further purification with *Ulex europaeus* agglutinin (a lectin-recognizing endothelial cells), cells expressed several specific endothelial markers (von Willebrand factor, CD146, CD105, E-selectin, VCAM-1 and VE-cadherin) [80]. Several studies have used animal models to examine neovascular development in response to exogenous administration of various agents as well as targeted mutations [81, 82].

Bone Marrow-Derived Cells Participate in Normal Maintenance and Repair of the Endothelium

As mentioned earlier, circulating BM-derived cells participate in normal maintenance of the endothelium [75, 83–87]. Approximately 1–12% of endothelial cells in blood vessels are BM derived;

however, BM-derived cell integration into the endothelium varies among vascular beds [88–91]. The contribution of BM to the endothelium of injured tissue ranges from 1% to as high as 50% of vessels [75, 84–86]. These data strongly suggest that the magnitude of recruitment of EPC may be organ-specific and dependent on the extent of vascular injury and remodeling.

Recruitment of specific subsets of HSCs may be essential for the proper repair and incorporation into locally derived endothelium. Compelling evidence suggests that unique subsets of proangiogenic HSCs support angiogenesis postnatally not only by incorporating into the vascular lumen but by delivering bioavailable angiogenic factors including VEGF, matrix metalloproteases (MMPs) and angiopoietins to the neovessels [92–98]. Monocyte precursors of EPC such as CD14+ cells contribute to neoangiogenesis by releasing MMP-9 [99] and MMP-12 [100].

Methods for Studying Stem/Progenitor Cell Behavior

Much of the work in characterizing the contribution of HSCs has been with the use of chimeric animals where the BM cells from a donor are labeled for tracking using either transgenic fluorescent proteins or an overexpressed protein that can be detected immunologically, such as LacZ. Similarly, male BM cells transplanted into female recipients can be detected by fluorescence in situ hybridization to the Y-chromosome. In any case, the donor cells are given to recipient animals whose own BM has been ablated either chemically or by high-dose irradiation.

Alternatively, either HSCs or EPCs may be administered directly into the circulation without BM ablation of the recipient in a method known as adoptive transfer. This technique has been extremely useful, specifically to examine the contribution of specific stem cell subpopulations to repair. It has been used therapeutically with adoptive transfer of EPCs to restore blood flow and increase capillary density, resulting in decreased loss of limbs and recovery from myocardial ischemia [101–107]. EPCs can be ex vivo-expanded and then infused and have been shown to improve neovascularization in hind limb ischemia models [108] and improve ejection fractions and end-systolic volumes, indicating better cardiac function in myocardial infarction models [84, 106, 107]. Several clinical studies showed similar effects [109].

Factors Regulating Stem and Progenitor Cell Involvement in Angiogenesis

Numerous hypoxia-regulated factors have been implicated in angiogenesis. VEGF is by far the most well studied [110–113]. Even minor states of hypoxia can promote VEGF expression through a family of hypoxia-inducible transcription factors that bind to a hypoxia response element in the VEGF promoter [114]. Six isoforms of VEGF exist including placental growth factor (PlGF). PlGF can stimulate angiogenesis in vivo [115], migration of endothelial cells in vitro, potentiate the effect of VEGF on permeability, and induce chemotaxis of monocytes [92, 116–119]. Other isoforms, VEGF-A and VEGF-B, are highly expressed in EPCs as compared to human umbilical vein endothelial cells and human microvascular endothelial cells [120]. VEGF receptors, VEGFR-1, VEGFR-2 and VEGFR-3 only bind certain isoforms of VEGF. Ligands for VEGFR-1 include VEGF-A, -B and PlGF; ligands for VEGFR-2 include VEGF-A, -C, -D, and -E, while ligands for VEGFR-3 are VEGF-C and -D. Thus, PlGF uniquely binds VEGFR-1, and VEGF-E uniquely binds VEGFR-2. By using these specific ligands, the activities of these receptors can be dissected [121, 122].

VEGFR-2 expression is upregulated by hypoxia and possibly by VEGF-A, and it is accepted as the receptor that mediates functional VEGF signaling in endothelial cells [123]. The role of VEGFR-1 is less clear as it may function as a negative regulator of VEGFR-2 [124]. VEGFR-1 signaling may also be involved in migration of monocytes and endothelial cells induced by PlGF and VEGF-A, due to its ability to induce tissue factor [117]. PlGF regulates inter- and intramolecular crosstalk between VEGFR-1 and VEGFR-2 tyrosine kinases. Activation of VEGFR-1 by PlGF resulted in intermolecular transphosphorylation of VEGFR-2, thereby amplifying VEGF-driven angiogenesis through VEGFR-2 [125]. These studies show the complexity of the VEGF signaling mechanisms. Furthermore, aspects of signaling of these receptors may be context-dependent as well as cell type specific. Most of what is known about these receptors in HSCs is their surface expression as determined by flow cytometry analysis. Less is known about their characterization in vivo.

SDF-1 is the principal chemokine responsible for the localization of HSCs to the BM niche and subsequent mobilization to the circulation. Together with VEGF, SDF-1 not only stimulates the migration of mature endothelial cells but also acts as the main chemoattractant to promote homing and tissue invasion of endothelial and progenitor cells [126]. SDF-1 expression is increased in response to tissue ischemia and its expression is regulated by VEGF. We demonstrated that SDF-1 is elevated in the vitreous fluid of diabetic patients and correlates with vitreous VEGF levels and with retinopathy severity [127]. Blocking SDF-1 prevents recruitment of HSCs and EPCs to the retina [65] and choroid [68] following injury of these areas, and thus prevents development of neovascularization. Overexpression of SDF-1 promoted neovascularization of ischemic tissues [128].

Picomolar concentrations of SDF-1, similar to those found in the vitreous of patients with proliferative diabetic retinopathy (PDR), increase CD34+ cell migration [129] and promote nondiabetic CD34+ cell differentiation into endothelial cells by increasing VEGFR-2 surface expression [Grant, unpubl. studies]. Exposure of CD34+ cells to SDF-1 at a concentration of 0.1 ng/ml results in a rapid increase in VEGFR-2 expression with a gradual return to baseline over a 6-hour period and no change in VEGFR-1 expression. In contrast, a high concentration of SDF-1 (100 ng/ml) results in a sustained increase in VEGFR-2 expression and no change in VEGFR-1 levels. This suggests that SDF-1 is mediating its effects in CD34+ cells via VEGFR-2 activation, whereas pigment epithelium-derived factor inhibits VEGFR-2-induced angiogenesis via VEGFR-1 [130].

Insulin-like growth factor (IGF)-1 is a potent antiapoptotic protein and promotes angiogenesis in different models [131, 132]. Urbich and Dimmeler [106] and Urbich et al. [133] found that IGF-1 mRNA was highly expressed in CD34+ cells when compared to mature endothelial cells or CD14+ monocytes, which produce approximately 10-fold less IGF-1 mRNA. IGF-1 is needed for survival of EPC populations in culture [133]. IGF-1 is regulated by a series of binding proteins (BPs); IGFBP is the most abundant BP in serum. Finally, Liu et al. [134] showed using in vitro cell proliferation assays that the addition of exogenous IGFBP-3 to cultures of purified CD34+/–CD38–Lin– cells stimulates the proliferation of primitive hematopoietic cells with CD34+CD38– phenotype, suggesting that IGFBP-3 is capable of expanding primitive human blood cells. Our data show that IGFBP-3 stimulates migration, tube formation and differentiation of CD34+ cells into endothelial cells in a dose-dependent manner [135].

The expression of IGF-1 in EPC has been shown. Urbich et al. [136] analyzed the expression profile of cytokines in human peripheral blood-derived EPC, human umbilical vein endothelial cell, human microvascular endothelial cell and CD14+ monocytes by microarray technology. These authors found that IGF-1 mRNA was highly expressed in EPC when compared to mature endothelial cells or CD14+ monocytes which produce approximately 10-fold less IGF-1 mRNA. These results suggest that progenitor cells may promote neovascularization-releasing factors, which act in a paracrine manner to support local angiogenesis and mobilize tissue-residing progenitor cells. Hanley et al. [137] identified specific targets of IGF-1 within human fetal BM (FBM). These authors found that IGF-1 stimulated the expansion of primitive multilineage CD34+CD38– hematopoietic progenitor cells and increased yields of several hematopoietic subpopulations, including CD34+CD38+CD10+ lymphoid progenitor cells. Additionally, IGF-1 had direct effects on FBM stromal elements, inducing the expansion of myeloid-like CD45+CD14+ FBM stromal cells and enhancing production of the hematopoietic cytokine interleukin-3 by fibroblast-like CD45-CD10+ FBM stromal cells.

In addition, Kim et al. [133] demonstrated that AC133–CD14+ cells from human umbilical cord blood are able to develop endothelial phenotype with expression of endothelial-specific surface markers and form cord- and tubular-like structures in vitro. The AC133-CD14+ cells were grown in medium supplemented with fetal bovine serum, VEGF, basic fibroblast growth factor and IGF-1. After 14 days, the cells formed cord- and tubular-like structures, and showed a strong increase in the endothelial marker P1H12 over time. In addition, CD14 decreased, and CD45 did not change. The cells also expressed endothelial markers von Willebrand's factor, platelet/endothelial cell adhesion molecule-1 (CD31), VEGFR-1, VEGFR-2, eNOS and VE-cadherin, but did not express Tie-2 after 7 days of culture. Finally, Liu et al. [134] showed in in vitro cell proliferation assays that the addition of an exogenous IGFBP-3 to cultures of purified CD34+/–CD38–Lin– cells stimulates the proliferation of primitive hematopoietic cells with CD34+CD38– phenotype, suggesting that IGFBP-3 is capable of expanding primitive human blood cells.

SDF-1 and IGF-1 released from EPCs which have already been recruited into the ischemic tissue may promote vascular remodeling of resident cells [104, 138]. The release of factors from EPCs involved in neovascularization is a dynamic process, and it is very likely that the expression pattern of angiogenic factors by EPCs may regulate their differentiation and may change during different EPC activities such as homing versus vascular incorporation in ischemic tissue.

The role of monocyte chemoattractant protein (MCP)-1 and its receptor (CCR2) in repair has also been examined. Sakai et al. [139] showed that human peripheral CD14+ cells contribute directly to fibrogenesis by an MCP-1/CCR2-dependent amplification loop. These authors investigated the effect of MCP-1 on the expression of MCP-1, CCR2, transforming growth factor-β1 (TGF-β1) and type I collagen in circulating human CD14+ cells. They found that the stimulation of CD14+ cells with MCP-1 increased mRNA and protein levels of TGF-β1 and a pro-α_1-chain of type I collagen. Similarly, the expression of MCP-1 and CCR2 was enhanced by the stimulation with MCP-1 in dose- and time-dependent manners. Umland et al. [140] showed that CD34+ BM cells stimulated by TNF-α also show enhanced secretion of MCP-1. Awad et al. [108] demonstrated that at least some progenitor-induced healing is probably mediated through increased sensitivity to VEGF and increases in MCP-1, and possibly modulation of angiopoietins. These authors showed that injection of CD14+ and CD34+ cells into mice improved healing and vessel growth associated with the expression of VEGF and MCP-1 proteins. Nakajima et al. [141] found that in the pathogenesis of multiple sclerosis (MS), the CD14+CCR2+ blood monocytes may play an important role in the shift from active disease to a state in which MS is in remission. These authors found that expression of CCR2 and CD14 on the monocytes in the MS patients was markedly decreased, and there was a significant negative correlation between the Th1/Th2 ratio [CD4+CXCR3+ cells (Th1), CD4+CCR4+ cells (Th2)] and the CCR2 and CD14 expression on monocytes. However, despite all these studies, the magnitude and temporal sequence of MCP-1 expression in relation to tissue injury and regeneration following ischemic injury remains unknown. Shireman et al. [142] found that the transient increases and selective tissue distribution of MCP-1 during early inflammation and muscle regeneration, in a mouse model of femoral artery excision, support the hypothesis that this cytokine participates in the early reparative events preceding the restoration of vascular perfusion following ischemic injury.

CD34+ and CD14+ Cells in Diabetes

CD34+ Cells from Diabetic Patients Have Impaired Migration

As discussed previously, one marker that has been extensively used to identify the origin of human EPCs among hematopoietic cells is CD34 [143–147]. There is considerable disagreement in the literature as to whether CD34 is found on HSCs or whether it is expressed by more differentiated HSC progeny such as EPCs [145, 148–151]. Angiogenesis can be amplified by injection of CD34+ cells [77]. Among those who feel that CD34 is expressed by less differentiated stem cells, it has been hypothesized that the presence of CD34 may represent an activated state of the stem cell [152, 153]. These data indicate that CD34+ cells are involved in stem/progenitor cell identification and angiogenesis; however, the precise mechanisms of (inter)action have yet to be determined.

Defective CD34+ function is associated with diseases such as diabetes [88, 90, 154–163]. Diabetes is associated with reduced mobilization of CD34+ cells from the BM, reduced numbers of CD34+ in the circulation, reduced migration of CD34+ cells into areas of ischemia, reduced incorporation of these cells into capillaries and reduced differentiation into endothelial cells [83, 161, 162, 164, 165]. Blood glucose control also correlates with CD34+ cell counts, with better control associated with higher numbers [161, 162]. However, diabetic CD34+ cell growth defects are not reversed by cultivation in normoglycemic medium, suggesting that the impairment of CD34+ cells is not reversible by glucose correction alone [162].

We have demonstrated that CD34+ cells isolated from diabetic individuals have defective migration in response to SDF-1 [129]. We have since studied the migration of CD34+ cells isolated from patients with type 1 or type 2 diabetes in response to VEGF and IGF-1 and have found that the diabetic CD34+ cells have defective migration to these factors. These data suggest that the defect in migration of diabetic CD34+ cells is a generalized defect to all hypoxia-regulated factors. We have characterized the mechanism of this defect in diabetic CD34+ cells by measuring intracellular, bioavailable NO using diaminofluorescein-FM [129]. Diabetic CD34+ cells inherently have diminished NO compared to CD34+ cells isolated from healthy controls. This does not appear to be the case in CD14+ cells of diabetic and nondiabetic origin, and these cells migrate to MCP-1.

Human nondiabetic blood-derived CD34+ cells promoted revascularization of skin wounds in mice with type 1 diabetes [160]. In a nude mouse model of hind limb ischemia, exogenous nondiabetic blood-derived CD34+ cells profoundly accelerated blood flow restoration in type 1 diabetic mice [163]. Lambiase et al. [165] demonstrated that reduced numbers of CD34+ cells with impaired chemotactic and proangiogenic activity exist in type 1 diabetics and that when infused result in reduced formation of collateral vessels.

CD14+ Monocytes Participate in Capillary Formation

Traditionally, monocytes were considered a homogenous class of blood mononuclear cells, behaving mostly as acute-phase phagocytes and as precursors of tissue macrophages. With the recent progress in the understanding of their true heterogeneity in the blood, the very notion of 'monocyte' [166], as well as the whole 'mononuclear phagocyte system' seems to have outlived its usefulness [167]. In particular, monocytes and their descendants in culture were repeatedly shown to acquire endothelial properties when exposed to appropriate growth factors [168, 169]. In vivo, incorporation of monocyte descendants into neovessels is more and more accepted [170, 171].

Moldovan and coworkers demonstrated that monocytes and macrophages participate in neovascularization by staging a pattern for development of new capillaries. To better understand this process, they developed in vitro and in vivo models of extracellular matrix invasion by monocytes, identified either by their origin, or by the F8/40 marker [172].

These cells form tubular, low-density domains (tunnels) in the Matrigel, are often at the 'tips' of new capillaries and pave the way for subsequent vascular maturation by providing a conduit to revascularization. In vitro, they confirmed both formation of tunnels and the adoption of a cylindrical shape by many cells, consistent with a *trans*cellular lumen [173]. The polarized matrix dissolution and stepwise development of macrophage-generated intracellular vacuoles, culminating with formation of lumen is remarkably similar to lumen formation in endothelial cells. Moreover, macrophages in their in vivo experimental model also formed a lumen and generated branching patterns, supporting the recent suggestion that macrophages could control the branching of capillaries [99].

The many different metabolic perturbations typically associated with diabetes including excess free fatty acids, insulin resistance, oxidative stress, PKC activation and others may impact EPC behavior. In addition, vascular basement membranes including those of the retinal capillaries are heavily modified by advanced glycation end products' crosslink formation [174, 175] and the impact of these changes on EPC behavior has not yet been characterized.

It is well-recognized that cellular phenotype and response to exogenous factors are highly dependent on receptor expression; however, receptor expression in EPCs has been mostly used to classify the EPC population rather than characterize cell function. VEGF receptors, VEGFR-1 and VEGFR-2, and the SDF-1 receptor CXCR4 are expressed on CD34+ and CD14+ cells. However, quantitation of receptor number in health and disease and regulation of receptor expression by their appropriate ligands remains largely unknown. The differential interplay between VEGF receptors, CXCR4 and other growth factor receptors in these two cell populations will determine their ability to differentiate into endothelial cells. In addition, these receptor-ligand interactions will regulate the production of cytokines by activated CD34+ and CD14+ cells and orchestrate their complex behavior in vascular remodeling.

Diabetic CD34+ cells are defective and less able to repair ischemic regions associated with acellular capillaries. These defects could manifest themselves as reduced attachment, differentiation and invasive potential by CD34+ cells. The repair of injured vessels will require the EPCs to first attach, migrate through any thrombus/matrix in the region and finally differentiate into endothelium. The incorporation of EPCs into pre-existing vessels relies not only on growth factor gradients and recruitment factors but also on appropriate interaction with the underlying vascular basement membrane that is exposed after endothelial cell death.

CD34+ cells of patients with type 2 diabetes show impaired adhesion to the endothelium, decreased proliferation and aberrant tubule formation [161]. Murine Sca-1+ HSCs dramatically improved vascularization of skin wounds in obese type 2 diabetic *Lepr*^{db} but not in congenic lean nondiabetic C57Bl/6 mice [155]. Moreover, when skin wounds of $Lepr^{db}$ mice were treated with $Lepr^{db}$-derived Sca-1+ HSC-enriched BM cells, wound vascularization was severely inhibited [155]. Awad et al. [156] demonstrated that the obese type 2 diabetes syndrome induces intrinsic defects in CD34+ EPCs but not in CD14+ monocytic cells. The defects in CD34+ cells were evident in vitro by decreases in CD34+ cell-derived endothelial cells after stress and in vivo in nondiabetic mice by the reduction in vascular growth in skin wounds and exacerbation of ischemia-induced tissue damage in limb muscle. The behavior of BM cells in diabetic and nondiabetic environments may differ [154, 155], and there may be negative synergism between the diabetic environment and diabetic BM-derived cells.

MCP-1 is the primary chemokine that induces CD14+ cell migration. Interestingly, blocking p38 MAPK in CD14+ cells promoted endothelial differentiation [176]. Therapy with CD14+ cells improved healing and vessel growth, although not as rapidly or effectively as CD34+ cells. Cell treatments with either cell type modulated local expression of VEGF, MCP-1 and angiopoietin. Most importantly, in diabetes CD14+ cells are not hindered in their angiogenic activity as are CD34+ cells [108]. Intramuscularly injected freshly isolated CD14+ cells, CD34+ cells, or the combination of the two increased arteriolar density and promoted muscle salvage in the diabetic mouse ischemic hind limb. All cell treatments also accelerated blood flow restoration, but with different kinetics. Western analysis showed distinct patterns of proangiogenic factor expression in CD34+ and CD14+ cell-treated limbs [108]. CD34+ cells isolated from umbilical cord blood and exposed to VEGF showed increased expression of CD14 and rapid differentiated into endothelial cells in vitro. These studies suggest that when CD34+ cells differentiate towards the more mature CD14+ cell, they become less vulnerable to the adverse conditions associated with diabetes.

CD34+ and CD14+ EPCs and the Retina

Data support that CD14+ and CD34+ cells participate in neovascularization, are affected by the disease state of the retina, and are likely to participate in both normal homeostasis and pathology in retinal vasculature. The unique responses of CD34+ and CD14+ cells may be dependent on distinctive VEGFR-1/VEGFR-2 interactions and further modified by exposure to SDF-1 acting through its receptor CXCR4. Our and other studies suggest that the VEGFR-1/VEGFR-2 interaction may affect the angiogenic phenotype. We have already demonstrated that in the most hypoxic regions of the retina, the new vascular tufts are composed exclusively of EPCs; however, we have not characterized the EPC population forming these tufts.

CD14+ cells are a heterogeneous class of progenitors that can generate dendritic cells, macrophages, fibroblasts and endothelial cells as part of vascular maintenance. CD34+ cells can become CD14+ cells, but CD34+ cells usually become endothelial cells without transitioning through a CD14+ phenotype. CD34+ cells can assist the CD14+ cells in acquiring full endothelial function (fig. 2) [108, 177]. In the context of repair and maintenance of the retinal vasculature, if any ischemia or vascular injury occurs in a nondiabetic individual, CD34+ cells would quickly be recruited to the ischemic/injured retinal vasculature to promote repair of any injured endothelium. In diabetes, this does not occur, and acellular capillaries, extracellular matrix tubes with no cellular components, develop instead. In this context, we also postulate that in the event of proper repair, i.e. re-endothelialization and re-perfusion of ischemic retina by CD34+ cells, minimal CD14+ cell contribution would occur. The CD14+ response to vascular repair is predominately initiated when the CD34+ cell response is impaired.

Numerous studies demonstrate that CD14+ cells can differentiate into endothelial-like cells [173, 178–182] and participate in

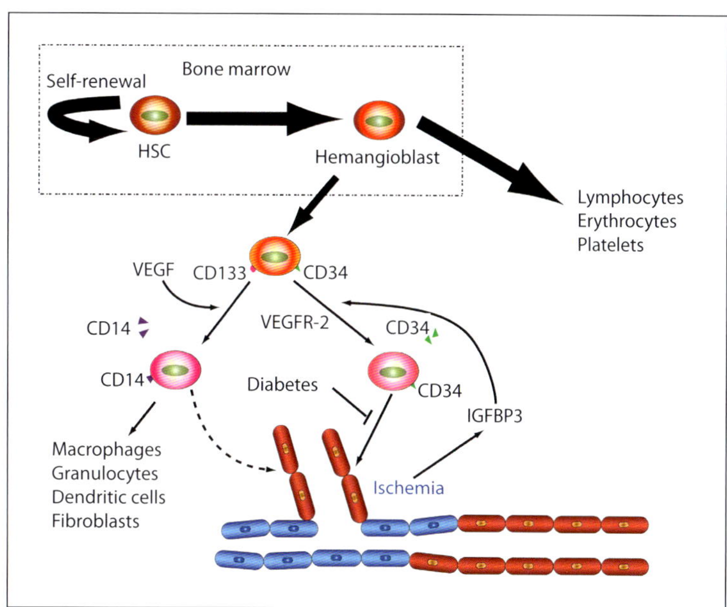

Fig. 2. Vascular mimicry by CD14+ progenitors. The self-renewing HSC in the BM can show hemangioblast activity, which is defined as the capacity to differentiate into all of the components of the vascular system. One of the progeny, the CD133+CD34+ common macrophage granulocyte precursor can then lead to either mature CD14+ progenitor, which normally becomes either a macrophage, or granulocyte, dendritic cell, fibroblast, or supposedly remain a CD34+ EPC. There is a large body of evidence indicating that the diabetic milieu negatively affects the CD34+ EPC, inhibiting its ability to restore or repair damaged vasculature. In such a case, the CD14 progenitor, in a process known as vascular mimicry, can provide compensatory re-endothelialization or repair. Unfortunately, since the CD14+ progenitor is already a committed cell, the process is aberrant and can result in preretinal neovascularization. Any stem cell therapy designed to correct this would have to include the restoration of the functions of CD34+ cell.

neovascularization in experimental models [179, 182]. These studies suggest that these cells need priming to differentiate into endothelial cells and promote vascular growth. This should not be surprising as monocytes require activation to perform virtually every function with which they are associated [108]. Diabetes is associated with inflammation implicated in the pathogenesis of macrovascular complications [183]. There is a growing body of evidence that the ability of BM-derived cells to promote vascular growth is altered by diabetes, although exactly which BM cells are impaired and the precise nature of the impairment remains unknown.

In diabetic retinopathy, monocytes contribute to capillary occlusion and nonperfusion [184]. Leukostasis of circulating monocytes promotes endothelial apoptosis [184, 185]. The contribution of monocytes to pathological retinal neovascularization, however, has not been studied. Circulating CD14+ monocytes change towards an increased inflammatory phenotype in patients with type 2 diabetes [186] displaying increased CD36 cell surface expression, increased uptake of oxidized low-density lipoprotein, increased attachment to endothelial monolayers [187] and increased MCP-1 gene expression.

The death of pericytes and endothelial cells is a hallmark of diabetic retinopathy and leads to the formation of acellular capillaries [188, 189]. The inability of acellular capillaries to support blood flow leads to irreversible retinal ischemia, increased expression of angiogenic growth factors and subsequent retinal neovascularization. The collective evidence indicates that the loss of retinal microvascular cells, a critical early step in diabetic retinopathy, may be due not only to increased cell death but also to dysfunctional repair mechanisms.

Hypoxia is known to regulate the ligand and receptor activities for angiogenic factors in vascular endothelial cells, thus determining angiogenic outcome. Hypoxia can similarly regulate receptor expression in CD34+ cells. Hypoxia (pO_2 = 20 mm Hg) increases CXCR4, VEGFR-2 and IGF-1R mRNA expression but dramatically increases (4- to 8-fold) in CD34+ cells [Grant, unpubl. results]. In CD14+ cells, hypoxia increases CXCR4 (2-fold) and VEGFR-1 (14-fold) and reduces IGF-1R and VEGFR-2 mRNA expression. We postulate that the hypoxia-induced differential interplay between VEGFR-1, VEGFR-2, CXCR4 and IGF-1R in the different cell populations will determine their cellular response and ultimate fate.

Conclusion

While ES cells have long been heralded for their therapeutic potential, it is only recently that adult stem cells have been identified as existing and playing a role in normal physiology. While it was initially thought that adult stem cells might have less therapeutic potential than ES cells because of presumed loss of plasticity, newer investigations have demonstrated robust differentiation potential of these adult cells.

The adult HSCs, because of their abundance and relative ease of isolation from a variety of laboratory animals, have been among the most studied of the adult stem cells. These cells have shown at times an amazing capacity to differentiate into seemingly disparate tissues, such as blood, liver, muscle and neural tissue. At the same time these same cells, in the hands of others, have failed to differentiate into other than their most accepted progeny, i.e. blood, blood components and, most recently, vasculature. These disparate results should not be interpreted as a failure of the therapeutic potential of adult stem cells, but rather as an indication of how little is known about the complex processes required for canonical and noncanonical differentiation.

One of the most promising areas for adult stem cell therapy is that of vascular biology. The evidence presented in this review has shown that adult HSCs and their EPC progeny most certainly play an important role in vascular maintenance as well as pathological neovascularization. Diabetic retinopathy is among the most intensely studied neovascular diseases. Its prevalence and its devastating life changes have made it a target of intense investigation. This neovascular disease is thus a prime objective for developing stem cell-base therapies. Initially, it was thought that preventing stem cell involvement in PDR would be sufficient to reduce or eliminate preretinal neovascularization. Further investigation, however, has drawn a much more complicated picture. It is becoming evident that not only are different molecular mechanisms involved in the progression of PDR, but also different types of precursor cells may contribute to the degree of pathology. Because of these recent findings, the complex interactions among the biochemical pathways and cell types need to be explored in more depth.

The state of knowledge in adult stem cell research today stands at a point similar to that of molecular biology at the discovery of the structure of DNA. Only now are the tools being discovered and assembled that will allow a deeper understanding of the processes involved in stem cell physiology, and it is the hope that that understanding will lead to perhaps miraculous stem cell-based therapies.

References

1 McLaren A: Ethical and social considerations of stem cell research. Nature 2001;414:129–131.
2 Donovan PJ, Gearhart J: The end of the beginning for pluripotent stem cells. Nature 2001;414:92–97.
3 Herzog EL, Chai L, Krause DS: Plasticity of marrow-derived stem cells. Blood 2003;102:3483–3493.
4 de Rooij DG: Stem cells in the testis. Int J Exp Pathol 1998;79:67–80.
5 de Rooij DG, Grootegoed JA: Spermatogonial stem cells. Curr Opin Cell Biol 1998;10:694–701.
6 Spradling A, Drummond-Barbosa D, Kai T: Stem cells find their niche. Nature 2001;414:98–104.
7 Huttmann A, Li CL, Duhrsen U: Bone marrow-derived stem cells and 'plasticity'. Ann Hematol 2003;82:599–604.
8 Preston SL, Alison MR, Forbes SJ, Direkze NC, Poulsom R, Wright NA: The new stem cell biology: something for everyone. Mol Pathol 2003;56:86–96.
9 Toma JG, Akhavan M, Fernandes KJ, Barnabe-Heider F, Sadikot A, Kaplan DR, Miller FD: Isolation of multipotent adult stem cells from the dermis of mammalian skin. Nat Cell Biol 2001;3:778–784.
10 Ferrari G, Cusella-De Angelis G, Coletta M, Paolucci E, Stornaiuolo A, Cossu G, Mavilio F. Muscle regeneration by bone marrow-derived myogenic progenitors. Science 1998;279:1528–1530.
11 Gussoni E, Soneoka Y, Strickland CD, Buzney EA, Khan MK, Flint AF, Kunkel LM, Mulligan RC: Dystrophin expression in the mdx mouse restored by stem cell transplantation. Nature 1999;401:390–394.
12 Mezey E, Chandross KJ, Harta G, Maki RA, McKercher SR: Turning blood into brain: cells bearing neuronal antigens generated in vivo from bone marrow. Science 2000;290:1779–1782.
13 Brazelton TR, Rossi FM, Keshet GI, Blau HM: From marrow to brain: expression of neuronal phenotypes in adult mice. Science 2000;290:1775–1779.
14 Eglitis MA, Mezey E: Hematopoietic cells differentiate into both microglia and macroglia in the brains of adult mice. Proc Natl Acad Sci USA 1997;94:4080–4085.
15 Petersen BE, Bowen WC, Patrene KD, Mars WM, Sullivan AK, Murase N, Boggs SS, Greenberger JS, Goff JP: Bone marrow as a potential source of hepatic oval cells. Science 1999;284:1168–1170.
16 Theise ND, Badve S, Saxena R, Henegariu O, Sell S, Crawford JM, Krause DS: Derivation of hepatocytes from bone marrow cells in mice after radiation-induced myeloablation. Hepatology 2000;31:235–240.
17 Theise ND, Nimmakayalu M, Gardner R, Illei PB, Morgan G, Teperman L, Henegariu O, Krause DS: Liver from bone marrow in humans. Hepatology 2000;32:11–16.
18 Lagasse E, Connors H, et al: Purified hematopoietic stem cells can differentiate into hepatocytes in vivo. Nat Med 2000;6:1229–1234.
19 Alison MR, Poulsom R, et al: Hepatocytes from non-hepatic adult stem cells. Nature 2000;406:257.
20 Poulsom R, Forbes SJ, et al: Bone marrow contributes to renal parenchymal turnover and regeneration. J Pathol 2001;195:229–235.
21 Imasawa T, Utsunomiya Y, Kawamura T, Zhong Y, Nagasawa R, Okabe M, Maruyama N, Hosoya T, Ohno T: The potential of bone marrow-derived cells to differentiate to glomerular mesangial cells. J Am Soc Nephrol 2001;12:1401–1409.
22 Krause DS, Theise ND, Collector MI, Henegariu O, Hwang S, Gardner R, Neutzel S, Sharkis SJ: Multi-organ, multi-lineage engraftment by a single bone marrow-derived stem cel. Cell 2001;105:369–377.
23 Jackson KA, Majka SM, et al: Regeneration of ischemic cardiac muscle and vascular endothelium by adult stem cells. J Clin Invest 2001;107:1395–1402.
24 Orlic D, Kajstura J, et al: Bone marrow cells regenerate infarcted myocardium. Nature 2001;410:701–705.
25 Orlic D, Kajstura J, et al: Mobilized bone marrow cells repair the infarcted heart, improving function and surviva.l Proc Natl Acad Sci USA 2001;98:10344–10349.
26 Grant MB, May WS, et al: Adult hematopoietic stem cells provide functional hemangioblast activity during retinal neovascularization. Nat Med 2002;8:607–612.
27 Morshead CM, Benveniste P, Iscove NN, van der Kooy D: Hematopoietic competence is a rare property of neural stem cells that may depend on genetic and epigenetic alterations. Nat Med 2002;8:268–273.
28 Wagers AJ, Sherwood RI, Christensen JL, Weissman IL: Little evidence for developmental plasticity of adult hematopoietic stem cells. Science 2002;297:2256–2259.
29 Priller J, Persons DA, Klett FF, Kempermann G, Kreutzberg GW, Dirnagl U: Neogenesis of cerebellar Purkinje neurons from gene-marked bone marrow cells in vivo. J Cell Biol 2001;155:733–738.
30 Weimann JM, Charlton CA, Brazelton TR, Hackman RC, Blau HM: Contribution of transplanted bone marrow cells to Purkinje neurons in human adult brains. Proc Natl Acad Sci USA 2003;100:2088–2093.
31 Tsai RY, Kittappa R, McKay RD: Plasticity, niches, and the use of stem cells. Dev Cell 2002;2:707–712.

32 Ying QL, Nichols J, Evans EP, Smith AG: Changing potency by spontaneous fusion. Nature 2002;416:545–548.
33 Terada N, Hamazaki T, et al: Bone marrow cells adopt the phenotype of other cells by spontaneous cell fusion. Nature 2002;416:542–545.
34 Spees JL, Olson SD, Ylostalo J, Lynch PJ, Smith J, Perry A, Peister A, Wang MY, Prockop DJ: Differentiation, cell fusion, and nuclear fusion during ex vivo repair of epithelium by human adult stem cells from bone marrow stroma. Proc Natl Acad Sci USA 2003;100:2397–2402.
35 Cattaneo E, McKay R: Proliferation and differentiation of neuronal stem cells regulated by nerve growth factor. Nature 1990;347:762–765.
36 Temple S: Division and differentiation of isolated CNS blast cells in microculture. Nature 1989;340:471–473.
37 Stemple DL, Anderson DJ: Isolation of a stem cell for neurons and glia from the mammalian neural crest. Cell 1992;71:973–985.
38 Kilpatrick TJ, Bartlett PF: Cloning and growth of multipotential neural precursors: requirements for proliferation and differentiation. Neuron 1993;10:255–265.
39 Reynolds BA, Tetzlaff W, Weiss S: A multipotent EGF-responsive striatal embryonic progenitor cell produces neurons and astrocytes. J Neurosci 1992;12:4565–4574.
40 Reynolds BA, Weiss S: Generation of neurons and astrocytes from isolated cells of the adult mammalian central nervous system. Science 1992;255:1707–1710.
41 Temple S: The development of neural stem cells. Nature 2001;414:112–117.
42 Tropepe V, Hitoshi S, Sirard C, Mak TW, Rossant J, van der Kooy D: Direct neural fate specification from embryonic stem cells: a primitive mammalian neural stem cell stage acquired through a default mechanism. Neuron 2001;30:65–78.
43 Tropepe V, Coles BL, Chiasson BJ, Horsford DJ, Elia AJ, McInnes RR, van der Kooy D: Retinal stem cells in the adult mammalian eye. Science 2000;287:2032–2036.
44 Prockop DJ: Marrow stromal cells as stem cells for nonhematopoietic tissues. Science 1997;276:71–74.
45 Friedenstein AJ, Chailakhyan RK, Gerasimov UV: Bone marrow osteogenic stem cells: in vitro cultivation and transplantation in diffusion chambers. Cell Tissue Kinet 1987;20:263–272.
46 Friedenstein AJ: Precursor cells of mechanocytes. Int Rev Cytol 1976;47:327–359.
47 Ashton BA, Allen TD, Howlett CR, Eaglesom CC, Hattori A, Owen M: Formation of bone and cartilage by marrow stromal cells in diffusion chambers in vivo. Clin Orthop 1980;151:294–307.
48 Ashton BA, Smith R: Plasma alpha 2HS-glycoprotein concentration in Paget's disease of bone: its possible significance. Clin Sci (Lond) 1980;58:435–438.
49 Spruance SL, Ashton BN, Smith CB: Preparation and characterization of high-specific activity radiolabeled 50 S measles virus RNA. J Virol Methods 1980;1:223–228.
50 Pittenger MF, Mackay AM, et al: Multilineage potential of adult human mesenchymal stem cells. Science 1999;284:143–147.
51 Goodwin HS, Bicknese AR, Chien SN, Bogucki BD, Quinn CO, Wall DA: Multilineage differentiation activity by cells isolated from umbilical cord blood: expression of bone, fat, and neural markers. Biol Blood Marrow Transplant 2001;7:581–588.
52 Simmons PJ, Torok-Storb B: Identification of stromal cell precursors in human bone marrow by a novel monoclonal antibody, STRO-1. Blood 1991;78:55–62.
53 Reyes M, Dudek A, Jahagirdar B, Koodie L, Marker PH, Verfaillie CM: Origin of endothelial progenitors in human postnatal bone marrow. J Clin Invest 2002;109:337–346.
54 Jiang Y, Jahagirdar BN, et al: Pluripotency of mesenchymal stem cells derived from adult marrow. Nature 2002;418:41–49.
55 Sabin F: Studies on the origin of blood-vessels and of red blood-corpuscles as seen in the living blastoderm of chicks during the second day of incubation. Contrib Embryol 1920:215–262.
56 Kallianpur AR, Jordan JE, Brandt SJ: The SCL/TAL-1 gene is expressed in progenitors of both the hematopoietic and vascular systems during embryogenesis. Blood 1994;83:1200–1208.
57 Young PE, Baumhueter S, Lasky LA: The sialomucin CD34 is expressed on hematopoietic cells and blood vessels during murine development. Blood 1995;85:96–105.
58 Bernex F, De Sepulveda P, Kress C, Elbaz C, Delouis C, Panthier JJ: Spatial and temporal patterns of c-kit-expressing cells in WlacZ/+ and WlacZ/WlacZ mouse embryos. Development 1996;122:3023–3033.
59 Yano M, Iwama A, Nishio H, Suda J, Takada G, Suda T. Expression and function of murine receptor tyrosine kinases, TIE and TEK, in hematopoietic stem cells. Blood 1997;89:4317–4326.
60 Eichmann A, Corbel C, Nataf V, Vaigot P, Breant C, Le Douarin NM: Ligand-dependent development of the endothelial and hemopoietic lineages from embryonic mesodermal cells expressing vascular endothelial growth factor receptor 2. Proc Natl Acad Sci USA 1997;94:5141–5146.
61 Wright DE, Wagers AJ, Gulati AP, Johnson FL, Weissman IL: Physiological migration of hematopoietic stem and progenitor cells. Science 2001;294:1933–1936.
62 Brouard N, Chapel A, Neildez-Nguyen TM, Granotier C, Khazaal I, Peault B, Thierry D: Transplantation of stromal cells transduced with the human IL3 gene to stimulate hematopoiesis in human fetal bone grafts in non-obese, diabetic-severe combined immunodeficiency mice. Leukemia 1998;12:1128–1135.
63 Dorshkind K: Regulation of hemopoiesis by bone marrow stromal cells and their products. Annu Rev Immunol 1990;8:111–137.
64 Reya T, Morrison SJ, Clarke MF, Weissman IL: Stem cells, cancer, and cancer stem cells. Nature 2001;414:105–111.
65 Butler JM, Guthrie SM, et al: SDF-1 is both necessary and sufficient to promote proliferative retinopathy. J Clin Invest 2005;115:86–93.
66 Espinosa-Heidmann DG, Caicedo A, Hernandez EP, Csaky KG, Cousins SW: Bone marrow-derived progenitor cells contribute to experimental choroidal neovascularization. Invest Ophthalmol Vis Sci 2003;44:4914–4919.

67 Sengupta N, Caballero S, Mames RN, Butler JM, Scott EW, Grant MB: The role of adult bone marrow-derived stem cells in choroidal neovascularization. Invest Ophthalmol Vis Sci 2003;44:4908–4913.

68 Sengupta N, Caballero S, Mames RN, Timmers AM, Saban D, Grant MB: Preventing stem cell incorporation into choroidal neovascularization by targeting homing and attachment factors. Invest Ophthalmol Vis Sci 2005;46:343–348.

69 Mikkola HK, Klintman J, Yang H, Hock H, Schlaeger TM, Fujiwara Y, Orkin SH: Haematopoietic stem cells retain long-term repopulating activity and multipotency in the absence of stem-cell leukaemia SCL/tal-1 gene. Nature 2003;421:547–551.

70 George F, Poncelet P, Laurent JC, Massot O, Arnoux D, Lequeux N, Ambrosi P, Chicheportiche C, Sampol J: Cytofluorometric detection of human endothelial cells in whole blood using S-Endo 1 monoclonal antibody. J Immunol Methods 1991;139:65–75.

71 Woywodt A, Streiber F, Regelsberger H, de Groot K, Haller H, Haubitz M: Detection of circulating endothelial cells in ANCA-associated small-vessel vasculitis. World Congr Nephrol, San Francisco, 2001.

72 Mutin M, Canavy I, Blann A, Bory M, Sampol J, Dignat-George F: Direct evidence of endothelial injury in acute myocardial infarction and unstable angina by demonstration of circulating endothelial cells. Blood 1999;93:2951–2958.

73 Bertolini F, Mancuso P, Kerbel RS: Circulating endothelial progenitor cells. N Engl J Med 2005;353:2613–2616; author reply 2613–2616.

74 Mancuso P, Rabascio C, Bertolini F: Strategies to investigate circulating endothelial cells in cancer. Pathophysiol Haemost Thromb 2003;33:503–506.

75 Crosby JR, Kaminski WE, Schatteman G, Martin PJ, Raines EW, Seifert RA, Bowen-Pope DF: Endothelial cells of hematopoietic origin make a significant contribution to adult blood vessel formation. Circ Res 2000;87:728–730.

76 Asahara T, Takahashi T, Masuda H, Kalka C, Chen D, Iwaguro H, Inai Y, Silver M, Isner JM: VEGF contributes to postnatal neovascularization by mobilizing bone marrow-derived endothelial progenitor cells. EMBO J 1999;18:3964–3972.

77 Asahara T, Murohara T, Sullivan A, Silver M, van der Zee R, Li T, Witzenbichler B, Schatteman G, Isner JM: Isolation of putative progenitor endothelial cells for angiogenesis. Science 1997;275:964–967.

78 Peichev M, Naiyer AJ, et al: Expression of VEGFR-2 and AC133 by circulating human CD34+ cells identifies a population of functional endothelial precursors. Blood 2000;95:952–958.

79 Gehling UM, Ergun S, et al: In vitro differentiation of endothelial cells from AC133-positive progenitor cells. Blood 2000;95:3106–3112.

80 Quirici N, Soligo D, Caneva L, Servida F, Bossolasco P, Deliliers GL: Differentiation and expansion of endothelial cells from human bone marrow CD133+ cells. Br J Haematol 2001;115:186–194.

81 Brooks SE, Gu X, Samuel S, Marcus DM, Bartoli M, Huang PL, Caldwell RB: Reduced severity of oxygen-induced retinopathy in eNOS-deficient mice. Invest Ophthalmol Vis Sci 2001;42:222–228.

82 D'Amato R, Wesolowski E, Smith LE: Microscopic visualization of the retina by angiography with high- molecular-weight fluorescein-labeled dextrans in the mouse. Microvasc Res 1993;46:135–142.

83 Hill JM, Zalos G, Halcox JP, Schenke WH, Waclawiw MA, Quyyumi AA, Finkel T: Circulating endothelial progenitor cells, vascular function, and cardiovascular risk. N Engl J Med 2003;348:593–600.

84 Kocher AA, Schuster MD, Szabolcs MJ, Takuma S, Burkhoff D, Wang J, Homma S, Edwards NM, Itescu S: Neovascularization of ischemic myocardium by human bone-marrow-derived angioblasts prevents cardiomyocyte apoptosis, reduces remodeling and improves cardiac function. Nat Med 2001;7:430–436.

85 Lagaaij EL, Cramer-Knijnenburg GF, van Kemenade FJ, van Es LA, Bruijn JA, van Krieken JH: Endothelial cell chimerism after renal transplantation and vascular rejection. Lancet 2001;357:33–37.

86 Quaini F, Urbanek K, Beltrami AP, Finato N, Beltrami CA, Nadal-Ginard B, Kajstura J, Leri A, Anversa P: Chimerism of the transplanted heart. N Engl J Med 2002;346:5–15.

87 Schmidt-Lucke C, Rossig L, Fichtlscherer S, Vasa M, Britten M, Kamper U, Dimmeler S, Zeiher AM: Reduced number of circulating endothelial progenitor cells predicts future cardiovascular events: proof of concept for the clinical importance of endogenous vascular repair. Circulation 2005;111:2981–2987.

88 Schatteman GC: Adult bone marrow-derived hemangioblasts, endothelial cell progenitors, and EPCs. Curr Top Dev Biol 2004;64:141–180.

89 Schatteman GC, Awad O: Hemangioblasts, angioblasts, and adult endothelial cell progenitors. Anat Rec 2004;276A:13–21.

90 Jiang S, Walker L, Afentoulis M, Anderson DA, Jauron-Mills L, Corless CL, Fleming WH: Transplanted human bone marrow contributes to vascular endothelium. Proc Natl Acad Sci USA 2004;101:16891–16896.

91 Peters BA, Diaz LA, et al: Contribution of bone marrow-derived endothelial cells to human tumor vasculature. Nat Med 2005;11:261–262.

92 Luttun A, Carmeliet G, Carmeliet P: Vascular progenitors: from biology to treatment. Trends Cardiovasc Med 2002;12:88–96.

93 Rafii S, Meeus S, Dias S, Hattori K, Heissig B, Shmelkov S, Rafii D, and Lyden D Contribution of marrow-derived progenitors to vascular and cardiac regeneration Semin Cell Dev Biol 2002 13(1) p 61–7

94 Hiratsuka S, Nakamura K, Iwai S, Murakami M, Itoh T, Kijima H, Shipley JM, Senior RM, Shibuya M: MMP9 induction by vascular endothelial growth factor receptor-1 is involved in lung-specific metastasis. Cancer Cell 2002;2:289–300.

95 Coussens LM, Tinkle CL, Hanahan D, Werb Z: MMP-9 supplied by bone marrow-derived cells contributes to skin carcinogenesis. Cell 2000;103:481–490.

96 Coussens LM, Raymond WW, Bergers G, Laig-Webster M, Behrendtsen O, Werb Z, Caughey GH, Hanahan D: Inflammatory mast cells up-regulate angiogenesis during squamous epithelial carcinogenesis. Genes Dev 1999;13:1382–1397.
97 Pipp F, Heil M, et al: VEGFR-1-selective VEGF homologue PlGF is arteriogenic: evidence for a monocyte-mediated mechanism. Circ Res 2003;92:378–385.
98 Cursiefen C, Chen L, et al: VEGF-A stimulates lymphangiogenesis and hemangiogenesis in inflammatory neovascularization via macrophage recruitment. J Clin Invest 2004;113:1040–1050.
99 Johnson C, Sung HJ, Lessner SM, Fini ME, Galis ZS: Matrix metalloproteinase-9 is required for adequate angiogenic revascularization of ischemic tissues: potential role in capillary branching. Circ Res 2004;94:262–268.
100 Moldovan NI, Goldschmidt-Clermont PJ, Parker-Thornburg J, Shapiro SD, Kolattukudy PE: Contribution of monocytes/macrophages to compensatory neovascularization: the drilling of metalloelastase-positive tunnels in ischemic myocardium. Circ Res 2000;87:378–384.
101 Lee IG, Chae SL, Kim JC: Involvement of circulating endothelial progenitor cells and vasculogenic factors in the pathogenesis of diabetic retinopathy. Eye 2005.
102 Asahara T, Murohara T, Sullivan A, Silver M, van der Zee R, Li T: Isolation of putative progenitor endothelial cells for angiogenesis. Science 1997;275:964–967.
103 Shi Q, Rafii S, et al: Evidence for circulating bone marrow-derived endothelial cells. Blood 1998;92:362–367.
104 Kalka C, Masuda H, Takahashi T, Kalka-Moll WM, Silver M, Kearney M, Li T, Isner JM, Asahara T: Transplantation of ex vivo expanded endothelial progenitor cells for therapeutic neovascularization. Proc Natl Acad Sci USA 2000;97:3422–3427.
105 Murohara T, Ikeda H, Duan J, Shintani S, Sasaki K, Eguchi H, Onitsuka I, Matsui K, Imaizumi T: Transplanted cord blood-derived endothelial precursor cells augment postnatal neovascularization. J Clin Invest 2000;105:1527–1536.
106 Urbich C, Dimmeler S: Endothelial progenitor cells: Characterization and role in vascular biology. Circ Res 2004;95:343–353.
107 Urbich C, Dimmeler S: Endothelial progenitor cells functional characterization. Trends Cardiovasc Med 2004;14:318–322.
108 Awad O, Dedkov E, Jiao C, Bloomer S, Tomanek RJ, Schatteman GC: Differential healing activities of CD34+ and CD14+ endothelial cell progenitors. Arterioscler Thromb Vasc Biol 2006;26:758–764.
109 Losordo DW, Vale PR, Isner JM: Gene therapy for myocardial angiogenesis. Am Heart J 1999;138(2 Pt 2):132–141.
110 Adamis AP, Miller JW, Bernal MT, D'Amico DJ, Folkman J, Yeo TK, Yeo KT: Increased vascular endothelial growth factor levels in the vitreous of eyes with proliferative diabetic retinopathy. Am J Ophthalmol 1994;118:445–450.
111 Aiello LP, Avery RL, et al: Vascular endothelial growth factor in ocular fluid of patients with diabetic retinopathy and other retinal disorders. N Engl J Med 1994;331:1480–1487.
112 Malecaze F, Clamens S, Simorre-Pinatel V, Mathis A, Chollet P, Favard C, Bayard F, Plouet J: Detection of vascular endothelial growth factor messenger RNA and vascular endothelial growth factor-like activity in proliferative diabetic retinopathy. Arch Ophthalmol 1994;112:1476–1482.
113 Ferrara N: Vascular endothelial growth factor: basic science and clinical progress. Endocr Rev 2004;25:581–611.
114 Semenza GL: HIF-1:using two hands to flip the angiogenic switch. Cancer Metastasis Rev 2000;19:59–65.
115 Ziche M, Maglione D, et al: Placenta growth factor-1 is chemotactic, mitogenic, and angiogenic. Lab Invest 1997;76:517–531.
116 Odorisio T, Schietroma C, Zaccaria ML, Cianfarani F, Tiveron C, Tatangelo L, Failla CM, Zambruno G: Mice overexpressing placenta growth factor exhibit increased vascularization and vessel permeability. J Cell Sci 2002;115 (Pt 12):2559–2567.
117 Clauss M, Weich H, Breier G, Knies U, Rockl W, Waltenberger J, Risau W: The vascular endothelial growth factor receptor Flt-1 mediates biological activities. Implications for a functional role of placenta growth factor in monocyte activation and chemotaxis. J Biol Chem 1996;271:17629–17634.
118 Sawano A, Iwai S, Sakurai Y, Ito M, Shitara K, Nakahata T, Shibuya M: Flt-1, vascular endothelial growth factor receptor 1, is a novel cell surface marker for the lineage of monocyte-macrophages in humans. Blood 2001;97:785–791.
119 Simpson DA, Murphy GM, Bhaduri T, Gardiner TA, Archer DB, Stitt AW: Expression of the VEGF gene family during retinal vaso-obliteration and hypoxia. Biochem Biophys Res Commun 1999;262:333–340.
120 Walter DH, Dimmeler S: Endothelial progenitor cells: regulation and contribution to adult neovascularization. Herz 2002;27:579–588.
121 Ogawa S, Oku A, Sawano A, Yamaguchi S, Yazaki Y, Shibuya M: A novel type of vascular endothelial growth factor, VEGF-E (NZ-7 VEGF), preferentially utilizes KDR/Flk-1 receptor and carries a potent mitotic activity without heparin-binding domain. J Biol Chem 1998;273:31273–31282.
122 Meyer M, Clauss M, et al: A novel vascular endothelial growth factor encoded by Orf virus, VEGF-E, mediates angiogenesis via signalling through VEGFR-2 (KDR) but not VEGFR-1 (Flt-1) receptor tyrosine kinases. EMBO J 1999;18:363–374.
123 Kremer C, Breier G, Risau W, Plate KH: Up-regulation of flk-1/vascular endothelial growth factor receptor 2 by its ligand in a cerebral slice culture system. Cancer Res 1997;57:3852–3859.
124 Witmer AN, Vrensen GF, Van Noorden CJ, Schlingemann RO: Vascular endothelial growth factors and angiogenesis in eye disease. Prog Retin Eye Res 2003;22:1–29.
125 Autiero M, Waltenberger J, et al: Role of PlGF in the intra- and intermolecular cross talk between the VEGF receptors Flt1 and Flk1. Nat Med 2003;9:936–943.

126 Aiuti A, Webb IJ, Bleul C, Springer T, Gutierrez-Ramos JC: The chemokine SDF-1 is a chemoattractant for human CD34+ hematopoietic progenitor cells and provides a new mechanism to explain the mobilization of CD34+ progenitors to peripheral blood. J Exp Med 1997;185:111–120.
127 Brooks HL Jr, Caballero S Jr, Newell CK, Steinmetz RL, Watson D, Segal MS, Harrison JK, Scott EW, Grant MB: Vitreous levels of vascular endothelial growth factor and stromal-derived factor 1 in patients with diabetic retinopathy and cystoid macular edema before and after intraocular injection of triamcinolone. Arch Ophthalmol 2004;122:1801–1807.
128 Yamaguchi J, Kusano KF, et al: Stromal cell-derived factor-1 effects on ex vivo expanded endothelial progenitor cell recruitment for ischemic neovascularization. Circulation 2003;107:1322–1328.
129 Segal MS, Shah R, et al: Nitric oxide cytoskeletal-induced alterations reverse the endothelial progenitor cell migratory defect associated with diabetes. Diabetes 2006;55:102–109.
130 Cai J, Jiang WG, Grant MB, Boulton M: Pigment epithelium-derived factor inhibits angiogenesis via regulated intracellular proteolysis of vascular endothelial growth factor receptor 1. J Biol Chem 2006;281:3604–3613.
131 Grant MB: Insulinlike growth factor-I in diabetic vascular complications. Curr Opin Endocr Diabetes 1996;3:335–345.
132 Delafontaine P, Song YH, Li Y: Expression, regulation, and function of IGF-1, IGF-1R, and IGF-1 binding proteins in blood vessels. Arterioscler Thromb Vasc Biol 2004;24:435–444.
133 Kim SY, Park SY, et al: Differentiation of endothelial cells from human umbilical cord blood AC133-CD14+ cells. Ann Hematol 2005;84:417–422.
134 Liu B, Sun Y, Jiang F, Zhang S, Wu Y, Lan Y, Yang X, Mao N: Disruption of Smad5 gene leads to enhanced proliferation of high-proliferative potential precursors during embryonic hematopoiesis. Blood 2003;101:124–133.
135 Grant MB, Prabakaran SL, K. Chang AA, LiCalzi S, Segal MS, Boulton ME: Endothelial precursor cells (EPCs) of diabetic and nondiabetic origin are differentally modulated by hypoxia inducible factors present in serum; in Annu Meet Assoc Res Vision Ophthalmol 2006, Ft Lauderdale.
136 Urbich C, Aicher A, Heeschen C, Dernbach E, Hofmann WK, Zeiher AM, Dimmeler S: Soluble factors released by endothelial progenitor cells promote migration of endothelial cells and cardiac resident progenitor cells. J Mol Cell Cardiol 2005;39:733–742.
137 Hanley MB, Napolitano LA, McCune JM: Growth hormone-induced stimulation of multilineage human hematopoiesis. Stem Cells 2005;23:1170–1179.
138 Asahara T, Masuda H, Takahashi T, Kalka C, Pastore C, Silver M, Kearne M, Magner M, Isner JM: Bone marrow origin of endothelial progenitor cells responsible for postnatal vasculogenesis in physiological and pathological neovascularization. Circ Res 1999;85:221–228.
139 Sakai N, Wada T, et al: MCP-1/CCR2-dependent loop for fibrogenesis in human peripheral CD14-positive monocytes. J Leukoc Biol 2006;79:555–563.
140 Umland O, Heine H, Miehe M, Marienfeld K, Staubach KH, Ulmer AJ: Induction of various immune modulatory molecules in CD34(+) hematopoietic cells. J Leukoc Biol 2004;75:671–679.
141 Nakajima H, Sugino M, Kimura F, Hanafusa T, Ikemoto T, Shimizu A: Decreased CD14+CCR2+ monocytes in active multiple sclerosis. Neurosci Lett 2004;363:187–189.
142 Shireman PK, Contreras-Shannon V, Reyes-Reyna SM, Robinson SC, McManus LM: MCP-1 parallels inflammatory and regenerative responses in ischemic muscle. J Surg Res 2006.
143 Jones RJ, Collector MI, et al: Characterization of mouse lymphohematopoietic stem cells lacking spleen colony-forming activity. Blood 1996;88:487–491.
144 Osawa M, Hanada K, Hamada H, Nakauchi H: Long-term lymphohematopoietic reconstitution by a single CD34-low/negative hematopoietic stem cell. Science 1996;273:242–245.
145 Goodell MA, Brose K, Paradis G, Conner AS, Mulligan RC: Isolation and functional properties of murine hematopoietic stem cells that are replicating in vivo. J Exp Med 1996;183:1797–1806.
146 Morel F, Szilvassy SJ, Travis M, Chen B, Galy A: Primitive hematopoietic cells in murine bone marrow express the CD34 antigen. Blood 1996;88:3774–3784.
147 Krause DS, Ito T, Fackler MJ, Smith OM, Collector MI, Sharkis SJ, May WS: Characterization of murine CD34, a marker for hematopoietic progenitor and stem cells. Blood 1994;84:691–701.
148 Bhatia M, Bonnet D, Murdoch B, Gan OI, Dick JE: A newly discovered class of human hematopoietic cells with SCID-repopulating activity. Nat Med 1998;4:1038–1045.
149 Zanjani ED, Almeida-Porada G, Livingston AG, Flake AW, Ogawa M: Human bone marrow CD34– cells engraft in vivo and undergo multilineage expression that includes giving rise to CD34+ cells. Exp Hematol 1998;26:353–360.
150 Civin CI, Strauss LC, Brovall C, Fackler MJ, Schwartz JF, Shaper JH: Antigenic analysis of hematopoiesis. III. A hematopoietic progenitor cell surface antigen defined by a monoclonal antibody raised against KG-1a cells. J Immunol 1984;133:157–165.
151 Donnelly DS, Krause DS: Hematopoietic stem cells can be CD34+ or CD34. Leuk Lymphoma 2001;40:221–234.
152 Sato T, Laver JH, Ogawa M: Reversible expression of CD34 by murine hematopoietic stem cells. Blood 1999;94:2548–2554.
153 Nakamura Y, Ando K, Chargui J, Kawada H, Sato T, Tsuji T, Hotta T, Kato S: Ex vivo generation of CD34+ cells from CD34– hematopoietic cells. Blood 1999;94:4053–4059.
154 Schatteman GC, Hanlon HD, Jiao C, Dodds SG, Christy BA: Blood-derived angioblasts accelerate blood-flow restoration in diabetic mice. J Clin Invest 2000;106:571–578.
155 Stepanovic V, Awad O, Jiao C, Dunnwald M, Schatteman GC: Leprdb diabetic mouse bone marrow cells inhibit skin wound vascularization but promote wound healing. Circ Res 2003;92:1247–1253.

156 Awad O, Jiao C, Ma N, Dunnwald M, Schatteman GC: Obese diabetic mouse environment differentially affects primitive and monocytic endothelial cell progenitors. Stem Cells 2005;23:575–583.
157 Stefanec T: How the endothelium and its bone marrow-derived progenitors influence development of disease. Med Hypotheses 2004;62:247–251.
158 Schatteman GC, Ma N: Old bone marrow cells inhibit skin wound vascularization. Stem Cells 2006;24:717–721.
159 Vasa M, Fichtlscherer S, Aicher A, Adler K, Urbich C, Martin H, Zeiher AM, Dimmeler S: Number and migratory activity of circulating endothelial progenitor cells inversely correlate with risk factors for coronary artery disease. Circ Res 2001;89:E1–E7.
160 Sivan-Loukianova E, Awad OA, Stepanovic V, Bickenbach J, Schatteman GC: CD34+ blood cells accelerate vascularization and healing of diabetic mouse skin wounds. J Vasc Res 2003;40:368–377.
161 Tepper OM, Galiano RD, Capla JM, Kalka C, Gagne PJ, Jacobowitz GR, Levine JP, Gurtner GC: Human endothelial progenitor cells from type II diabetics exhibit impaired proliferation, adhesion, and incorporation into vascular structures. Circulation 2002;106:2781–2786.
162 Loomans CJ, de Koning EJ, et al: Endothelial progenitor cell dysfunction: a novel concept in the pathogenesis of vascular complications of type 1 diabetes. Diabetes 2004;53:195–199.
163 Tamarat R, Silvestre JS, Le Ricousse-Roussanne S, Barateau V, Lecomte-Raclet L, Clergue M, Duriez M, Tobelem G, Levy BI: Impairment in ischemia-induced neovascularization in diabetes: bone marrow mononuclear cell dysfunction and therapeutic potential of placenta growth factor treatment. Am J Pathol 2004;164:457–466.
164 Galiano RD, Tepper OM, Pelo CR, Bhatt KA, Callaghan M, Bastidas N, Bunting S, Steinmetz HG, Gurtner GC: Topical vascular endothelial growth factor accelerates diabetic wound healing through increased angiogenesis and by mobilizing and recruiting bone marrow-derived cells. Am J Pathol 2004;164:1935–1947.
165 Lambiase PD, Edwards RJ, Anthopoulos P, Rahman S, Meng YG, Bucknall CA, Redwood SR, Pearson JD, Marber MS: Circulating humoral factors and endothelial progenitor cells in patients with differing coronary collateral support. Circulation 2004;109:2986–2992.
166 Moldovan NI: Current priorities in the research of circulating pre-endothelial cells. Adv Exp Med Biol 2003;522:1–8.
167 Hume DA: The mononuclear phagocyte system. Curr Opin Immunol 2006;18:49–53.
168 Havemann K, Pujol BF, Adamkiewicz J: In vitro transformation of monocytes and dendritic cells into endothelial like cells. Adv Exp Med Biol 2003;522:47–57.
169 Sharifi BG, Zeng Z, Wang L, Song L, Chen H, Qin M, Sierra-Honigmann MR, Wachsmann-Hogiu S, Shah PK: Pleiotrophin induces transdifferentiation of monocytes into functional endothelial cells. Arterioscler Thromb Vasc Biol 2006;26:1273–1280.
170 Conejo-Garcia JR, Buckanovich RJ, Benencia F, Courreges MC, Rubin SC, Carroll RG, Coukos G: Vascular leukocytes contribute to tumor vascularization. Blood 2005;105:679–681.
171 Maruyama K, Ii M, et al: Inflammation-induced lymphangiogenesis in the cornea arises from CD11b-positive macrophages. J Clin Invest 2005;115:2363–2372.
172 Gordon S: Macrophage-restricted molecules: role in differentiation and activation. Immunol Lett 1999;65:5–8.
173 Anghelina M, Krishnan P, Moldovan L, Moldovan NI: Monocytes/macrophages cooperate with progenitor cells during neovascularization and tissue repair: conversion of cell columns into fibrovascular bundles. Am J Pathol 2006;168:529–541.
174 Bailey AJ: Molecular mechanisms of ageing in connective tissues. Mech Ageing Dev 2001;122:735–755.
175 Gardiner TA, Anderson HR, Stitt AW: Inhibition of advanced glycation endproducts protects against retinal capillary basement membrane expansion during long-term diabetes. J Pathol 2003;201:328–333.
176 Seeger FH, Haendeler J, et al: p38 mitogen-activated protein kinase downregulates endothelial progenitor cells. Circulation 2005;111:1184–1191.
177 Yoon CH, Hur J, et al: Synergistic neovascularization by mixed transplantation of early endothelial progenitor cells and late outgrowth endothelial cells: the role of angiogenic cytokines and matrix metalloproteinases. Circulation 2005;112:1618–1627.
178 Polverini PJ, Cotran PS, Gimbrone MA Jr, Unanue ER: Activated macrophages induce vascular proliferation. Nature 1977;269:804–806.
179 Kamihata H, Matsubara H, et al: Implantation of bone marrow mononuclear cells into ischemic myocardium enhances collateral perfusion and regional function via side supply of angioblasts, angiogenic ligands, and cytokines. Circulation 2001;104:1046–1052.
180 Hur J, Yoon CH, Kim HS, Choi JH, Kang HJ, Hwang KK, Oh BH, Lee MM, Park YB: Characterization of two types of endothelial progenitor cells and their different contributions to neovasculogenesis. Arterioscler Thromb Vasc Biol 2004;24:288–293.
181 Badorff C, Brandes RP, et al: Transdifferentiation of blood-derived human adult endothelial progenitor cells into functionally active cardiomyocytes. Circulation 2003;107:1024–1032.
182 Wollert KC, Meyer GP, et al: Intracoronary autologous bone-marrow cell transfer after myocardial infarction: the BOOST randomised controlled clinical trial. Lancet 2004;364:141–148.
183 Fogelstrand L, Hulthe J, Hulten LM, Wiklund O, Fagerberg B: Monocytic expression of CD14 and CD18, circulating adhesion molecules and inflammatory markers in women with diabetes mellitus and impaired glucose tolerance. Diabetologia 2004;47:1948–1952.
184 Joussen AM, Poulaki V, et al: A central role for inflammation in the pathogenesis of diabetic retinopathy. FASEB J 2004;18:1450–1452.
185 Ishida S, Usui T, et al: VEGF164-mediated inflammation is required for pathological, but not physiological, ischemia-induced retinal neovascularization. J Exp Med 2003;198:483–489.
186 Patino R, Ibarra J, Rodriguez A, Yague MR, Pintor E, Fernandez-Cruz A, Figueredo A: Circulating monocytes in patients with diabetes mellitus, arterial disease, and increased CD14 expression. Am J Cardiol 2000;85:1288–1291.

187 Cipolletta C, Ryan KE, Hanna EV, Trimble ER: Activation of peripheral blood CD14+ monocytes occurs in diabetes. Diabetes 2005;54:2779–2786.

188 Engerman RL, Kern TS: Retinopathy in animal models of diabetes. Diabetes Metab Rev 1995;11:109–120.

189 Mizutani M, Kern TS, Lorenzi M: Accelerated death of retinal microvascular cells in human and experimental diabetic retinopathy. J Clin Invest 1996;97:2883–2890.

Maria B. Grant, MD
Department of Pharmacology and Therapeutics
University of Florida, PO Box 100267
Gainesville, FL 32610-0267 (USA)
Tel. +1 352 846 0978, Fax +1 352 392 9696, E-Mail grantma@ufl.edu

Hammes H-P, Porta M (eds): Experimental Approaches to Diabetic Retinopathy.
Front Diabetes. Basel, Karger, 2010, vol 20, pp 194–202

Role of Pericytes in Vascular Biology

Annika Armulik[a] · Christer Betsholtz[a,b]

[a]Vascular Biology Laboratory, Division of Matrix Biology, Department of Medical Biochemistry and Biophysics, and [b]Department of Medicine, Karolinska Institutet, Stockholm, Sweden

Abstract

Pericytes are obligatory constituents of blood microvessels and important regulators of blood vessel development and function. Analysis of mouse genetic mutants for factors that regulate pericyte recruitment has demonstrated the importance of pericytes for vessel remodeling, maturation and stabilization. Such studies have also shown that impairments of one vessel wall cell type, endothelial or pericyte, will inevitably affect the other. However, we still lack a detailed understanding of the identity of pericyte-derived signals and their mechanism of action. Recent evidence suggests that pericytes may also have important homeostatic functions in the adult vasculature. In the present review, we summarize work that has broadened our understanding of the role of pericytes in vascular biology.

Pericytes Are Cells with a Unique Position in the Microvascular Wall

Several cell types such as astrocytes in the central nervous system (CNS) and podocytes in the kidney glomeruli contact the microvascular basement membrane (BM) in different microvascular beds and communicate with the endothelial cells in order to help determine and maintain local microvessel identity and function. Among these cells, pericytes are unique by their obligatory presence in the microvessel wall, by their distribution and relationship with the microvascular BM, as well as by the type of contacts they form with the endothelial cells [1].

True pericytes are embedded within the endothelial BM of blood capillaries, precapillary arterioles, and postcapillary and collecting venules (fig. 1a). This distinguishes pericytes from classical vascular smooth muscle cells (vSMCs) of large arteries and veins, in which vSMCs are separated from the endothelium by a layer of mesenchymal cells and extracellular matrix – the intima. In addition, cell morphology, and to some extent marker expression, differs between vSMCs and pericytes. For example, α-smooth muscle actin (SMA) is not expressed by skin or CNS pericytes in mice under normal circumstances, but becomes upregulated in these cells during retinopathy and in subcutaneously transplanted tumors [2]. Pericytes also make different types of cell-cell contacts with the endothelium. However, the distinction between pericyte and vSMC morphology and location is not absolute. Rather, there exists a continuum of phenotypes, ranging from the classical vSMC to the typical pericyte, distributed along intermediate-size to small vessels, i.e. between arteriole, capillaries and venules. It has also been suggested that a population of pericytes may reside subjacent to the endothelium of large vessels (fig. 1a).

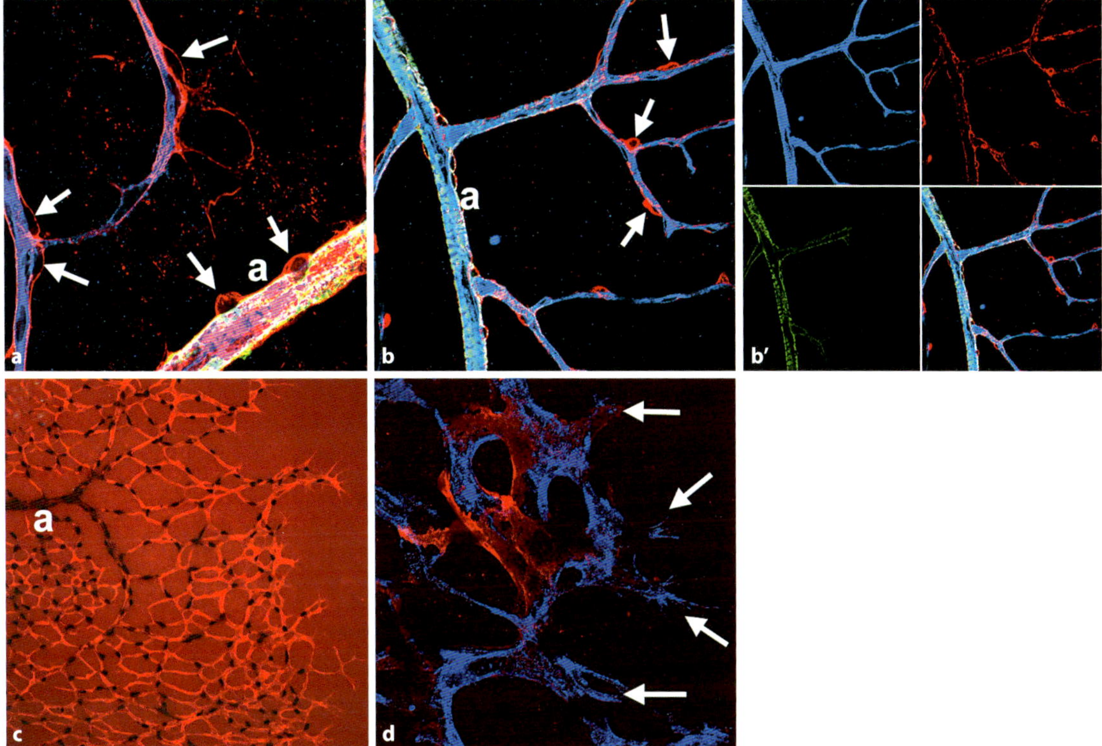

Fig. 1. **a** Retinal vasculature of a 6-day-old mouse. Vessels are visualized using anti-CD31 mAb (blue); vSMCs surrounding an artery (a) are stained with anti-ASMA mAb (green/yellow), and the BM is visualized using anti-collagen IV Ab (red). Arrows indicate pericytes lining the vessels. **b** Retinal vasculature of a 5-week-old mouse. Vessels are visualized using anti-CD31 mAb (blue); vSMCs surrounding an artery (a) are stained with anti-ASMA mAb (green), and pericytes (arrows) are visualized using anti-NG-2 Ab (red). **c** Angiogenic vascular plexus in the retina of a 6-day-old XlacZ4 promoter trap transgenic mouse. Vessels are visualized using anti-CD31 mAb (red) and mural cells expressing β-galactosidase in the nucleus are visualized using X-gal staining. Note the X-gal-positive cells that line around a developing artery (a). **d** Leading edge of the retinal vascular plexus of a 6-day-old mouse. Endothelial tip cells (anti-CD31; blue; arrows) are contacted by pericytes (anti-NG2 Ab; red).

Identification of Pericytes

The heterogeneous morphology and marker expression make unambiguous identification of pericytes a challenge. However, in the mouse retina, pericytes can be identified relatively easily by their expression of desmin, NG-2 (chondroitin sulfate proteoglycan 4), platelet-derived growth factor (PDGF) receptor-β, and the promoter trap transgene XlacZ4 [2]. These markers are also expressed by vSMCs, which contrary to the pericytes also express SMA (fig. 1b′, c). The expression of pericyte/vSMC markers is dynamic and varies between organs and developmental stage. For example, SMA is not appreciably expressed by retinal vSMCs until a few days after birth. In addition, we have found that expression of XlacZ4 in retinal mural cells in adult animals is often mosaic. Another pericyte marker, regulator of G-protein signaling 5 is upregulated in pericytes in vasculature undergoing angiogenic remodeling, such as during development or in tumors [3, 4].

Most pericyte markers identified and used to date have provided little insights into the *functions* of pericytes. However, recently identified additional pericyte markers in the CNS; ATP-sensitive potassium channel Kir6.1 and sulfonylurea receptor 2, which are both part of the same potassium channel complex, and delta homologue 1, could potentially broaden our understanding of pericyte function [5]. Genetic ablation of Kir6.1 in mice shows that Kir6.1 is critical in regulating vascular tonus. These mice die prematurely due to arrhythmia caused by spontaneous cardiac ischemia [6].

Functions of Pericytes

Our current understanding about the pericyte functions is limited. The first evidence for a role of pericytes in embryonic blood vessel morphogenesis during embryonic development was published more than 10 years ago [7]. Numerous subsequent studies have underscored the importance of pericytes in the formation of stable and durable blood vessels by regulating proliferation and maturation of endothelial cells. In addition, the presence of pericytes is needed for proper vessel BM deposition. A single pericyte often contacts several endothelial cells, and they may therefore integrate and coordinate neighboring endothelial cell responses. Apart from being important for blood vessel morphogenesis and durability, pericytes have been suggested to regulate blood flow in microvessels. Recent studies have added strength to this idea, which for many years remained controversial. This is further discussed below.

Among microvascular beds, The CNS microvasculature shows the highest pericyte coverage, which may imply that CNS pericytes have special functions. It has, for example, been proposed that pericytes contribute to the formation of blood-brain barrier (BBB). Several studies indicate that in the adult organism pericyte coverage might be needed for vessel maintenance, and dropout of pericytes from the microvessel wall might play a role in the pathogenesis of certain conditions, e.g. diabetic microangiopathy and retinopathy. However, our limited knowledge about the normal developmental and homeostatic functions of pericytes is an obstacle in the study of pathogenic roles of pericyte loss or dysfunction. Because we know so little about pericytes, the specific changes in the microvasculature caused by defective pericytes may go unnoticed in most types of analyses. As discussed further below, there is for example a need for deepening and refinement of the phenotypic analysis of various pericyte-deficient animal models.

Blood Vessel Morphogenesis and Vessel Stability

Studies on mouse mutants where pericytes are missing or not in proper contact with endothelial cells have demonstrated that pericyte-endothelial interactions are necessary for the formation of durable vessels. The list of molecules affecting pericyte association with endothelium is long, indicating complex networks of signaling pathways/interactions needed for proper association and interaction between endothelial cells and pericytes [8]. Surprisingly, these interactions do not seem to be redundant as often lack of only a single one of these pathways has catastrophic consequences for vascular development. PDGF-B, transforming growth factor-β (TGF-β), angiopoietin-1 and ephrinB2, their respective receptors, as well as some of their downstream signaling molecules, are examples of factors required for proper pericyte and vSMC recruitment to blood vessels during developmental angiogenesis. Several of these factors have their primary role in the endothelium, and their deficiency compromises the endothelium's ability to recruit pericytes. PDGF-B is an example of an endothelium-derived ligand that triggers signaling through PDGFR-β expressed by pericytes or their progenitors. The PDGF-B/PDGFR-β pathway was the first one demonstrated to be directly involved in pericyte recruitment to newly formed vessels [7, 9]. Knockout studies of PDGF-B/PDGFR-β mice show identical perinatal lethal phenotypes – microvascular leakage and hemorrhage. The primary cause of the lethality is lack of pericytes, particularly noticeable around CNS microvessels. The lack of pericyte recruitment has immediate secondary consequences for the endothelium, which becomes hyperplastic, shows excessive luminal membrane folds, and immature inter-endothelial junctions [10]. Upregulation of VEGF-A in *pdgfb* and *pdgfrb* knockouts is likely a secondary consequence of impaired microvessel function leading to tissue hypoxia, which may nevertheless reinforce some of the vessel abnormalities, such as the vascular leakage. Induction of pericytes in the immature mesenchyme surrounding the larger axial vessels takes place independently of PDGF-B, but in the absence of PDGF-B or PDGFR-β the induced population of pericytes fails to expand and spread along the growing vessels. During angiogenesis, sprouting endothelial cells synthesize and secrete high levels of PDGF-B, which results in expansion and migration of pericytes particularly along sprouting or enlarging vessels. Various mouse mutants with partially impaired PDGF-B secretion or localization, or with partially impaired PDGFR-β signaling, show partial lack of pericytes, and reduced pericyte density or defective pericyte-endothelial association [11–13]. Tumor suppressor Arf-deficient mice develop an eye disease resembling persistent hyperplastic primary vitreous, caused by failed regression of hyaloid vessels [14]. In this case, increased PDGFR-β signaling in vitreous pericyte-like cells leads to excessive accumulation of these cells around hyaloid vessels, in turn preventing hyaloid vessel regression. Together, these data demonstrate that the amount of PDGF-B secreted and the strength of PDGFR-β signals need to be tightly controlled during development. Also, proper localization of PDGF-B is important for correct pericyte recruitment. Mice that lack the binding motif to heparin sulfate proteoglycans in PDGF-B, needed for localizing secreted PDGF-B close vicinity to vessels, show defective pericyte coverage, which in turn leads to vascular defects [15].

Not only pericyte-endothelium contacts are crucial for pericyte recruitment to newly formed blood vessels, but also pericyte contacts with surrounding matrix. α_4-integrin-deficient mouse embryos show wider cranial (but not caudal) vessel diameter and reduced pericyte cell coverage and abnormal distribution. At this stage of development, α_4 is expressed by mural cells, suggesting that that $\alpha_4\beta_1$ interaction with fibronectin is important for pericyte migration along developing cranial vessels [16]. $\alpha_4\beta_1$- and VCAM-1-mediated adhesion between endothelium and pericytes has recently been implicated in tumor angiogenesis [17], but in this case the $\alpha_4\beta_1$-integrin was found mainly on proliferating endothelial cells. The discrepant expression sites for $\alpha_4\beta_1$ indicate that angiogenesis in tumors and during the development might utilize partly different modes of endothelial/pericyte signaling.

The TGF-β signaling pathway is required for proper vessel development. Knockout of several genes in the TGF-β signaling pathway (e.g. endoglin and activin-receptor-like kinase 1, ALK1) in mice results in phenotypes that resemble human diseases caused by the mutations in the same genes [18, 19]. A number of studies analyzing the effect of lack of TGF-β1 and genes encoding its receptors, as well as downstream effectors have shown that TGF-β signaling has important primary functions in both endothelial cells and mural cells. TGF-β regulates several cellular processes: proliferation, differentiation and secretion of extracellular matrix proteins. In endothelial cells, TGF-β signaling is mediated by two receptors: TGF-β receptor I, which signals via ALK1-Smad5, and TGF-β receptor II, which signals via ALK5-Smad2/3 [19]. In addition, endothelial cells express type III TGF-β receptor – endoglin, which promotes ALK1 signaling and thus shifts the TGF-β response in endothelial cells towards proliferation. Even though the vasculature of mouse mutants for TGF-β signaling shows defects in mural cell coverage, the primary defect seems to occur primarily in the endothelium [20]. However, TGF-β signaling has been shown to be required also for vSMC differentiation in vitro and in vivo. TGF-β secreted by endothelium induces vSMC formation in the perivascular mesenchyme, possibly via the ALK5-Smad2/3 pathway. Defective TGF-β signaling in endothelial cells appears to promote defective TGF-β signaling also in surrounding mesenchyme, which inhibits vSMC differentiation. Failure of neural crest cells to differentiate into SMC has been described in mouse knockouts of TGF-β receptor II in neural crest cells, indicating that TGF-β signaling is indeed important for SMC differentiation. It is not known what signal shifts TGF-β signaling in endothelium from proliferation (ALK1-Smad1 pathway) towards differentiation (ALK5-Smad2/3 pathway), but it remains an interesting possibility that it is pericyte derived. Genetic ablation of Man1, an inner nuclear membrane protein antagonizing bone morphogenetic protein signaling, leads to death at mid-gestation due to defects in vasculature [21]. In Man1-deficient embryos TGF-β1 signaling is upregulated and shifted towards Smad2/3 pathway in endothelium. Also in these embryos, differentiation of vSMCs around dorsal aorta does not take place. Increased apoptosis, especially in mesenchymal tissues, was observed in Man1 knockout embryos, which might contribute to the defective vSMC coverage [21].

What are the pericyte-derived signals to endothelium that result in vessel stabilization? Angiopoietins (Ang1 and Ang2) signal via Tie2 receptors expressed by the endothelium. Ang1, expressed by perivascular cells, promotes autophosphorylation of Tie2 in endothelial cells, which leads to signals important for vessel maturation [22, 23]. Ang2, expressed by endothelial cells, is mainly an antagonistic Tie2 ligand. It inhibits Tie2 phosphorylation and leads to destabilization of vasculature. In a recent study, it was shown that Ang2 triggers endothelial responsiveness to pro-inflammatory stimuli, such as TNF-α [24]. Genetic deletion of *Ang1* and *Tie2* leads to death in utero around mid-gestation due to cardiovascular failure. The vasculature of those embryos shows reduced coverage of pericytes. In a recent study, Tachibana et al. [25] have shown that a mutation of one of major autophosphorylation sites (tyrosine 1,100 to phenylalanine) in Tie2 results in a similar phenotype as the full Tie2 knockout with one exception; even though $Tie2^{Y1100F/Y1100F}$ embryos died at the same time as Tie2-null embryos due to defects in heart development, they lacked hemorrhages in the head and displayed a normal pericyte coverage of the cranial vessels. Thus, signaling pathways emanating from other tyrosine residues in Tie2 than Y1100 may be involved in mural cell recruitment, but such putative pathway(s) remains to be identified. How is Ang1 expression switched on by pericytes? Studies on the role of EphB4 in vascular morphogenesis in tumor vasculature suggest that EphB4-mediated endothelial contact with mural cells, possibly via ephrinB2, leads via reverse signaling in mural cells to increased expression of the Ang1 mRNA [26]. Loss of the cytoplasmic domain of ephrinB2 has been shown to lead to reduced Ang1 expression [27]. Mural cell-specific knockout of ephrinB2 leads to vascular defects (edema and hemorrhaging) that correlate with a defective association between pericytes and the endothelium [28]. From cell culture experiments, the authors concluded that ephrinB2 has a cell-autonomous role in mural cells promoting cell migration and adhesion. It would be interesting to know whether these mice show defects in Ang1/Tie2 signaling in the endothelium.

Whereas pericytes appear to exert their primary function in vessel maturation and stabilization, recent data have clearly demonstrated that pericytes are present in association with actively sprouting and remodeling vessels (fig. 1c, d). Imaging of angiogenesis in the retina and elsewhere in the CNS has demonstrated that pericytes accompany tip cells in angiogenic sprouts (fig. 1d). This is in agreement with the PDGF-B expression pattern in angiogenic vessels, where PDGF-B is particularly high in the tip cells [29]. Thus, pericytes are immediately recruited to new sprouts, but they do not seem to have a role in sprout formation and elongation as these processes occur normally in the absence of pericytes (in PDGF-B or PDGFR-β knockouts). However, there is accumulating evidence that pericytes regulate the density of the forming vascular plexus. Injection of neutralizing PDGFR-β antibodies into postnatal retina results in the formation of a sparse vascular bed with tortuous arteries and veins [30]. Analysis of the developing retinal capillary bed in PDGF-B retention motif knockouts has shown similar results [15, 31]. Likewise, mice that express lower than normal levels of PDGF-B in the endothelium, resulting in a 70–80% reduction in the pericyte density in the CNS also develop a sparse and disorganized vasculature in the CNS [Armulik and Betsholtz, unpubl. data]. Presently, it is unclear what kind of mechanism(s) lies behind the reduced capillary density. i.e. whether it is the result of defective vessel formation or exaggerated vessel pruning. On the other hand, the mere presence of pericytes does not protect vessels from regression. It has been demonstrated that certain vascular beds regress after VEGF-A blockade independently of the presence of pericytes [32]. Interestingly, pericytes without endothelium do not survive, indicating that endothelium supplies pericytes with essential survival factor(s).

Regulation of Blood Flow

In the CNS, blood flow is rapidly regulated in response to neuronal activity. The blood flow is primarily thought to be regulated by arteries and arterioles that are located upstream of the capillary bed, but there is now a growing body of evidence suggesting that pericyte-covered microvessels participate in blood flow regulation, at least in the CNS. Early electron microscopy studies indicate the presence of grooves in CNS capillary walls, which may represent constrictions caused by mural cells [33, 34]. Many studies have shown that pericytes contract in response to vasoactive stimuli. In addition, presence of ATP-sensitive potassium channels, which when activated (opened) have vasodilating effects, has been demonstrated on CNS pericytes by electrophysiology and in situ hybridization, indicating that pericytes have the machinery needed for blood flow regulation [5, 35, 36]. However, it has been difficult to prove that pericytes regulate blood flow in vivo. A recent study by Peppiatt et al. [37] provides convincing evidence that the blood flow in the CNS can be regulated by pericytes in response to neuronal stimuli. These authors show that pericytes in brain and retinal tissue explants contract and relax in response to stimulation, leading to changes in capillary diameter. They also observed that stimulation of one pericyte often causes contraction of nearby pericytes. Wu et al. [36] have investigated how an electrical signal is propagated between pericytes. They showed that there is a relatively inefficient electrotonic transmission via pericyte/endothelial gap junctions in isolated rat retinal vessel. Instead, they propose that it is the endothelium that provides efficient transmission and thus functionally links contractile pericytes, thereby coordinating vasomotor response [36].

Blood-Brain and Blood-Retina Barriers

Blood vessels in the CNS show specific features referred to as the BBB which controls entry of blood-borne substances into the brain tissue. Brain endothelial cells are connected via tight junctions and they lack fenestrations. As mentioned above, the CNS blood vessels also show a very high pericyte coverage. In addition, blood vessels in the CNS are covered by astrocyte end-foot processes. The role of astrocytes in the BBB has been investigated extensively, which has led to the suggestion that astrocytes play an active role in promoting endothelial BBB formation [38]. Much less is known about whether pericytes contribute to the formation and maintenance of BBB. Brain injury is often accompanied by microvessel leakage. Dore-Duffy et al. [39] showed that pericytes migrate away from the endothelium in response to brain injury and in association with BBB disruption. Whether dissociation of pericytes from the CNS microvessel plays a causal role in BBB disruption needs further investigation. Viable pericyte-deficient mouse models will be valuable tools for such studies. It has been suggested using in vitro assays that pericyte-derived Ang1 and TGF-β induce expression of components crucial for formation of the tight junction between capillary endothelial cells [40]. TGF-β signaling is important for maintenance or formation of the BBB. In this respect, it is interesting that gap junctions between endothelial cells and pericytes appear to be needed for activation of latent TGF-β [41]. As mentioned above, pericyte-derived angiopoietin-1 signaling via Tie2 is thought to mediate vessel stabilization, implicating a direct role in the regulation of endothelial junctions and the BBB. Overexpression of angiopoietin-1 in mice results in partially leakage-resistant vessels [42].

Maintenance of the Adult Vasculature

PDGF-B mutants have made us realize that pericytes have important functions not only during development but also in adult homeostasis and pathological processes, such as tumor angiogenesis [43]. It has been observed that loss of pericytes along retinal microvessels is one of the earliest cellular changes occurring as a result of diabetes, and hence potentially constituting a key step in the pathogenesis of diabetic retinopathy [44, 45]. Indeed, several studies in mice have suggested that pericyte dropout might have a causal role in diabetic retinopathy. Endothelial-specific knockout of PDGF-B leads to severely reduced pericyte numbers along microvessels. Animals where pericyte numbers were reduced by more than 90% in the CNS compared to control animals developed retinopathy without diabetes [46]. On the other hand, diabetic animals lacking one *pdgfb* allele showed increased pericyte loss compared to diabetic wild-type mice, indicating that PDGF-B might be an important survival factor for pericytes during diabetic challenge [47]. Mice that express retention motif-deficient PDGF-B have abnormal pericyte coverage with pericytes partially detached from the abluminal vessel surface. Also these mice develop severe retinopathy, showing that not only presence of pericytes but also the proper association between pericytes and endothelial cells is important for vessel protection [15].

There are indications that pericytes regulate deposition of BM. Thickening of BM around blood vessels is observed in diseased conditions and in aging animals [48]. Mice expressing retention motif-deficient PDGF-B show abnormal deposition of collagen IV in the BM around aorta [31]. Age-related thickening of the BM around vessels coincides with reduced pericyte number and altered association with endothelium in rat retina [48]. Altered thickness of vessel BM is also observed in diabetes. Ultrastructural studies of skin microvessels of patients with lipoid proteinosis also indicate that pericytes contribute to excess deposition of BM [49].

Acknowledgements

We acknowledge research support from the Karolinska Institute, The Ludwig Institute for Cancer Research, The Swedish Cancer Foundation, The Inga-Britt and Arne Lundberg, Knut and Alice Wallenberg and Ragnar Söderberg Foundations and the Association for International Cancer Research (UK).

References

1 Sims DE: The pericyte – A review. Tissue and Cell 1986;18:153–174.
2 Gerhardt H, Betsholtz C: Endothelial-pericyte interactions in angiogenesis. Cell Tissue Res 2003;22:15–23.
3 Bondjers C, Kalen M, Hellstrom M, Scheidl SJ, Abramsson A, Renner O, Lindahl P, Cho H, Kehrl J, Betsholtz C: Transcription profiling of platelet-derived growth factor-B-deficient mouse embryos identifies RGS5 as a novel marker for pericytes and vascular smooth muscle cells. Am J Pathol 2003;162:721–729.
4 Song S, Ewald AJ, Stallcup WB, Werb Z, Bergers G: PDGFRb+ perivascular cells in tumours regulate pericyte differentiation and vascular survival. Nat Cell Biol 2005;7:870–879.
5 Bondjers C, He L, Takemoto M, Norlin J, Asker N, Hellstrom M, Lindahl P, Betsholtz C: Microarray analysis of blood microvessels from PDGF-B and PDGF-Rb mutant mice identifies novel markers for brain pericytes. FASEB J 2006;20:E1005–E1012.
6 Miki T, Suzuki M, Shibasaki T, Uemura H, Sato TN, Yamaguchi K, KOseki H, Iwanaga T, Nakaya H, Seino S: Mouse model of Prinzmetal angina by disruption of the inward rectifier Kir6.1. Nat Med 2002;8:466–472.
7 Lindahl P, Johansson BR, Levéen P, Betsholtz C: Pericyte loss and microaneurysm formation in PDGF-B-deficient mice. Science 1997;277:242–245.
8 Armulik A, Abramsson A, Betsholtz C: Endothelial/Pericyte interactions. Circ Res 2005;97:512–523.
9 Hellstrom M, Kalen M, Lindahl P, Abramsson A, Betsholtz C: Role of PDGF-B and PDGFR-beta in recruitment of vascular smooth muscle cells and pericytes during embryonic blood vessel formation in the mouse. Development 1999;126:3047–3055.
10 Hellström M, Gerhardt H, Kalén M, Li X, Eriksson U, Wolburg H, Betsholtz C: Lack of pericytes leads to endothelial hyperplasia and abnormal vascular morphogenesis. J Cell Biol 2001;153:543–553.
11 Tallquist MD, French WJ, Soriano P: Additive effects of PDGF receptor beta signaling pathways in vascular smooth muscle cell development. PLoS Biol 2003;1:E52.
12 Hoch RV, Soriano P: Roles of PDGF in animal development. Development 2003;130:4769–4784.
13 Betsholtz C, Lindblom P, Gerhardt H: Role of pericytes in vascular morphogenesis. EXS 2005;115–125.
14 Silva RL, Thornton JD, Matrin AC, Rehg JE, Bertwistle D, Zindy F, Skapek SX: Arf-dependent regulation of Pdgf signaling in perivascular cells in the developing mouse eye. EMBO J 2005;24:2803–2814.
15 Lindblom P, Gerhardt H, Liebner S, Abramsson A, Enge M, Hellstrom M, Backstrom G, Fredriksson S, Landegren U, Nystrom HC, Bergstrom G, Dejana E, Ostman A, Lindahl P, Betsholtz C: Endothelial PDGF-B retention is required for proper investment of pericytes in the microvessel wall. Genes Dev 2003;17:1835–1840.
16 Grazioli A, Alves CS, Konstantopoulos K, Yang JT: Defective blood vessel development and pericyte/pvSMC distribution in alpha 4 integrin-deficient mouse embryos. Dev Biol 2006;293:165–177.
17 Garmy-Susini B, Jin H, Zhu Y, Sung R-J, Hwang R, Varner J: Integrin a4b1-VCAM-1-mediated adhesion between endothelial cells and mural cells is required for blood vessel maturation. J Clin Invest 2005;115:1542–1551.
18 Bobik A: Transforming growth factor-betas and vascular disorders. Arterioscler Thromb Vasc Biol 2006;26:1712–1720.
19 Bertolino P, Deckers M, Lebrin F, ten Dijke P: Transforming growth factor-β signal transduction in angiogenesis and vascular disorders. Chest 2005;128:585S–590S.
20 Lebrin F, Deckers M, Bertolino P, ten Dijke P: TGF-beta receptor function in the endothelium. Cardiovasc Res 2005;65:599–608.
21 Ishimura A, Ng JK, Taira M, Young SG, Osada S: Man1, an inner nuclear membrane protein, regulates vascular remodeling by modulating transforming growth factor beta signaling. Development 2006;133:3919–3928.
22 Brindle NP, Saharinen P, Alitalo K: Signaling and functions of angiopoietin-1 in vascular protection. Circ Res 2006;98:1014–1023.
23 Li LY, Barlow KD, Metheny-Barlow LJ: Angiopoietins and Tie2 in health and disease. Pediatr Endocrinol Rev 2005;2:399–408.
24 Fiedler U, Reiss Y, Scharpfenecker M, Grunow V, Koidl S, Thurston G, Gale NW, Witzenrath M, Rosseau S, Suttorp N, Sobke A, Herrmann M, Preissner KT, Vajkoczy P, Augustin HG: Angiopoietin-2 sensitizes endothelial cells to TNF-alpha and has a crucial role in the induction of inflammation. Nat Med 2006;12:235–239.
25 Tachibana K, Jones N, Dumont DJ, Puri MC, Bernstein A: Selective role of a distinct tyrosine residue in Tie2 in heart development and early hematopoiesis. Mol Cell Biol 2005;25:4693–4702.
26 Erber R, Eichelsbacher U, Powajbo V, Korn T, Djonov V, Lin J, Hammes HP, Grobholz R, Ullrich A, Vajkoczy P: EphB4 controls blood vascular morphogenesis during postnatal angiogenesis. EMBO J 2006;25:628–641.
27 Adams RH, Diella F, Hennig S, Helmbacher F, Deutsch U, Klein R: The cytoplasmic domain of the ligand ephrinB2 is required for vascular morphogenesis but not cranial neural crest migration. Cell 2001;104:57–69.
28 Foo SS, Turner CJ, Adams S, Compagni A, Aubyn D, Kogata N, Lindblom P, Shani M, Zicha D, Adams RH: Ephrin-B2 controls cell motility and adhesion during blood-vessel-wall assembly. Cell 2006;124:161–173.
29 Gerhardt H, Golding M, Fruttiger M, Ruhrberg C, Lundkvist A, Abramsson A, Jeltsch M, Mitchell C, Alitalo K, Shima D, Betsholtz C: VEGF guides angiogenic sprouting utilizing endothelial tip-cell filopodia. J Cell Biol 2003;161:1163–1177.
30 Uemura A, Ogawa M, Hirashima M, Fujiwara T, Koyama S, Takagi H, Honda Y, Wiegand SJ, Yancopoulos GD, Nishikawa S: Recombinant angiopoietin-1 restores higher-order architecture of growing blood vessels in mice in the absence of mural cells. J Clin Invest 2002;110:1619–1628.

31 Nyström HC, Lindblom P, Wickman A, Andersson I, Norlin J, Fäldt J, Lindahl P, Skott O, Bjarnegård M, Fitzgerald SM, Caidahl K, Gan L-m, Betsholtz C, Bergström G: Platelet-derived growth factor B retention is essential for development of normal structure and function of conduit vessels and capillaries. Cardiovasc Res 2006;71:557–565.
32 Inai T, Mancuso M, Hashizume H, Baffert F, Haskell A, Baluk P, HU-Lowe DD, Shallinsky DR, Thurston G, Yancopoulos GD, McDonald DM: Inhibition of vascular endothelial growth factor (VEGF) signaling in cancer causes loss od endothelial fenestrations, regression of tumor vessels, and appearance of basement membrane ghosts. Am J Pathol 2004;165:35–52.
33 Toribatake Y, Tomita K, Kawahara N, Baba H, Ohnari H, Tanaka S: Regulation of vasomotion of arterioles and capillaries in the cat spinal cord: role of alpha actin and endothelin-1. Spinal Cord 1997;35:26–32.
34 Harrison RV, Harel N, Panesar J, Mount RJ: Blood capillary distribution correlates with hemodynamic-based functional imaging in cerebral cortex. Cereb Cortex 2002;12:225–233.
35 Kawamura H, Sugiyama T, Wu DM, Kobayashi M, Yamanishi S, Katsumura K, Puro DG: ATP: a vasoactive signal in the pericyte-containing microvasculature of the rat retina. J Physiol 2003;551:787–799.
36 Wu DM, Minami M, Kawamura H, Puro DG: Electrotonic transmission within pericyte-containing retinal microvessels. Microcirculation 2006;13:353–363.
37 Peppiatt CM, Howarth C, Mobbs P, Attwell D: Bidirectional control of CNS capillary diameter by pericytes. Nature 2006;443:700–704.
38 Abbott NJ, Rönnbäck L, Hansson E: Astrocyte-endothelial interactions at the blood-brain barrier. Nat Rev Neurosci 2006;7:41–53.
39 Dore-Duffy P, Owen C, Balabanov R, Murphy S, Beaumont T, Rafols JA: Pericyte migration from the vascular wall in response to traumatic brain injury. Microvasc Res 2000;60:55–69.
40 Hori S, Ohtsuki K, Hosoya E, Nakashima T, Terasaki A: A pericyte-derived angiopoietin-1 multimeric complex induces occludin gene expression in brain capillary endothelial cells through Tie-2 activation in vitro. J Neurochem 2004;89:503–513.
41 Hirschi KK, Burt JM, Hirschi KD, Dai C: Gap junction communication mediates transforming growth factor-b activation and endothelial-induced mural cell differentiation. Circ Res 2003;93:429–437.
42 Thurston G, Suri C, Smith K, McClain J, Sato TN, Yancopoulos GD, McDonald DM: Leakage-resistant blood vessels in mice transgenically overexpressing angiopoietin-1. Science 1999;286:2511–2514.
43 Abramsson A, Lindblom P, Betsholtz C: Endothelial and non-endothelial sources of PDGF-B regulate pericyte recruitment and influence vascular pattern formation in tumors. J Clin Invest 2003;112:1142–1151.
44 Cogan DG, Toussaint D, Kuwabara T: Retinal vascular patterns. IV. Diabetic retinopathy. Arch Opthalmol 1961;66:366–378.
45 Buzney SM, Frank RN, Varma SD, Tanishima T, Gabbay KH: Aldose reductase in retinal mural cells. Invest Ophtal Vis Sci 1977;16:392–396.
46 Enge M, Bjarnegård M, Gerhardt H, Gustafsson E, Kalén M, Asker N, Hammes H-P, Shani M, Fässler R, Betsholtz C: Endothelium-specific platelet-derived growth factor-B ablation mimics diabetic retinopathy. EMBO J 2002;21:4307–4316.
47 Hammes H-P, Lin J, Renner O, Shani M, Lundqvist A, Betsholtz C, Brownlee M, Deutsch U: Pericytes and the pathogenesis of diabetic retinopathy. Diabetes 2002;51:3107–3112.
48 Hughes S, Gardiner T, Hu P, Baxter L, Rosinova E, Chan-Ling T: Altered pericyte-endothelial relations in the rat retina during aging: implications for vessel stability. Neurobiol Aging 2006;27:1838–1847.
49 Mirancea N, Hausser I, Beck R, Metze D, Fusenig NE, Breitkreutz D: Vascular anomalities in lipoid proteinosis (hyalinosis cutis et mucosae): basement membrane components and ultrastructure. J Dermatol Sci 2006;42:231–239.

Dr. Christer Betsholtz
Department of Medical Biochemistry and Biophysics, Karolinska Institutet
Scheeles Väg 2
SE–17177 Stockholm (Sweden)
Tel. +46 8 52487960, Fax +46 8 31 34 45, E-Mail christer.betsholtz@ki.se

Hammes H-P, Porta M (eds): Experimental Approaches to Diabetic Retinopathy.
Front Diabetes. Basel, Karger, 2010, vol 20, pp 203–219

Current Approaches to Retinopathy as a Predictor of Cardiovascular Risk

Ning Cheung[a] · Gerald Liew[b] · Tien Y. Wong[a,c]

[a]Centre for Eye Research Australia, Royal Victorian Eye and Ear Hospital, University of Melbourne, Melbourne, Vic., [b]Centre for Vision Research, University of Sydney, Sydney, N.S.W., Australia; [c]Singapore Eye Research Institute, Yong Loo Lin School of Medicine, National University of Singapore, Singapore, Singapore

Abstract

Current guidelines emphasize the need for regular eye screening to detect retinopathy signs in patients with diabetes. This presents clinicians with a unique opportunity to visualize, assess and monitor the direct effects of diabetes and hyperglycemia on the microcirculation. Although the adverse impact of diabetic retinopathy on vision is well known, its clinical significance beyond the eye is less well recognized. Recent studies show that patients with diabetic retinopathy are more likely to have subclinical cardiovascular disease, and the presence of retinopathy signs is associated with increased risk of clinical stroke, coronary heart disease, heart failure and mortality. There is also emerging evidence to suggest that diabetic retinopathy may share common genetic linkages with many vascular diseases. These new data support the theory that retinopathy signs may reflect widespread microcirculatory disease not only in the eye but also in vital organs elsewhere in the body. Being a specific and noninvasive measure of diabetic microvascular damage, retinopathy signs may therefore also have a role in improving cardiovascular risk prediction in patients with diabetes.

Diabetic retinopathy is the most common and specific microvascular complication of diabetes and a leading cause of blindness in working aged adult people around the world. While its adverse impact on vision is well known, the importance and significance of retinopathy signs beyond ocular morbidity is less well recognized. Two decades ago, the Framingham Heart and Eye Study proposed that diabetic retinopathy signs may reflect generalized microangiopathic processes that affect not only the eyes but also organs elsewhere in the body [1]. In recent years, with the use of standardized assessment of retinopathy signs based on retinal photographs [2], studies have more precisely quantified the associations of diabetic retinopathy with a range of subclinical and clinical cardiovascular diseases, suggesting that retinal assessment may have a role in improving cardiovascular risk prediction in patients with diabetes.

This chapter summarizes the evidence regarding the systemic associations of diabetic retinopathy and discusses their potential clinical and research implications.

Diabetic Retinopathy and Mortality

It has long been observed that in persons with diabetes, the presence of retinopathy is associated with poorer survival [3]. Newer studies have provided further insights into this association. There is now good evidence that this association is more consistently seen in patients with type 2 as compared to type 1 diabetes, reflecting older age and possibly higher prevalence of cardiovascular risk factors in type 2 diabetes.

In persons with type 2 diabetes, the Wisconsin Epidemiological Study of Diabetic Retinopathy (WESDR) demonstrated that both nonproliferative (NPDR) and proliferative (PDR) diabetic retinopathies were associated with a 30–90% excess risk of death after 16 years of follow-up [4]. Importantly, this association was independent of age, sex, diabetes duration, glycemic control and other survival-related risk factors. Consistent with this finding are subsequent publications from other studies, mostly in Caucasian populations [5–9], but also in Asians [10] and Mexican-Americans [11].

In persons with type 1 diabetes, although some studies suggest that retinopathy also predicts mortality risk, the association may be chiefly explained by concomitant cardiovascular risk factors [4, 12, 13]. In the Early Treatment Diabetic Retinopathy Study, a large clinical trial with a relatively short follow-up, retinopathy was shown to have no association with mortality in type 1 diabetes [9]. Some [14, 15], but not all [8], investigators suggest that coexisting nephropathy (e.g. end-stage renal disease) is a major factor for the poorer survival in type 1 diabetic patients with retinopathy.

The association of diabetic retinopathy with mortality is mainly driven by an increased risk of cardiovascular disease in persons with retinopathy. The World Health Organization Multinational Study of Vascular Disease in Diabetes (WHO-MSVDD) consists of a large cohort of type 1 and 2 diabetic persons who were followed up for 12 years for incidence of fatal and nonfatal cardiovascular outcomes [16]. In the WHO-MSVDD, the presence of diabetic retinopathy predicted higher risk of cardiovascular disease and mortality [16]. This association remained significant even after adjusting for traditional cardiovascular risk factors, and was stronger in women than in men, and again confined to persons with type 2, but not type 1, diabetes [16].

While the presence of retinopathy itself seems to signify an increased mortality risk, studies have also shown a 'dose-dependent' association between increasing severity of diabetic retinopathy and increasing cardiovascular disease risk [5–8, 13, 17–20].

Diabetic Retinopathy and Cerebrovascular Disease

Stroke is a major source of morbidity and mortality in people with diabetes. The significant progress made in stroke prevention and treatment has been confined to the management of strokes that are caused by large vessel disease (e.g. carotid atherosclerosis). However, up to one third of symptomatic strokes are now thought to be attributable to disease of the small arteries/arterioles in the cerebral circulation [21], and this is especially so in people with diabetes [22–26]. However, relatively little is known about these small vessel pathologies due to the paucity of simple and noninvasive methods to study the cerebral microcirculation [27, 28].

Since the retinal and cerebral vasculatures share similar embryological origin, anatomical features and physiological properties [29, 30], retinopathy lesions in persons with diabetes may mirror similar pathological disease processes in the cerebral microcirculation. Indeed, there is now a strong and consistent level of evidence that retinopathy signs are associated with both clinical and subclinical stroke, independent of cerebrovascular risk factors.

Dating back to the 1970s, physicians documented that the presence of retinopathy is associated with stroke, particularly in persons with hypertension [31–37]. Newer population-based studies, using standardized photographic

Table 1. Selected studies on the association of diabetic retinopathy and stroke

Study	Retinal status	Associations[1]	Population	Follow-up years
WESDR [12]	PDR in T1DM PDR in T2DM	+++ +++	996 T1DM 1,370 T2DM	4
WESDR [4]	Mild NPDR PDR	+ (NS) ++	1,370 T2DM	16
WESDR [15]	DR severity	++	996 T1DM	20
ARIC [38, 40]	Any DR	++	1,617 T2DM	8
WHO-MSVDD [16]	DR in T1DM men DR in T1DM women DR in T2DM men DR in T2DM women	+ (NS) + (NS) +++ +++	1,126 T1DM 3,179 T2DM	12

T1DM = Type 1 diabetes mellitus; T2DM = type 2 diabetes mellitus; DR = diabetic retinopathy; NS = not statistically significant.
[1] Adjusted hazard rate or relative risk <1.5 (+), 1.5–2.0 (++), >2.0 (+++).

evaluation of retinal images to ascertain retinopathy lesions, have confirmed these early observations (table 1). In the WESDR, PDR was associated with incident stroke mortality in both type 1 and 2 diabetes, independent of diabetes duration, glycemic control and other risk factors [4, 12, 15]. In type 1 diabetes, increasing retinopathy severity was also associated with higher stroke risk [15]. These findings are consistent with data from the WHO-MSVDD in both men and women with type 2 diabetes [16].

More recently, the Atherosclerosis Risk in Communities (ARIC) study, a large prospective cohort study of 1,617 middle-aged white and black Americans with type 2 diabetes, showed that the presence of NPDR, even of the mildest phenotype (presence of retinal microaneurysms and/or retinal hemorrhages only, level 14 or 15 on the ETDRS scale), was associated with a two- to three-fold higher risk of ischemic stroke (fig. 1) [38, 39]. In a substudy of the ARIC cohort in which participants had cranial magnetic resonance imaging (MRI) scans, a synergistic interaction between the presence of retinopathy and the presence of MRI-defined cerebral white matter lesions on subsequent risk of clinical stroke development was seen. Participants with retinopathy or white

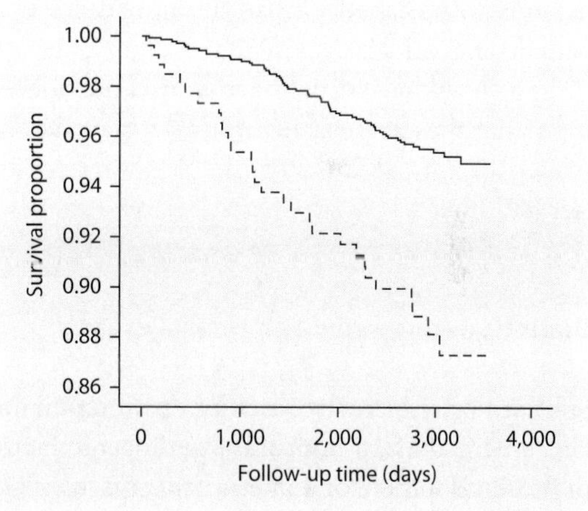

Fig. 1. Stroke-free survival in participants with (dashed line) and without (solid line) diabetic retinopathy [38].

matter lesions alone had about two-fold increase in stroke risk, but participants with both retinopathy and white matter lesions had more than eighteen times higher stroke risk than those without either finding [40]. This supports the theory that subclinical cerebrovascular disease may be more severe or extensive in persons with both cerebral and retinal markers of microvascular pathology compared to those without these markers. Findings from the ARIC study are further reinforced by the Cardiovascular Health Study (an older population) [41] and other studies reported similar findings [37, 42–44]. Finally, there is new evidence that retinopathy signs are associated with stroke risk even in persons without clinical diabetes [45] and in persons with impaired glucose tolerance [46].

The importance of these reported associations is that they directly support a possible contribution of small vessel disease, evident in the retina, in the pathogenesis of cerebrovascular disease in persons with diabetes. In addition, because diabetic retinopathy is usually the result of a disruption in the blood-retinal barrier, it is possible to infer that these cerebral conditions may also be related to a breakdown of the blood-brain barrier [47].

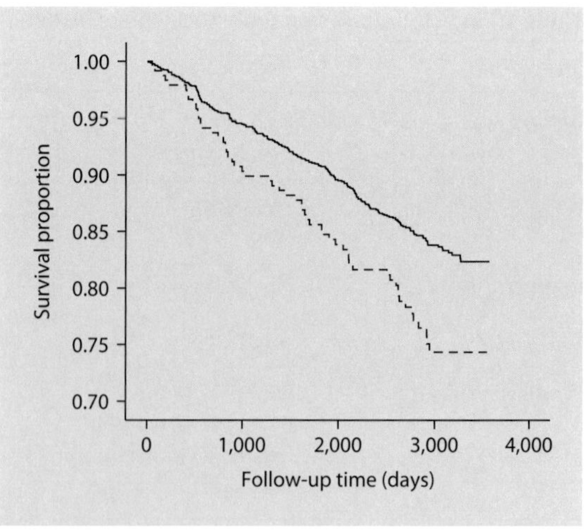

Fig. 2. Coronary heart disease-free survival in participants with (dashed line) and without (solid line) diabetic retinopathy [59].

Diabetic Retinopathy and Heart Disease

Similar to stroke, microvascular dysfunction has also emerged as an important pathogenic factor in the development of diabetic heart disease [48]. However, there are no simple and noninvasive techniques for the assessment of coronary microcirculation [49], and studies that have traditionally evaluated the role of coronary microvascular dysfunction in diabetic heart disease have been limited to small clinic-based samples using highly specialized and invasive methods [50–54].

Data from the Framingham Heart and Eye Study conducted two decades ago suggest that retinopathy signs may reflect a generalized microangiopathic process that affects the myocardium in people with diabetes [1]. This hypothesis is supported by earlier studies, based on ophthalmoscopic examinations, linking retinopathy signs with ischemic T-wave changes on electrocardiogram [55, 56], severity of coronary artery stenosis on angiography [57], histological evidence of microvascular disease in the myocardium [50], and incident clinical coronary heart disease events [58].

Recent epidemiological studies using standardized photographic grading of retinopathy have produced more robust evidence in support of previous observations. It is now clear that diabetic retinopathy signs are associated with an increased risk of not only coronary artery disease (fig. 2) but also its major complication, congestive heart failure (fig. 3; table 2). The ARIC study showed that the presence of any retinopathy signs was associated with two-fold higher risk of incident coronary heart disease (and myocardial infarction), three-fold higher risk of fatal coronary heart disease, and four-fold higher risk of heart

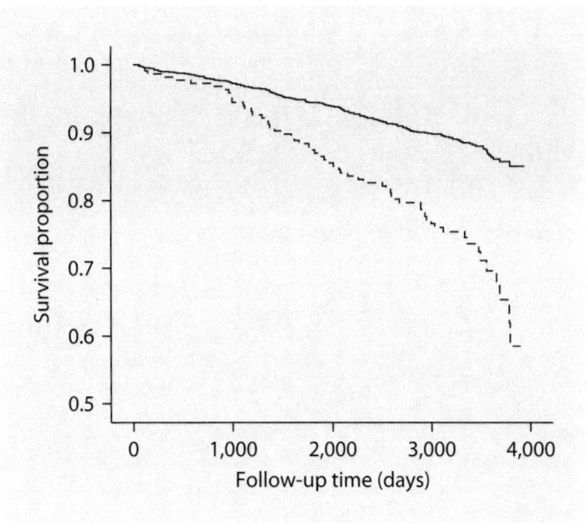

Fig. 3. Heart failure-free survival in participants with (dashed line) and without (solid line) diabetic retinopathy [Cheung, unpubl. data; the ARIC Study].

failure, independent of diabetes duration, glycemic control, smoking, lipid profile and other risk factors [59–61]. The population-attributable risk of retinopathy to heart failure has been estimated to be about 30% in people with diabetes without a previous history of myocardial infarction and hypertension. Thus, if retinopathy signs are a perfect reflection of coronary small vessel pathology, nearly one third of diabetic cardiomyopathy cases could be related to microvascular dysfunction [60]. There is a graded, dose-dependent association of increasing diabetic retinopathy severity with increasing coronary heart disease risk [59]. These findings are consistent with data from the WHO-MSVDD [16] and other studies showing associations of not only NPDR but also PDR with ischemic heart disease [7, 62, 63].

In addition to population-based studies, there are clinical studies that suggest the presence of retinopathy can be used as an indicator of silent myocardial ischemia and help guide investigative approaches and potentially treatment in diabetic patients with suspected heart disease [64–69]. For example, retinopathy may be a valuable prognostic predictor for diabetic patients undergoing cardiac revascularization procedures. Studies show that compared to patients without diabetic retinopathy, patients with retinopathy are more likely to sustain major adverse cardiac events or complications (e.g. death, myocardial infarction, heart failure, in-stent restenosis) after percutaneous coronary intervention or coronary artery bypass surgery, even after factoring in effects of age, gender, diabetes duration, insulin use and other factors that may affect prognosis after these procedures [70–73]. Thus, it may be important to assess retinopathy status to assist in clinical decision-making for revascularization strategies in diabetic patients with established coronary heart disease [74].

The association of retinopathy with clinical heart disease is well supported by the observed links between diabetic retinopathy and subclinical coronary micro- and macrovascular pathology. Pathological and radiological studies have shown that persons with retinopathy are more likely to have myocardial arteriolar abnormalities [50], coronary perfusion defects [69, 75, 76], poorer coronary flow reserve [77] and lower coronary collateral score [78], than those without retinopathy. The presence of retinopathy signs has also been associated with higher degrees of coronary artery calcification [79, 80] and more diffuse/severe coronary artery stenosis on angiograms [68], two established measures of subclinical coronary atherosclerotic burden.

Retinal Venules and Cardiovascular Disease

Dilatation of the retinal venules has long been recognized as a characteristic clinical sign of severe diabetic retinopathy and as a possible marker of retinopathy progression [81]. However, this vascular feature has been less well described in comparison to other morphologically more distinct retinopathy lesions (e.g. microaneurysms,

Table 2. Selected studies on the relationship of diabetic retinopathy and heart disease

Study	Retinal status	Associations[1]	Population	Follow-up years
ARIC [59]	Any DR	++ (CHD)	1,524 T2DM	8
ARIC [60]	Any DR	+++ (CHF)	627 T2DM	7
WHO-MSVDD [16]	DR in T1DM men DR in T1DM women DR in T2DM men or women	+++ ++ ++	1,126 T1DM 3,179 T2DM	12
Finnish [7]	NPDR in men NPDR in women PDR in men or women	+ (NS) ++ +++	824 T2DM	18
Finnish [62]	NPDR PDR	+ (NS) +++	1,040 T2DM	7
WESDR [15]	DR severity	+	996 T1DM	20
BMES [130]	Any DR	++	199 T2DM	12

BMES = Blue Mountains Eye Study; CHD = coronary heart disease; CHF = congestive heart failure.
[1] Adjusted hazard rate or relative risk <1.5 (+), 1.5–2.0 (++), >2.0 (+++).

blot hemorrhages, soft exudates), largely because of difficulties in quantifying retinal venular dilation based on clinical examination.

Recent advances in retinal image-analytical techniques have allowed precise measurements of retinal vascular caliber from retinal photographs [2, 82, 83]. Using this new approach, wider (or dilated) retinal venular caliber has been associated with higher risks of diabetic retinopathy progression and incident PDR in the WESDR [84, 85]. Furthermore, there is now evidence that wider retinal venules may also have associations with major cardiovascular outcomes [86–91]. Wider retinal venular caliber has been shown to predict higher risks of stroke and coronary heart disease in several population-based studies, even after factoring the effects of concomitant risk factors [87–89, 91, 92]. In addition, data from these new studies suggest that wider retinal venular caliber is a marker of early retinal as well as systemic microvascular damage caused by hyperglycemia-related processes (e.g. impaired vascular tone autoregulation, inflammation, endothelial dysfunction) [93, 94]. These findings provide further support for the link between early retinal vascular changes and cardiovascular disease.

Pathogenic Links between Retinopathy and Cardiovascular Disease

Despite the increasingly abundant evidence from epidemiological and clinical studies that diabetic retinopathy is associated with cardiovascular disease, the underlying pathophysiological mechanisms remain uncertain [95]. This reflects, at least in part, an incomplete understanding of the pathogenesis of diabetic retinopathy itself [81]. Nevertheless, several mechanisms have been hypothesized.

First, in people with type 2 diabetes, the presence of retinopathy may simply indicate a more adverse cardiovascular risk profile. It is known that compared to those without retinopathy, diabetic persons with retinopathy are more likely to have concomitant cardiovascular risk factors, such as hypertension and dyslipidemia, which can all increase their cardiovascular risk [18, 96–98]. However, this is unlikely the sole reason as many studies have demonstrated that traditional cardiovascular risk factors cannot fully explain the observed associations [4, 7, 15, 38, 59, 62], suggesting the existence of other biological mechanisms.

Second, it has been suggested that retinopathy is a manifestation of generalized vascular dysfunction caused by endothelial dysfunction or genetically determined alterations in the basement membrane metabolism associated with hyperglycemia (the Steno hypothesis) [99, 100]. These vascular effects increase arterial or arteriolar wall permeability and leakage. Therefore, in small arteriolar or capillary beds, retinopathy and nephropathy may develop as a result. In large arterial wall, increased permeability facilitates entry and accumulation of lipids, thus promoting the pathogenic cascade of atherosclerosis formation.

Third, another possibility is that microvascular disease, evident as retinopathy lesions in the eye, may be present in other tissues and play a causal role in the development of atherosclerotic disease in people with diabetes. This is based on the observations that diabetic retinopathy is related not only to classic microvascular complications (e.g. nephropathy), but also complications of predominantly macrovascular etiology (e.g. coronary heart disease; table 2). There is now a large body of literature indicating that retinopathy is associated with several direct subclinical measures of large artery atherosclerosis, including carotid artery intima-media thickness or carotid plaque, arterial stiffness, coronary artery calcification as well as atherosclerotic lesions detected on angiograms [18, 41, 68, 79, 80, 101]. Based on the complex pathophysiological interactions between diabetic microvascular and macrovascular disease [95, 102], a possible mechanism that may causally link retinopathy to the development of atherosclerosis is shown in figure 4 [103].

Finally, there is a circulatory mechanism hypothesis that may also provide a causal link for diabetic retinopathy and cardiovascular disease [104, 105]. Microvascular disease is known to play an important role in the pathogenesis of diabetic cardiomyopathy, a complex and unique disease entity that is independent of coronary atherosclerosis and hypertension [106]. Recently, in the Multi-Ethnic Study of Atherosclerosis, diabetic retinopathy was found to be associated with left ventricular concentric remodeling, a known precursor for heart failure development [104]. This finding is consistent with the ARIC study, which demonstrated a strong association of retinopathy with clinical congestive heart failure in people with diabetes [60]. Both studies offer good support for a pathogenic link between diabetic retinopathy and cardiomyopathy. It is possible that diabetic retinopathy may represent widespread systemic microcirculatory (resistance vessel) disease, which places an increased impedance burden, in part through reflected pulse waves, on the diabetic heart. The excess load may in turn compromise the efficiency of cardiac performance (e.g. ventricular emptying and cardiac contractility), predisposing the development and manifestation of diabetic cardiomyopathy [104, 105].

Genetic Links between Retinopathy and Cardiovascular Disease

There is a great deal of interest in identifying genetic factors involved in the development of cardiovascular disease, as knowledge of these genes

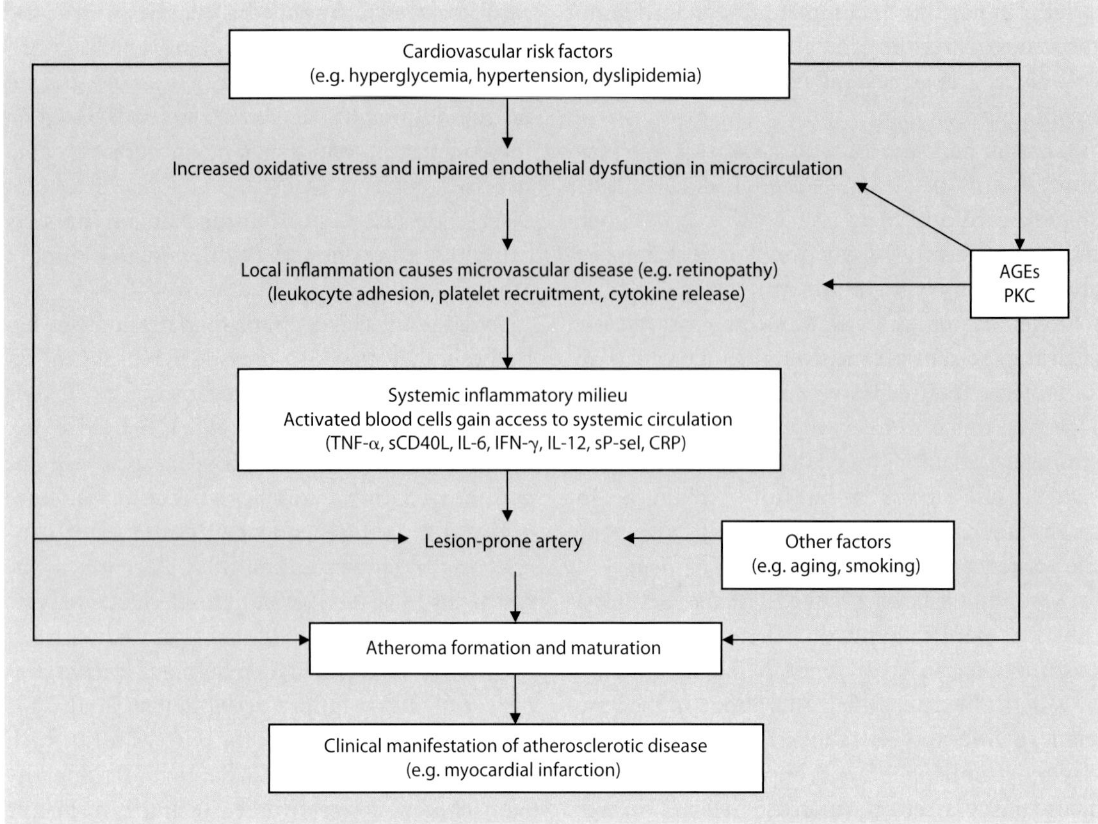

Fig. 4. Potential mechanisms linking diabetic microvascular (retinopathy) to macrovascular (atherosclerosis) disease. Cardiovascular risk factors increase oxidative stress which activates the endothelial cells lining the microvasculature. The resultant imbalance between superoxide and nitric oxide leads to endothelial dysfunction, which is further augmented by advanced glycation end-products (AGEs) and protein kinase C (PKC) activation. This promotes the expression of adhesion molecules, leukocyte and platelet recruitment, and subsequent generation of inflammatory mediators. These mediators, along with activated leukocytes and platelets, gain access into the systemic circulation, where they prime, initiate or exacerbate an inflammatory response in those lesion-prone large arteries that are rendered vulnerable to oxidative stress and inflammation due to chronic exposure to flow disturbances or cardiovascular risk factors. The inflammatory mediators derived from the microcirculation work in concert with other immune cells within the wall of lesion-prone arteries, leading to development of the nascent atheroma, which continues to mature and give rise to clinical manifestation of atherosclerotic disease.

may open new avenues for preventative and therapeutic strategies. However, previous studies have largely focused on the genetic associations of large vessel atherosclerotic disease [107, 108]. There is less research on the genetic determinants of small vessel microvascular disease. Thus, understanding the genetic basis of diabetic retinopathy may uncover important insights into the genetic etiology of systemic diabetic microangiopathy.

Twin studies and family-based analyses of diabetic populations have shown significant familial aggregation in retinopathy risk. Ethnic variations in retinopathy frequency do not appear to be solely attributable to environmental and biological risk factors [109–113]. In addition, previous studies have found associations of some genetic markers with the presence or absence of diabetic retinopathy [103]. These findings indicate the existence of genetic determinants for predisposition or resistance to retinopathy development in people with diabetes. Importantly, several candidate genes associated with diabetic retinopathy have also been implicated in the pathogenesis of cardiovascular disease [Gerald, in press]. Further research in this field is needed to determine whether retinopathy is a useful vascular phenotype for genetic association studies of cardiovascular disease.

Implications

Clinical Implications

Understanding the relationships of diabetic retinopathy with cardiovascular disease is clinically important not only to ophthalmologists, but also to physicians and others who treat and counsel patients with diabetes.

The assessment of cardiovascular risk in persons with diabetes is a key component of clinical care. It allows early implementation of targeted preventive treatments for patients who are asymptomatic but at high risk of systemic vascular complications. However, current cardiovascular risk prediction for diabetic populations is inaccurate and unsatisfactory [114–118]. A recent systematic review of data from more than 70,000 participants showed that the Framingham risk scores significantly underestimate the absolute risk of cardiovascular disease in diabetic populations [117]. Therefore, there is clearly a need to identify additional predictors and biomarkers of cardiovascular disease risk in people with diabetes [118]. A major clinical challenge in risk prediction is that individual susceptibility to cardiovascular disease varies greatly. While some diabetic patients are particularly prone to develop vascular complications, others appear to have a degree of 'vascular resilience' despite long duration of disease. Therefore, to improve risk prediction, merely assessing traditional cardiovascular risk factors is inadequate, and a personalized and specific marker of underlying vascular disease may be more useful [119].

Being a common, specific and noninvasively assessable measure of diabetic microangiopathic burden, retinopathy could serve as a useful biomarker to improve cardiovascular risk stratification in people with diabetes. This is supported by good biological rationale and consistent associations of diabetic retinopathy with both subclinical and clinical cardiovascular diseases in epidemiological and clinical studies. Thus, incorporating retinal assessment into the currently available cardiovascular risk prediction tools [120, 121] may improve the precision of cardiovascular risk prediction for people with, and possibly also without, diabetes [88, 122, 123]. In fact, as discussed, in certain clinical settings, this is already the case. For example, retinopathy may guide preoperative assessment and counseling of diabetic patients planning for elective cardiac revascularization procedures [70–74].

Finally, photographic evaluation of retinopathy signs has also been found to be a cost-effective means to enhance health outcomes for Australians with diabetes (pers. commun. with Wong TY, Access Economic Report 2008). Adding in retinopathy assessment to the Framingham equation to predict coronary heart disease, stroke and other health outcomes could save almost up to USD 500 millions and 700 quality-adjusted life years over a 10-year period.

Apart from people with diabetes, there is emerging evidence that typical signs of early diabetic retinopathy (e.g. microaneurysms, blot hemorrhages, hard exudates and cotton wool spots) are relatively common in people who do not fit the current diagnostic criteria for diabetes.

Studies have reported high prevalence (up to 14%) and incidence (6–10%) rates of these retinopathy signs in nondiabetic populations [124–127]. Retinopathy signs in people without diabetes have also been associated with a similar spectrum of cardiovascular diseases, including stroke [39, 45, 128], ischemic heart disease [129, 130] and congestive heart failure [60]. Additionally, these retinopathy signs may also signify an increased risk of diabetes, especially among those with a family history of diabetes [131–133]. These 'non-diabetic' retinopathy signs may therefore reflect the adverse influences of long-standing but subtle abnormalities in glucose metabolism, blood pressure dysregulation and other processes on the systemic circulatory system. Further research is needed to delineate the pathogenic basis and prognostic significance of these retinopathy signs in people without diabetes.

Therapeutic Implications

The close relationship between diabetic retinopathy and cardiovascular disease may also allow the development and use of common therapeutic strategies. The effectiveness of targeting cardiovascular risk factors in the prevention of diabetic retinopathy has been clearly demonstrated in several landmark randomized clinical trials, such as the Diabetes Control and Complications Trial, in which controlling traditional cardiovascular risk factors (e.g. hyperglycemia, hypertension, dyslipidemia) reduces both the risk of retinopathy and cardiovascular disease in people with diabetes [134–140].

However, it remains uncertain whether specific therapies targeted at the microcirculation level may have additional benefits in reducing retinopathy beyond improvement in traditional risk factors (e.g. blood pressure). The EURODIAB Controlled Trial of Lisinopril in Insulin-Dependent Diabetes Mellitus (EUCLID) evaluated the effects of the angiotensin-converting enzyme (ACE) inhibitor lisinopril on diabetic retinopathy progression in normotensive, normoalbuminuric patients with type 1 diabetes. Lisinopril reduced the progression of diabetic retinopathy by 50% and progression to PDR by 80% over 2 years [141]. The authors speculated that ACE inhibitors may have an additional benefit on diabetic retinopathy progression independent of blood pressure lowering, although data from other studies did not find ACE inhibitors to be superior to nonspecific blood pressure medications [135, 142, 143].

Two new trials provide further insights. The DIRECT trials appear to show a modest benefit of angiotensin II inhibitors in reducing progression of early retinopathy [144, 145]. However, in the Action in Diabetes and Vascular disease: preterAx and diamicroN-MR Controlled Evaluation (ADVANCE) trial, routine administration of a fixed combination of angiogensin-converting enzyme inhibitor and diuretic reduced cardiovascular mortality but not retinopathy risk [146].

Concurrently, it is important for ophthalmologists and physicians to be aware of the potential systemic cardiovascular effects of new diabetic retinopathy treatments. In recent years, the development of agents used to suppress vascular endothelial growth factors (VEGF; e.g. pegaptanib, ranibizumab, bevacizumab) has revolutionized the management of neovascular age-related macular degeneration [147]. There is now emerging evidence that these anti-VEGF agents may also be useful in the management of diabetic retinopathy. Several clinical trials have demonstrated beneficial effects of anti-VEGF therapies for diabetic patients with macular edema [148–151] and neovascularization [152, 153]. Although these treatments may be poised for imminent clinical application, the long-term systemic safety of anti-VEGF agents remains uncertain [103, 147, 154], particularly in diabetic patients with already compromised circulatory systems.

Research Implications

Finally, the systemic vascular associations of diabetic retinopathy indicate several potential lines of future research. First, it remains inconclusive as to whether the associations of retinopathy with cardiovascular disease are indeed causal in nature. Most hypothesized mechanisms discussed herein are based on observational clinical studies, which provide little direct evidence for the underlying mechanistic pathways. Additional experimental studies are needed, preferably with a specific focus to elucidate the pathophysiology of diabetic retinopathy. A better understanding in this aspect may shed light into the complex pathogenesis of systemic vascular complications of diabetes.

Second, the literature clearly indicates that diabetic retinopathy signs are not confined exclusively to people with clinically diagnosed diabetes. Typical signs of early diabetic retinopathy are relatively common in people without diabetes or hypertension [124–127]. While there is some evidence that these retinopathy signs are associated with cardiovascular disease [129], including incident diabetes and hypertension [131, 132], data on this type of retinopathy remain relatively sparse. Further studies are needed to determine their pathophysiological basis and prognostic significance.

Third, as the review shows, the associations of diabetic retinopathy with cardiovascular disease appear to be most evident in middle-aged to older people with type 2 diabetes. Less consistent results have been seen in studies of younger people with type 1 diabetes. This could be due to a number of reasons related to methodological issues (e.g. insufficient length of follow-up to ascertain cardiovascular events and therefore lack of power to detect associations if present, or biological differences (e.g. better vascular profile in younger participants, variations in genetic susceptibility or resilience to systemic vascular complications). These areas deserve further exploration and research.

Finally, it remains unclear if retinopathy is a useful additional parameter to include in the currently available risk prediction tools for cardiovascular disease in persons with diabetes [117]. Assessing the integrity of the vasculature by screening for retinopathy lesions may offer a means to obtain more relevant and 'personalized' information regarding the patients' microvascular health. This 'personalized' information (presence or absence of retinopathy) may correlate more closely with and be incorporated into the assessment of individual susceptibility to cardiovascular disease [155], facilitating more precise quantification of the vascular effects of cardiovascular risk factors. Nevertheless, the value of retinopathy assessment in the prediction of cardiovascular risk is yet to be fully determined in clinical settings. There is a need for studies that are geared specifically to examine the ability of retinopathy signs to provide incremental predictive information above and beyond the currently available risk prediction models that may alter the cardiovascular management of patients with diabetes.

Conclusion

Diabetic retinopathy is a common microvascular complication that is not only a serious threat to vision, but may also signify an increased risk of morbidity and mortality attributable to cardiovascular disease. Both early and severe forms of diabetic retinopathy have been associated with increased risk of subclinical measures of cardiovascular disease and clinical cardiovascular events. These findings suggest that apart from being a manifestation of microvascular damage in the retina, retinopathy signs may also be considered as a noninvasively assessable risk marker for more generalized vascular disease. For ophthalmologists, physicians and other healthcare providers, it is therefore imperative not to overlook the broader associations and clinical implications of diabetic retinopathy.

References

1 Hiller R, Sperduto RD, Podgor MJ, Ferris FL 3rd, Wilson PW: Diabetic retinopathy and cardiovascular disease in type II diabetics. The Framingham Heart Study and the Framingham Eye Study. Am J Epidemiol 1988;128:402–409.

2 Hubbard LD, Brothers RJ, King WN, Clegg LX, Klein R, Cooper LS, Sharrett AR, Davis MD, Cai J: Methods for evaluation of retinal microvascular abnormalities associated with hypertension/sclerosis in the Atherosclerosis Risk in Communities Study. Ophthalmology 1999;106:2269–2280.

3 Berkow JW, Patz A, Fine S: A follow-up of blind diabetic patients. Ann Ophthalmol 1975;7:79–82.

4 Klein R, Klein BE, Moss SE, Cruickshanks KJ: Association of ocular disease and mortality in a diabetic population. Arch Ophthalmol 1999;117:1487–1495.

5 Van Hecke MV, Dekker JM, Nijpels G, Moll AC, Van Leiden HA, Heine RJ, Bouter LM, Stehouwer CD, Polak BC: Retinopathy is associated with cardiovascular and all-cause mortality in both diabetic and nondiabetic subjects: the hoorn study. Diabetes Care 2003;26:2958.

6 Henricsson M, Nilsson A, Heijl A, Janzon L, Groop L: Mortality in diabetic patients participating in an ophthalmological control and screening programme. Diabet Med 1997;14:576–583.

7 Juutilainen A, Lehto S, Ronnemaa T, Pyorala K, Laakso M: Retinopathy predicts cardiovascular mortality in type 2 diabetic men and women. Diabetes Care 2007;30:292–299.

8 Rajala U, Pajunpaa H, Koskela P, Keinanen-Kiukaanniemi S: High cardiovascular disease mortality in subjects with visual impairment caused by diabetic retinopathy. Diabetes Care 2000;23:957–961.

9 Cusick M, Meleth AD, Agron E, Fisher MR, Reed GF, Knatterud GL, Barton FB, Davis MD, Ferris FL 3rd, Chew EY: Associations of mortality and diabetes complications in patients with type 1 and type 2 diabetes: early treatment diabetic retinopathy study report no. 27. Diabetes Care 2005;28:617–625.

10 Sasaki A, Uehara M, Horiuchi N, Hasegawa K, Shimizu T: A 15-year follow-up study of patients with non-insulin-dependent diabetes mellitus (NIDDM) in Osaka, Japan. Factors predictive of the prognosis of diabetic patients. Diabetes Res Clin Pract 1997;36:41–47.

11 Hanis CL, Chu HH, Lawson K, Hewett-Emmett D, Barton SA, Schull WJ, Garcia CA: Mortality of Mexican Americans with NIDDM. Retinopathy and other predictors in Starr County, Texas. Diabetes Care 1993;16:82–89.

12 Klein R, Klein BE, Moss SE: Epidemiology of proliferative diabetic retinopathy. Diabetes Care 1992;15:1875–1891.

13 van Hecke MV, Dekker JM, Stehouwer CD, Polak BC, Fuller JH, Sjolie AK, Kofinis A, Rottiers R, Porta M, Chaturvedi N: Diabetic retinopathy is associated with mortality and cardiovascular disease incidence: the EURODIAB prospective complications study. Diabetes Care 2005;28:1383–1389.

14 Torffvit O, Lovestam-Adrian M, Agardh E, Agardh CD: Nephropathy, but not retinopathy, is associated with the development of heart disease in Type 1 diabetes: a 12-year observation study of 462 patients. Diabet Med 2005;22:723–729.

15 Klein BE, Klein R, McBride PE, Cruickshanks KJ, Palta M, Knudtson MD, Moss SE, Reinke JO: Cardiovascular disease, mortality, and retinal microvascular characteristics in type 1 diabetes: Wisconsin epidemiologic study of diabetic retinopathy. Arch Intern Med 2004;164:1917–1924.

16 Fuller JH, Stevens LK, Wang SL: Risk factors for cardiovascular mortality and morbidity: the WHO Mutinational Study of Vascular Disease in Diabetes. Diabetologia 2001;44(suppl 2):S54–S64.

17 Targher G, Bertolini L, Tessari R, Zenari L, Arcaro G: Retinopathy predicts future cardiovascular events among type 2 diabetic patients: The Valpolicella Heart Diabetes Study. Diabetes Care 2006;29:1178.

18 Klein R, Marino EK, Kuller LH, Polak JF, Tracy RP, Gottdiener JS, Burke GL, Hubbard LD, Boineau R: The relation of atherosclerotic cardiovascular disease to retinopathy in people with diabetes in the Cardiovascular Health Study. Br J Ophthalmol 2002;86:84–90.

19 Jager A, van Hinsbergh VW, Kostense PJ, Emeis JJ, Nijpels G, Dekker JM, Heine RJ, Bouter LM, Stehouwer CD: Prognostic implications of retinopathy and a high plasma von Willebrand factor concentration in type 2 diabetic subjects with microalbuminuria. Nephrol Dial Transplant 2001;16:529–536.

20 Targher G, Bertolini L, Zenari L, Lippi G, Pichiri I, Zoppini G, Muggeo M, Arcaro G: Diabetic retinopathy is associated with an increased incidence of cardiovascular events in Type 2 diabetic patients. Diabet Med 2008;25:45–50.

21 Greenberg SM: Small vessels, big problems. N Engl J Med 2006;354:1451–1453.

22 Fisher CM: Lacunes: small, deep cerebral infarcts. Neurology 1965;15:774–784.

23 Fisher CM: The arterial lesions underlying lacunes. Acta Neuropathol (Berl) 1968;12:1–15.

24 Alex M, Baron EK, Goldenberg S, Blumenthal HT: An autopsy study of cerebrovascular accident in diabetes mellitus. Circulation 1962;25:663–673.

25 Aronson SM: Intracranial vascular lesions in patients with diabetes mellitus. J Neuropathol Exp Neurol 1973;32:183–196.

26 Bell DS: Stroke in the diabetic patient. Diabetes Care 1994;17:213–219.

27 Bamford JM, Warlow CP: Evolution and testing of the lacunar hypothesis. Stroke 1988;19:1074–1082.

28 Wardlaw JM, Dennis MS, Warlow CP, Sandercock PA: Imaging appearance of the symptomatic perforating artery in patients with lacunar infarction: occlusion or other vascular pathology? Ann Neurol 2001;50:208–215.

29 Wong TY: Is retinal photography useful in the measurement of stroke risk? Lancet Neurol 2004;3:179–183.

30 Patton N, Aslam T, Macgillivray T, Pattie A, Deary IJ, Dhillon B: Retinal vascular image analysis as a potential screening tool for cerebrovascular disease: a rationale based on homology between cerebral and retinal microvasculatures. J Anat 2005;206:319–348.

31 Okada H, Horibe H, Yoshiyuki O, Hayakawa N, Aoki N: A prospective study of cerebrovascular disease in Japanese rural communities, Akabane and Asahi. Part 1: evaluation of risk factors in the occurrence of cerebral hemorrhage and thrombosis. Stroke 1976;7:599–607.
32 Tanaka H, Hayashi M, Date C, Imai K, Asada M, Shoji H, Okazaki K, Yamamoto H, Yoshikawa K, Shimada T, et al: Epidemiologic studies of stroke in Shibata, a Japanese provincial city: preliminary report on risk factors for cerebral infarction. Stroke 1985;16:773–780.
33 Svardsudd K, Wedel H, Aurell E, Tibblin G: Hypertensive eye ground changes. Prevalence, relation to blood pressure and prognostic importance. The study of men born in 1913. Acta Med Scand 1978;204:159–167.
34 Nakayama T, Date C, Yokoyama T, Yoshiike N, Yamaguchi M, Tanaka H: A 15.5-year follow-up study of stroke in a Japanese provincial city. The Shibata Study. Stroke 1997;28:45–52.
35 Goto I, Katsuki S, Ikui H, Kimoto K, Mimatsu T: Pathological studies on the intracerebral and retinal arteries in cerebrovascular and noncerebrovascular diseases. Stroke 1975;6:263–269.
36 Schneider R, Rademacher M, Wolf S: Lacunar infarcts and white matter attenuation. Ophthalmologic and microcirculatory aspects of the pathophysiology. Stroke 1993;24:1874–1879.
37 Petitti DB, Bhatt H: Retinopathy as a risk factor for nonembolic stroke in diabetic subjects. Stroke 1995;26:593–596.
38 Cheung N, Rogers S, Couper DJ, Klein R, Sharrett AR, Wong TY: Is diabetic retinopathy an independent risk factor for ischemic stroke? Stroke 2007;38:398–401.
39 Wong TY, Klein R, Couper DJ, Cooper LS, Shahar E, Hubbard LD, Wofford MR, Sharrett AR: Retinal microvascular abnormalities and incident stroke: the Atherosclerosis Risk in Communities Study. Lancet 2001;358:1134–1140.
40 Wong TY, Klein R, Sharrett AR, Couper DJ, Klein BE, Liao DP, Hubbard LD, Mosley TH: Cerebral white matter lesions, retinopathy, and incident clinical stroke. JAMA 2002;288:67–74.
41 Wong TY, Klein R, Sharrett AR, Manolio TA, Hubbard LD, Marino EK, Kuller L, Burke G, Tracy RP, Polak JF, Gottdiener JS, Siscovick DS: The prevalence and risk factors of retinal microvascular abnormalities in older persons: The Cardiovascular Health Study. Ophthalmology 2003;110:658–666.
42 Wong TY, Klein R, Nieto FJ, Klein BE, Sharrett AR, Meuer SM, Hubbard LD, Tielsch JM: Retinal microvascular abnormalities and 10-year cardiovascular mortality: a population-based case-control study. Ophthalmology 2003;110:933–940.
43 Wong TY, Cheung N, Tay WT, Wang JJ, Aung T, Saw SM, Lim SC, Tai ES, Mitchell P: Prevalence and Risk Factors for Diabetic Retinopathy The Singapore Malay Eye Study. Ophthalmology 2008;115:1869–1875.
44 Qiu C, Cotch MF, Sigurdsson S, Garcia M, Klein R, Jonasson F, Klein BE, Eiriksdottir G, Harris TB, van Buchem MA, Gudnason V, Launer LJ: Retinal and cerebral microvascular signs and diabetes: the age, gene/environment susceptibility-Reykjavik study. Diabetes 2008;57:1645–1650.
45 Mitchell P, Wang JJ, Wong TY, Smith W, Klein R, Leeder SR: Retinal microvascular signs and risk of stroke and stroke mortality. Neurology 2005;65:1005–1009.
46 Wong TY, Barr EL, Tapp RJ, Harper CA, Taylor HR, Zimmet PZ, Shaw JE: Retinopathy in persons with impaired glucose metabolism: the Australian Diabetes Obesity and Lifestyle (AusDiab) study. Am J Ophthalmol 2005;140:1157–1159.
47 Wardlaw JM, Sandercock PA, Dennis MS, Starr J: Is breakdown of the blood-brain barrier responsible for lacunar stroke, leukoaraiosis, and dementia? Stroke 2003;34:806–812.
48 Camici PG, Crea F: Coronary microvascular dysfunction. N Engl J Med 2007;356:830–840.
49 Duran JR 3rd, Taffet G: Coronary microvascular dysfunction. N Engl J Med 2007;356:2324–2325; author reply 5.
50 Factor SM, Okun EM, Minase T: Capillary microaneurysms in the human diabetic heart. N Engl J Med 1980;302:384–388.
51 Di Carli MF, Janisse J, Grunberger G, Ager J: Role of chronic hyperglycemia in the pathogenesis of coronary microvascular dysfunction in diabetes. J Am Coll Cardiol 2003;41:1387–1393.
52 Miura H, Wachtel RE, Loberiza FR Jr, Saito T, Miura M, Nicolosi AC, Gutterman DD: Diabetes mellitus impairs vasodilation to hypoxia in human coronary arterioles: reduced activity of ATP-sensitive potassium channels. Circ Res 2003;92:151–158.
53 Li Q, Wang J, Sun Y, Cui YL, Juzi JT, Li HX, Qian BY, Hao XS: Efficacy of postoperative transarterial chemoembolization and portal vein chemotherapy for patients with hepatocellular carcinoma complicated by portal vein tumor thrombosis–a randomized study. World J Surg 2006;30:2004–2011; discussion 12–13.
54 Pitkanen OP, Nuutila P, Raitakari OT, Ronnemaa T, Koskinen PJ, Iida H, Lehtimaki TJ, Laine HK, Takala T, Viikari JS, Knuuti J: Coronary flow reserve is reduced in young men with IDDM. Diabetes 1998;47:248–254.
55 Breslin DJ, Gifford RW Jr, Fairbairn JF 2nd, Kearns TP: Prognostic importance of ophthalmoscopic findings in essential hypertension. JAMA 1966;195:335–338.
56 Breslin DJ, Gifford RW Jr, Fairbairn JF 2nd: Essential hypertension. A twenty-year follow-up study. Circulation 1966;33:87–97.
57 Michelson EL, Morganroth J, Nichols CW, MacVaugh H 3rd: Retinal arteriolar changes as an indicator of coronary artery disease. Arch Intern Med 1979;139:1139–1141.
58 Duncan BB, Wong TY, Tyroler HA, Davis CE, Fuchs FD: Hypertensive retinopathy and incident coronary heart disease in high risk men. Br J Ophthalmol 2002;86:1002–1006.
59 Cheung N, Wang JJ, Klein R, Couper DJ, Richey Sharrett AR, Wong TY: Diabetic retinopathy and the risk of coronary heart disease: the Atherosclerosis Risk in Communities Study. Diabetes Care 2007;30:1742–1746.
60 Wong TY, Rosamond W, Chang PP, Couper DJ, Sharrett AR, Hubbard LD, Folsom AR, Klein R: Retinopathy and risk of congestive heart failure. JAMA 2005;293:63–69.

61 Cheung N, Wang JJ, Rogers S, Brancati F, Klein R, Sharret AR, Wong TY: Diabetic retinopathy and risk of heart failure. J Am Coll Cardiol 2008;51:1573–1578.
62 Miettinen H, Haffner SM, Lehto S, Ronnemaa T, Pyorala K, Laakso M: Retinopathy predicts coronary heart disease events in NIDDM patients. Diabetes Care 1996;19:1445–1448.
63 Faglia E, Favales F, Calia P, Paleari F, Segalini G, Gamba PL, Rocca A, Musacchio N, Mastropasqua A, Testori G, Rampini P, Moratti F, Braga A, Morabito A: Cardiac events in 735 type 2 diabetic patients who underwent screening for unknown asymptomatic coronary heart disease: 5-year follow-up report from the Milan Study on Atherosclerosis and Diabetes (MiSAD). Diabetes Care 2002;25:2032–2036.
64 Araz M, Celen Z, Akdemir I, Okan V: Frequency of silent myocardial ischemia in type 2 diabetic patients and the relation with poor glycemic control. Acta Diabetol 2004;41:38–43.
65 Gokcel A, Aydin M, Yalcin F, Yapar AF, Ertorer ME, Ozsahin AK, Muderrisoglu H, Aktas A, Guvener N, Akbaba M: Silent coronary artery disease in patients with type 2 diabetes mellitus. Acta Diabetol 2003;40:176–180.
66 Janand-Delenne B, Savin B, Habib G, Bory M, Vague P, Lassmann-Vague V: Silent myocardial ischemia in patients with diabetes: who to screen. Diabetes Care 1999;22:1396–1400.
67 Naka M, Hiramatsu K, Aizawa T, Momose A, Yoshizawa K, Shigematsu S, Ishihara F, Niwa A, Yamada T: Silent myocardial ischemia in patients with non-insulin-dependent diabetes mellitus as judged by treadmill exercise testing and coronary angiography. Am Heart J 1992;123:46–53.
68 Norgaz T, Hobikoglu G, Aksu H, Guveli A, Aksoy S, Ozer O, Bolca O, Narin A: Retinopathy is related to the angiographically detected severity and extent of coronary artery disease in patients with type 2 diabetes mellitus. Int Heart J 2005;46:639–646.
69 Yoon JK, Lee KH, Park JM, Lee SH, Lee MK, Lee WR, Kim BT: Usefulness of diabetic retinopathy as a marker of risk for thallium myocardial perfusion defects in non-insulin-dependent diabetes mellitus. Am J Cardiol 2001;87:456–459, A6.
70 Briguori C, Condorelli G, Airoldi F, Manganelli F, Violante A, Focaccio A, Ricciardelli B, Colombo A: Impact of microvascular complications on outcome after coronary stent implantations in patients with diabetes. J Am Coll Cardiol 2005;45:464–466.
71 Kim YH, Hong MK, Song JM, Han KH, Kang DH, Song JK, Kim JJ, Park SW, Park SJ: Diabetic retinopathy as a predictor of late clinical events following percutaneous coronary intervention. J Invasive Cardiol 2002;14:599–602.
72 Ono T, Kobayashi J, Sasako Y, Bando K, Tagusari O, Niwaya K, Imanaka H, Nakatani T, Kitamura S: The impact of diabetic retinopathy on long-term outcome following coronary artery bypass graft surgery. J Am Coll Cardiol 2002;40:428–436.
73 Ono T, Ohashi T, Asakura T, Ono N, Ono M, Motomura N, Takamoto S: Impact of diabetic retinopathy on cardiac outcome after coronary artery bypass graft surgery: prospective observational study. Ann Thorac Surg 2006;81:608–612.
74 Ohno T, Ando J, Ono M, Morita T, Motomura N, Hirata Y, Takamoto S: The beneficial effect of coronary-artery-bypass surgery on survival in patients with diabetic retinopathy. Eur J Cardiothorac Surg 2006;30:881–886.
75 Giugliano D, Acampora R, De Rosa N, Quatraro A, De Angelis L, Ceriello A, D'Onofrio F: Coronary artery disease in type-2 diabetes mellitus: a scintigraphic study. Diabete Metab 1993;19:463–466.
76 Ioannidis G, Peppa M, Rontogianni P, Callifronas M, Papadimitriou C, Chrysanthopoulou G, Anthopoulos L, Kesse M, Thalassinos N: The concurrence of microalbuminuria and retinopathy with cardiovascular risk factors; reliable predictors of asymptomatic coronary artery disease in type 2 diabetes. Hormones (Athens) 2004;3:198–203.
77 Akasaka T, Yoshida K, Hozumi T, Takagi T, Kaji S, Kawamoto T, Morioka S, Yoshikawa J: Retinopathy identifies marked restriction of coronary flow reserve in patients with diabetes mellitus. J Am Coll Cardiol 1997;30:935–941.
78 Celik T, Berdan ME, Iyisoy A, Kursaklioglu H, Turhan H, Kilic S, Gulec M, Ozturk S, Isik E: Impaired coronary collateral vessel development in patients with proliferative diabetic retinopathy. Clin Cardiol 2005;28:384–388.
79 Wong TY, Cheung N, Islam AFM, Klein R, Criqui MH, Cotch MF, Carr JJ, Klein BE, Sharrett AR: The relationship of retinopathy to coronary artery calcification: the Multi-Ethnic Study of Atherosclerosis. Am J Epidemiol 2007; Epub ahead of print.
80 Yoshida M, Takamatsu J, Yoshida S, Tanaka K, Takeda K, Higashi H, Kitaoka H, Ohsawa N: Scores of coronary calcification determined by electron beam computed tomography are closely related to the extent of diabetes-specific complications. Horm Metab Res 1999;31:558–563.
81 Frank RN: Diabetic retinopathy. N Engl J Med 2004;350:48–58.
82 Patton N, Aslam TM, MacGillivray T, Deary IJ, Dhillon B, Eikelboom RH, Yogesan K, Constable IJ: Retinal image analysis: concepts, applications and potential. Prog Retin Eye Res 2006;25:99–127.
83 Wong TY, Knudtson MD, Klein R, Klein BE, Meuer SM, Hubbard LD: Computer-assisted measurement of retinal vessel diameters in the Beaver Dam Eye Study: methodology, correlation between eyes, and effect of refractive errors. Ophthalmology 2004;111:1183–1190.
84 Klein R, Klein BE, Moss SE, Wong TY, Sharrett AR: Retinal vascular caliber in persons with type 2 diabetes: the Wisconsin Epidemiological Study of Diabetic Retinopathy: XX. Ophthalmology 2006;113:1488–1498.
85 Klein R, Klein BE, Moss SE, Wong TY, Hubbard L, Cruickshanks KJ, Palta M: The relation of retinal vessel caliber to the incidence and progression of diabetic retinopathy: XIX: the Wisconsin Epidemiologic Study of Diabetic Retinopathy. Arch Ophthalmol 2004;122:76–83.
86 Wang JJ, Taylor B, Wong TY, Chua B, Rochtchina E, Klein R, Mitchell P: Retinal vessel diameters and obesity: a population-based study in older persons. Obesity (Silver Spring) 2006;14:206–214.
87 Wang JJ, Liew G, Wong TY, Smith W, Klein R, Leeder SR, Mitchell P: Retinal vascular calibre and the risk of coronary heart disease-related death. Heart 2006;92:1583–1587.

88 Wang JJ, Liew G, Klein R, Rochtchina E, Knudtson MD, Klein BE, Wong TY, Burlutsky G, Mitchell P: Retinal vessel diameter and cardiovascular mortality: pooled data analysis from two older populations. Eur Heart J 2007;28:1984–1992.

89 Wong TY, Kamineni A, Klein R, Sharrett AR, Klein BE, Siscovick DS, Cushman M, Duncan BB: Quantitative retinal venular caliber and risk of cardiovascular disease in older persons: the cardiovascular health study. Arch Intern Med 2006;166:2388–2394.

90 Cheung N, Saw SM, Islam FM, Rogers SL, Shankar A, de Haseth K, Mitchell P, Wong TY: BMI and retinal vascular caliber in children. Obesity (Silver Spring) 2007;15:209–215.

91 Klein R, Klein BE, Moss SE, Wong TY: Retinal Vessel Caliber and Microvascular and Macrovascular Disease in Type 2 Diabetes XXI: The Wisconsin Epidemiologic Study of Diabetic Retinopathy. Ophthalmology 2007;114:1884–1892.

92 Cheung N, Islam AFM, Jacobs DR, Sharrett AR, Klein R, Polak JF, Cotch MF, Klein BE, Ouyang P, Wong TY: Arterial compliance and retinal vascular caliber in cerebrovascular disease. Ann Neurol 2007;62:618–624.

93 Nguyen TT, Wong TY: Retinal vascular manifestations of metabolic disorders. Trends Endocrinol Metab 2006;17:262–268.

94 Nguyen TT, Wang JJ, Wong TY: Retinal vascular changes in pre-diabetes and pre-hypertension – new findings and their research and clinical implications. Diabetes Care 2007;30:2708–2715.

95 Krentz AJ, Clough G, Byrne CD: Interactions between microvascular and macrovascular disease in diabetes: pathophysiology and therapeutic implications. Diabetes Obes Metab 2007;9:781–791.

96 Klein R, Sharrett AR, Klein BE, Moss SE, Folsom AR, Wong TY, Brancati FL, Hubbard LD, Couper D, Group A: The association of atherosclerosis, vascular risk factors, and retinopathy in adults with diabetes: the atherosclerosis risk in communities study. Ophthalmology 2002;109:1225–1234.

97 Klein R, Klein BE, Moss SE, Davis MD, DeMets DL: The Wisconsin epidemiologic study of diabetic retinopathy. II. Prevalence and risk of diabetic retinopathy when age at diagnosis is less than 30 years. Arch Ophthalmol 1984;102:520–526.

98 Klein R, Klein BE, Moss SE, Davis MD, DeMets DL: The Wisconsin epidemiologic study of diabetic retinopathy. III. Prevalence and risk of diabetic retinopathy when age at diagnosis is 30 or more years. Arch Ophthalmol 1984;102:527–532.

99 Parving HH, Nielsen FS, Bang LE, Smidt UM, Svendsen TL, Chen JW, Gall MA, Rossing P: Macro-microangiopathy and endothelial dysfunction in NIDDM patients with and without diabetic nephropathy. Diabetologia 1996;39:1590–1597.

100 Deckert T, Feldt-Rasmussen B, Borch-Johnsen K, Jensen T, Kofoed-Enevoldsen A: Albuminuria reflects widespread vascular damage. The Steno hypothesis. Diabetologia 1989;32:219–226.

101 Rema M, Mohan V, Deepa R, Ravikumar R: Association of carotid intima-media thickness and arterial stiffness with diabetic retinopathy: the Chennai Urban Rural Epidemiology Study (CURES-2). Diabetes Care 2004;27:1962–1967.

102 Stokes KY, Granger DN: The microcirculation: a motor for the systemic inflammatory response and large vessel disease induced by hypercholesterolaemia? J Physiol 2005;562(Pt 3):647–653.

103 Cheung N, Wong TY: Diabetic retinopathy and systemic vascular complications. Prog Retin Eye Res 2008;27:161–176.

104 Cheung N, Bluemke DA, Klein R, Sharrett AR, Islam FM, Cotch MF, Klein BE, Criqui MH, Wong TY: Retinal arteriolar narrowing and left ventricular remodeling: the multi-ethnic study of atherosclerosis. J Am Coll Cardiol 2007;50:48–55.

105 Cheung N, Wong TY: Microvascular disease and cardiomyopathy. J Card Fail 2007;13:792.

106 Boudina S, Abel ED: Diabetic cardiomyopathy revisited. Circulation 2007;115:3213–3223.

107 Samani NJ, Erdmann J, Hall AS, Hengstenberg C, Mangino M, Mayer B, Dixon RJ, Meitinger T, Braund P, Wichmann HE, Barrett JH, Konig IR, Stevens SE, Szymczak S, Tregouet DA, Iles MM, Pahlke F, Pollard H, Lieb W, Cambien F, Fischer M, Ouwehand W, Blankenberg S, Balmforth AJ, Baessler A, Ball SG, Strom TM, Braenne I, Gieger C, Deloukas P, Tobin MD, Ziegler A, Thompson JR, Schunkert H: Genomewide association analysis of coronary artery disease. N Engl J Med 2007;357:443–453.

108 Nabel EG: Cardiovascular disease. N Engl J Med 2003;349:60–72.

109 Fong DS, Aiello L, Gardner TW, King GL, Blankenship G, Cavallerano JD, Ferris FL 3rd, Klein R: Diabetic retinopathy. Diabetes Care 2003;26:226–229.

110 Alcolado J: Genetics of diabetic complications. Lancet 1998;351:230–231.

111 Warpeha KM, Chakravarthy U: Molecular genetics of microvascular disease in diabetic retinopathy. Eye 2003;17:305–311.

112 Simonelli F, Testa F, Bandello F: Genetics of diabetic retinopathy. Semin Ophthalmol 2001;16:41–51.

113 Cunha-Vaz J, Bernardes R: Nonproliferative retinopathy in diabetes type 2. Initial stages and characterization of phenotypes. Prog Retin Eye Res 2005;24:355–377.

114 Brindle P, May M, Gill P, Cappuccio F, D'Agostino R Sr, Fischbacher C, Ebrahim S: Primary prevention of cardiovascular disease: a web-based risk score for seven British black and minority ethnic groups. Heart 2006;92:1595–1602.

115 Stephens JW, Ambler G, Vallance P, Betteridge DJ, Humphries SE, Hurel SJ: Cardiovascular risk and diabetes. Are the methods of risk prediction satisfactory? Eur J Cardiovasc Prev Rehabil 2004;11:521–528.

116 Guzder RN, Gatling W, Mullee MA, Mehta RL, Byrne CD: Prognostic value of the Framingham cardiovascular risk equation and the UKPDS risk engine for coronary heart disease in newly diagnosed Type 2 diabetes: results from a United Kingdom study. Diabet Med 2005;22:554–562.

117 Brindle P, Beswick A, Fahey T, Ebrahim S: Accuracy and impact of risk assessment in the primary prevention of cardiovascular disease: a systematic review. Heart 2006;92:1752–1759.

118 Jurgensen JS: The value of risk scores. Heart 2006;92:1713–1714.
119 Keenan HA, Costacou T, Sun JK, Doria A, Cavellerano J, Coney J, Orchard TJ, Aiello LP, King GL: Clinical factors associated with resistance to microvascular complications in diabetic patients of extreme disease duration: the 50-year medalist study. Diabetes Care 2007;30:1995–1997.
120 Lee ET, Howard BV, Wang W, Welty TK, Galloway JM, Best LG, Fabsitz RR, Zhang Y, Yeh J, Devereux RB: Prediction of coronary heart disease in a population with high prevalence of diabetes and albuminuria: the Strong Heart Study. Circulation 2006;113:2897–2905.
121 Donnan PT, Donnelly L, New JP, Morris AD: Derivation and validation of a prediction score for major coronary heart disease events in a U.K. type 2 diabetic population. Diabetes Care 2006;29:1231–1236.
122 St Clair L, Ballantyne CM: Biological surrogates for enhancing cardiovascular risk prediction in type 2 diabetes mellitus. Am J Cardiol 2007;99:80B-88B.
123 Duprez DA: The eye, the mirror of the heart. Eur Heart J 2007;28:1915–1916.
124 Cugati S, Cikamatana L, Wang JJ, Kifley A, Liew G, Mitchell P: Five-year incidence and progression of vascular retinopathy in persons without diabetes: the Blue Mountains Eye Study. Eye 2006;20:1239–1245.
125 Klein R, Klein BE, Moss SE: The relation of systemic hypertension to changes in the retinal vasculature: the Beaver Dam Eye Study. Trans Am Ophthalmol Soc 1997;95:329–348; discussion 48–50.
126 Chao JR, Lai MY, Azen SP, Klein R, Varma R: Retinopathy in persons without diabetes: The Los Angeles Latino Eye Study. Invest Ophthalmol Vis Sci 2007;48:4019–4025.
127 Yu T, Mitchell P, Berry G, Li W, Wang JJ: Retinopathy in older persons without diabetes and its relationship to hypertension. Arch Ophthalmol 1998;116:83–89.
128 Cooper LS, Wong TY, Klein R, Sharrett AR, Bryan RN, Hubbard LD, Couper DJ, Heiss G, Sorlie PD: Retinal microvascular abnormalities and MRI-defined subclinical cerebral infarction: the Atherosclerosis Risk in Communities Study. Stroke 2006;37:82–86.
129 Hirai FE, Moss SE, Knudtson MD, Klein BE, Klein R: Retinopathy and survival in a population without diabetes: The Beaver Dam Eye Study. Am J Epidemiol 2007;166:724–730.
130 Liew G, Wong T, Mitchell P, Cheung N, Wang JJ: Retinopathy predicts coronary heart disease mortality. Heart 2009;95:391–394.
131 Klein R, Klein BE, Moss SE, Wong TY: The relationship of retinopathy in persons without diabetes to the 15-year incidence of diabetes and hypertension: Beaver Dam Eye Study. Trans Am Ophthalmol Soc 2006;104:98–107.
132 Wong TY, Mohamed Q, Klein R, Couper DJ: Do retinopathy signs in non-diabetic individuals predict the subsequent risk of diabetes? Br J Ophthalmol 2006;90:301–303.
133 Cugati S, Mitchell P, Wang JJ: Do retinopathy signs in non-diabetic individuals predict the subsequent risk of diabetes? Br J Ophthalmol 2006;90:928–929.
134 Nathan DM, Cleary PA, Backlund JY, Genuth SM, Lachin JM, Orchard TJ, Raskin P, Zinman B: Intensive diabetes treatment and cardiovascular disease in patients with type 1 diabetes. N Engl J Med 2005;353:2643–2653.
135 Tight blood pressure control and risk of macrovascular and microvascular complications in type 2 diabetes: UKPDS 38. UK Prospective Diabetes Study Group. BMJ 1998;317:703–713.
136 Mohamed Q, Gillies MC, Wong TY: Management of diabetic retinopathy: a systematic review. JAMA 2007;298:902–916.
137 Keech A, Simes RJ, Barter P, Best J, Scott R, Taskinen MR, Forder P, Pillai A, Davis T, Glasziou P, Drury P, Kesaniemi YA, Sullivan D, Hunt D, Colman P, d'Emden M, Whiting M, Ehnholm C, Laakso M: Effects of long-term fenofibrate therapy on cardiovascular events in 9795 people with type 2 diabetes mellitus (the FIELD study): randomised controlled trial. Lancet 2005;366:1849–1861.
138 Wong TY, Klein R, Klein BEK: The epidemiology of diabetic retinopathy; in Scott I, Flynn H, Smiddy W (eds): Diabetic Retinopathy. Oxford, Oxford University Press, 2007.
139 Wong TY, Mitchell P: The eye in hypertension. Lancet 2007;369:425–435.
140 Mitchell P, Wong TY: DIRECT new treatments for diabetic retinopathy. Lancet 2008;372:1361–1363.
141 Chaturvedi N, Sjolie AK, Stephenson JM, Abrahamian H, Keipes M, Castellarin A, Rogulja-Pepeonik Z, Fuller JH: Effect of lisinopril on progression of retinopathy in normotensive people with type 1 diabetes. The EUCLID Study Group. EURODIAB Controlled Trial of Lisinopril in Insulin-Dependent Diabetes Mellitus. Lancet 1998;351:28–31.
142 Estacio RO, Jeffers BW, Gifford N, Schrier RW: Effect of blood pressure control on diabetic microvascular complications in patients with hypertension and type 2 diabetes. Diabetes Care 2000;23(suppl 2):B54–B64.
143 Schrier RW, Estacio RO, Jeffers B: Appropriate Blood Pressure Control in NIDDM (ABCD) Trial. Diabetologia 1996;39:1646–1654.
144 Chaturvedi N, Porta M, Klein R, Orchard T, Fuller J, Parving HH, Bilous R, Sjolie AK: Effect of candesartan on prevention (DIRECT-Prevent 1) and progression (DIRECT-Protect 1) of retinopathy in type 1 diabetes: randomised, placebo-controlled trials. Lancet 2008;372:1394–1402.
145 Sjolie AK, Klein R, Porta M, Orchard T, Fuller J, Parving HH, Bilous R, Chaturvedi N: Effect of candesartan on progression and regression of retinopathy in type 2 diabetes (DIRECT-Protect 2): a randomised placebo-controlled trial. Lancet 2008;372:1385–1393.
146 Patel A, MacMahon S, Chalmers J, Neal B, Woodward M, Billot L, Harrap S, Poulter N, Marre M, Cooper M, Glasziou P, Grobbee DE, Hamet P, Heller S, Liu LS, Mancia G, Mogensen CE, Pan CY, Rodgers A, Williams B: Effects of a fixed combination of perindopril and indapamide on macrovascular and microvascular outcomes in patients with type 2 diabetes mellitus (the ADVANCE trial): a randomised controlled trial. Lancet 2007;370:829–840.
147 Wong TY, Liew G, Mitchell P: Clinical update: new treatments for age-related macular degeneration. Lancet 2007;370:204–206.

148 Chun DW, Heier JS, Topping TM, Duker JS, Bankert JM: A pilot study of multiple intravitreal injections of ranibizumab in patients with center-involving clinically significant diabetic macular edema. Ophthalmology 2006;113:1706–1712.

149 Cunningham ET, Jr., Adamis AP, Altaweel M, Aiello LP, Bressler NM, D'Amico DJ, Goldbaum M, Guyer DR, Katz B, Patel M, Schwartz SD: A phase II randomized double-masked trial of pegaptanib, an anti-vascular endothelial growth factor aptamer, for diabetic macular edema. Ophthalmology 2005;112:1747–1757.

150 Arevalo JF, Fromow-Guerra J, Quiroz-Mercado H, Sanchez JG, Wu L, Maia M, Berrocal MH, Solis-Vivanco A, Farah ME: Primary intravitreal bevacizumab (Avastin) for diabetic macular edema: results from the Pan-American Collaborative Retina Study Group at 6-month follow-up. Ophthalmology 2007;114:743–750.

151 Scott IU, Edwards AR, Beck RW, Bressler NM, Chan CK, Elman MJ, Friedman SM, Greven CM, Maturi RK, Pieramici DJ, Shami M, Singerman LJ, Stockdale CR: A phase II randomized clinical trial of intravitreal bevacizumab for diabetic macular edema. Ophthalmology 2007;114:1860–1867.

152 Adamis AP, Altaweel M, Bressler NM, Cunningham ET Jr, Davis MD, Goldbaum M, Gonzales C, Guyer DR, Barrett K, Patel M: Changes in retinal neovascularization after pegaptanib (Macugen) therapy in diabetic individuals. Ophthalmology 2006;113:23–28.

153 Avery RL, Pearlman J, Pieramici DJ, Rabena MD, Castellarin AA, Nasir MA, Giust MJ, Wendel R, Patel A: Intravitreal bevacizumab (Avastin) in the treatment of proliferative diabetic retinopathy. Ophthalmology 2006;113:1695 e1–15.

154 Gillies MC, Wong TY: Ranibizumab for neovascular age-related macular degeneration. N Engl J Med 2007;356:748–749; author reply 9–50.

155 Turner ST, Schwartz GL, Boerwinkle E: Personalized medicine for high blood pressure. Hypertension 2007;50:1–5.

Tien Y. Wong, MD, PhD
Professor of Ophthalmology, National University of Singapore
Director, Singapore Eye Research Institute, Singapore National Eye Centre
11 Third Hospital Avenue, Singapore 168751 (Singapore)
Tel. +65 63224571, Fax +65 63231903, E-Mail ophwty@nus.edu.sg

Hammes H-P, Porta M (eds): Experimental Approaches to Diabetic Retinopathy.
Front Diabetes. Basel, Karger, 2010, vol 20, pp 220–227

From Bedside to Bench and Back: Open Problems in Clinical and Basic Research

Massimo Porta[a] · Hans-Peter Hammes[b]

[a]Department of Medicine, University of Turin, Turin, Italy; [b]Section of Endocrinology, 5th Medical Department, Mannheim Medical Faculty, University Hospital Mannheim, Ruprechts-Karls University Heidelberg, Mannheim, Germany

Abstract

Diabetic retinopathy remains a leading cause of visual loss in the working age population of industrialized countries. Many unsolved problems remain as diabetic patients are still going blind, and many patients in poor countries have no access to screening or effective treatment of diabetic retinopathy. In particular, macular edema is becoming more and more the problem of elderly patients, for which we lack effective, definitive treatments. Clinical trials testing proofs of concept developed from in vitro and animal experiments have so far produced mixed results. Optimizing blood glucose and pressure control, platelet-active agents and blockers of the renin-angiotensin system appear to slow down retinopathy at initial or mild stages, whereas more advanced presentations may not be affected by systemic medication. The only options for sight-threatening retinopathy are either destructive (laser photocoagulation) or invasive (intravitreous administration of steroids and VEGF antagonists). The many questions that remain to be addressed are discussed in this chapter.

Overlooking the last 40 years of research in diabetic retinopathy, it appears that the retina was at the core of studies aiming at the improvement of the outcome of a patient with diabetes. The devastating condition of a blind person dependent on multiple daily injections of insulin always put a major emphasis on finding a cure for diabetes and its complications.

It was the prevention and secondary intervention of diabetic retinopathy that the Diabetes Control and Complications Trial (DCCT) was primarily designed for, based on findings in diabetic dogs that intensified glucose lowering with insulin was capable of reducing retinopathy [1]. However, the effect of glucose treatment was not 100%, suggesting that even mildly elevated glucose levels would lead to microvascular damage in the eye. Epidemiologic data also suggest that there is a continuous relation between blood glucose and retinal lesions rather than a discontinuous one as indicated by the WHO cut-offs for the diagnosis of diabetes mellitus and impaired glucose tolerance [2].

Recent epidemiologic and daily clinical work suggests that there is a slight but noticeable reduction in incident sight-threatening retinopathy. However, it would be misleading to ease the efforts towards the aims of the St. Vincent Declaration which, at the beginning of the last decade of the 20th century called for a reduction in diabetes-related blindness by one third within the next 5 years. Many unsolved problems remain as diabetic patients are still going blind, and many patients in poor countries have no access to screening or effective treatment of diabetic retinopathy.

Proliferative retinopathy, although still a severe sight-threatening condition especially for people with type 1 diabetes can be controlled fairly well by scatter, or panretinal, photocoagulation [3], whereas breakdown of the blood-retinal barrier and the subsequent development of macular edema affects patients with both type 1 and 2 diabetes. Since type 2 diabetes is at least ten times more prevalent than type 1, macular edema is becoming more and more the sight-threatening problem of elderly patients, for which we lack effective, definitive treatments.

Clinicians and basic scientists embarking on research in retinopathy may wish to address some open problems: Why do retinal capillaries become leaky at some stage(s) of the disease? What triggers growth of new vessels, again at some stages and in some patients only? How does laser work for new vessels and how, as far as it does, in macular edema?

Rather than investigating what happens in advanced retinopathy, however, it is probably more sensible to research what initiates it. Hyperglycemia is necessary, though not sufficient, for diabetic retinopathy to develop, and much work has been directed at establishing how high glucose damages the capillaries and neuroretina. This very rational approach has revealed a number of biochemical alterations caused by high glucose/hyperglycemia and resulted in an elegant unifying hypothesis according to which excess production of reactive oxygen species through the Krebs cycle is at the basis of the four culprits of diabetes-induced tissue damage: accelerated polyol and hexosamine pathways, activation of protein kinase C, and increased advanced glycation end-product formation [4]. Almost as a corollary of this hypothesis, the demonstration that thiamine, by modulating at least three enzymes of glycolysis and the Krebs cycle, may correct metabolic imbalances induced by high glucose in vitro [5–7] and prevent microalbuminuria [8] and retinal capillary occlusions (though not pericyte loss) [6] in diabetic animals points to a possible simple, inexpensive way of preventing or treating retinopathy.

Food for thought here includes: Which are the first steps in the natural history of retinopathy? Is pericyte loss the earliest event, leading to other changes in a sort of cascade? If so, what microenvironmental changes are causative? If not, what precedes the loss of pericytes? At what stage is the whole process still reversible? Can a clinical trial on the effects of thiamine on retinopathy be organized and carried out?

What has translational research produced so far? Clinical trials testing proofs of concept developed from in vitro and animal experiments have produced mixed results. Inhibition of growth hormone and insulin-like growth factor-1 by a long-acting analogue of somatostatin, octreotide, administered in two dosages versus placebo, was unable to modify the progression of sight-threatening retinopathy and reduce the need for laser therapy. A selective inhibitor of PKCβ2, ruboxistaurin, produced marginal improvement in visual acuity in patients with incipient diabetic macular edema [9].

Evidence for involvement of the renin-angiotensin system (RAS) in retinopathy suggested an intraocular mechanism through which stimulation of AT-1 receptors in the retina might enhance the expression of VEGF, hence edema and angiogenesis. The EUCLID study [10] had suggested that an ACE inhibitor lisinopril reduced progression of retinopathy and the incidence of proliferative retinopathy in patients with type 1 diabetes, probably not driven by a rather small blood pressure reduction of only 3 mm Hg. However, EUCLID was designed to study microalbuminuria and was rather underpowered to address retinopathy; its results were further confounded by differences in HbA1c between the treatment groups.

Another trial, ADVANCE [11]/ADREM [12] showed nonsignificantly protective effects of blood pressure lowering with perindopril, also an ACE inhibitor, associated with a thiazide, indapamide, on progression of retinopathy in 1,241 patients with type 2 diabetes. DIRECT (DIabetic REtinopathy Candesartan Trials), was a program of 3 randomized controlled trials designed specifically to verify if an angiotensin receptor blocker, candesartan, 32 mg/day, administered to 5,231 normoalbuminuric, mostly normotensive patients would: (1) prevent incidence of retinopathy in patients with type 1 diabetes (DIRECT Prevent-1), (2) prevent its progression or cause regression in patients with type 1 diabetes (DIRECT Protect-1), and (3) prevent its progression or cause regression in patients with type 2 diabetes (DIRECT Protect-2) [13, 14]. Mean follow-up was 4.7 years. Overall, patients on active treatment ended the trial with less severe retinopathy than those on placebo. Candesartan reduced by 35% the risk of new retinopathy in type 1 diabetes (NNT = 18) and increased by 34% the odds of improvement in type 2 diabetes (NNT = 21), the first ever report of consistent retinopathy regression. The favorable effects of RAS blockade were confirmed by RASS [15], another study of 285 normotensive patients, in which enalapril 20 mg/day and losartan 100 mg/day administered versus placebo reduced the odds of retinopathy progression by 65 and 70%, respectively.

Platelet aggregation has long been suspected to play a role in capillary occlusions [16], but trials with aspirin, dipyridamole and ticlopidine showed a small, clinically nonsignificant reduction in microaneurysm turnover in early retinopathy [17, 18] and no effects in more advanced stages in which, however, aspirin did not increase the risk of bleeding from new vessels [19]. Another molecule with possible vasoactive properties, calcium dobesilate, was recently found to be devoid of therapeutic effect in macular edema [20].

With reference to other possible pathogenic mechanisms, a rather serendipitous result was reported by the FIELD study [21] in which fenofibrate 200 mg/day reduced progression of existing retinopathy, though not incidence of new retinopathy, and the need for laser treatment for both macular edema and proliferative retinopathy. However, the effect on retinopathy was a tertiary objective of the trial, assessed in only 1,012 out of 9,795 patients enrolled. The effect of fenofibrate was apparently independent of its metabolic action, and did not correlate with glucose, lipid levels or blood pressure.

All in all, the above trials suggest that mechanism-targeted interventions may work in mild rather than moderate or severe retinopathy, when damage of the capillary wall, and possibly the neuroretina, is far too advanced. Is there a 'point of no return' in the natural history of retinopathy? Platelet-active agents appeared to slow down retinopathy at a very initial stage, when only microaneurysms are present [17, 18]. In DIRECT Protect-2 [14], only minimal to mild retinopathy (i.e. microaneurysms with rare hemorrhages and occasional hard exudates or cotton wool spots) was found to regress, whereas more advanced presentations – though still classified as moderate non-proliferative – continued to progress, suggesting that RAS blockade may be effective earlier than previously thought, when capillary occlusions and leakage are not yet predominant. Does RAS blockade work through mechanisms different from VEGF, or does VEGF damage the retinal microcirculation earlier than imagined, and not just by inducing hyperpermeability and angiogenesis?

The results of FIELD [21], if confirmed, will suggest that pathogenesis may be stopped in its steps also in moderate to severe retinopathy. If, as can be hypothesized, different mechanisms preside over subsequent stages of retinopathy, which ones should one elect to study with the best chances of an effective treatment modality in mind?

A situation in which antagonizing VEGF seems definitely effective is when specific antibodies are administered intravitreously for the treatment of aggressive new vessels and severe macular edema. Several RCTs are currently evaluating three VEGF-suppressing agents: pegaptanib (Macugen; Pfizer) an aptamer which targets the 165 isoform of VEGF, and two antibodies, ranibizumab (Lucentis; Genentech) and bevacizumab (Avastin; Genentech). The latter is approved for the treatment of disseminated colorectal cancer but not licensed, hence used off-label, for intraocular use. VEGF inhibition is effective in reducing both new vessels and edema, which represents a good example of translation from bench to bedside, but so are corticosteroids with their potent anti-inflammatory and antiangiogenic effects. Intravitreal triamcinolone has been used for treatment of diabetic macular edema, with a number of RCTs demonstrating significant improvements in edema and visual acuity [22].

Why are intravitreal steroids effective, albeit temporarily, on both conditions: do edema and new vessels share an inflammatory component or do steroids act through mechanism(s) that are altogether different from their anti-inflammatory properties?

Another common opinion is that retinopathy can be prevented by optimizing blood glucose and blood pressure control. Probably as a result of continuously improving clinical attention, drug delivery technology and widespread availability of monitoring systems, some latest epidemiological surveys report decreasing incidence of proliferative retinopathy among patients who developed diabetes in the most recent years [23, 24]. Data from the DCCT/EDIC confirm that, 30 years after enrolment, the cumulative incidence of proliferative retinopathy in the patients who had been on intensive insulin treatment during the trial is 21%, compared to 50% in those who were on conventional treatment [25]. Although encouraging from a public health point of view, the true effects of such measures in individual patients may be less than ideal. Retinopathy may be delayed rather than reduced and, since improved treatment leads to prolonged life expectancy, the final result might be a shift of the curve, with cumulative incidence adding up later in life. In addition, as reported in a retrospective evaluation of all patients who participated in the DCCT, 10% of those who remained in the best quintile for control (i.e. with an HbA1c ≤6.87%), whether in the active or the control group, developed retinopathy, whereas 43% of those in the worst quintile (i.e. HbA1c ≥9.49%) did not develop any lesions over the study period [26]. This corroborates clinical wisdom and strongly suggests that other factors play a pivotal role in the pathogenesis of this complication. More possible subjects for investigative minds include the search for genetic determinants which might make patients especially prone, or resilient, to microangiopathy.

Another reason why it is not justified to sit smug on the large trials that proved a link between blood glucose levels and retinopathy is the difficulty with which optimized metabolic control is achieved in the diabetic population at large. Surveys from different countries prove that only a minor share of patients do achieve the targets set by scientific societies. In the US [27], France [28], UK (Gill, 2003), Italy [29] and other countries, the percentages of patients with an HbA1c lower than 7.0% are less than half, often less than one third. Patients on insulin do worse than those on oral agents, and both are worse than those on lifestyle intervention (diet) only [30]. Possible reasons include medical inertia, poor patient adherence to treatment, insufficient effect of lifestyle and pharmacological interventions, environmental and socioeconomic obstacles, but none of these appears to entirely account for the difficulty in optimizing metabolic control. Although physicians are not very reactive to abnormally high values of HbA1c or blood pressure [27], a clinic-based intervention study in Liverpool showed virtually no effect in proactively pursuing improved metabolic control, except in patients on diet only [30]. Individual patients may be 'set' on different degrees of diabetes severity, hence different levels of metabolic control, a pragmatic though perhaps slightly heretical suggestion. Among children the situation is even worse, with less than 5% of patients having an HbA1c less than 7.0% and more than 80% above 8.0% [31]. Maybe the therapeutic targets are too ambitious, at least for very young and very old patients. In terms of personal motivation, only exceptional and time-limited circumstances may be powerful enough, as in the case of pregnancy, when 80% of patients achieve levels of 6.5% or less [32]. In any case, data from the 1999–2004 National Health and Nutrition Examination Survey suggest that the percentage of patients with an HbA1c lower than 7.0 in the US is slowly increasing [33].

As optimized control is not always attained and, even when it is, not necessarily effective, the search must go on for a straightforward pathogenic mechanism that would explain the natural history of retinopathy and indicate clear-cut therapeutic targets. There are also solutions which need to be applied to the most urgent questions arising from clinical work with patients. The subsequent paragraphs will address a selection of items from recent roadmaps proposed by the NIH (http://www2.niddk.nih.gov/AboutNIDDK/ResearchAndPlanning/Type1Diabetes/). Similar activities are ongoing in the EU (http://www.diamap.eu).

(a) *Hyperglycemic Memory.* The DCCT demonstrated that good glycemic control in type 1 diabetes reduces the incidence and progression of retinopathy to a large extent. After completion of the trial, many patients formerly in the 'standard' therapy group intensified their metabolic control and thereby achieved better HbA1c levels. Patients formerly in the 'intensified' therapy group experienced a slight worsening of their HbA1c levels. Subsequent follow-up studies called EDIC demonstrated that despite similar post-DCCT HbA1c levels, patients in the former standard treatment group continued to have a higher rate of developing retinopathy, while members of the former well-controlled group remained protected [34]. This phenomenon is called metabolic memory, and the underlying molecular basis which is currently almost unexplored will help to identify possible targets for novel interventions, and answer the clinically important question of the 'point of no return' of retinopathy.

(b) *Vascular Repair Mechanisms.* In the past, much interest has been focused on the damaging mechanisms of chronic hyperglycemia. Adaptive responses had been largely ignored and were underrepresented. Since diabetic retinopathy is not only the result of tissue damage, but also inferior repair responses, much of the basis for improved treatment and prevention may lie in the therapeutic support of repair mechanisms. As in all other target tissues of diabetic complications, retinopathy starts with progressive vascular dropout. Angiogenic responses leading to proliferative diabetic retinopathy are only secondary and occur only in some patients. Repair of damaged vessels is partly promoted by cells from the bone marrow. In diabetic patients, these cells are reduced in number and dysfunctional [35]. The injection of progenitor cells of nondiabetic origin can correct this defect to a certain extent. It is proposed that research in this area will lead to novel drug- and cell-based therapies to restore proper vascular function, including the early lesions in the retina.

(c) *Epigenetic Factors.* The genetic make-up of an individual determines life span and disease susceptibility. Work over the past years has provided much more information on genetic risk for diabetic nephropathy than for diabetic retinopathy, although it is clear that there is a genetic background of retinopathy susceptibility, at least in type 1 diabetes [36, 37]. Recently, permanent molecular changes which can last through life have been identified that can, for example, explain phenotypic differences in identical twins [38]. These epigenetic changes result either from DNA methylation in which a methyltransferase attached a methyl group to DNA, which leads to gene silencing, or from histone acetylation in which a silenced gene is activated by acetyl modification of regulatory parts. These permanent modifications can be critical for diabetic retinopathy if hyperglycemia can cause them. Novel findings indicate that transient periods of hyperglycemia can permanently turn on genes that modify inflammatory signaling in target cells [39]. The propensity of glucose-derived epigenetic changes may also be relevant in different stages of retinopathy, as many adaptive and maladaptive factors are stage dependent. Therapeutic strategies targeting epigenetic changes are fascinating, as they would allow interventions beyond a specific point of no return.

(d) *New Animal Models.* Much of the delay in translating innovative therapies into clinically established treatments results from the paucity of animal models that represent human diseases adequately. In the case of diabetic retinopathy, this is particularly the case. There is no animal model that properly reflects hyperglycemia-induced proliferative diabetic retinopathy and diabetic maculopathy. Most of the animals used to investigate the effectiveness of specific treatments only reflect certain aspects of the complex human pathology. Moreover, it has been recently appreciated that even the genetic background of an experimental model – mostly mouse models – have a profound effect on the phenotype in a transgenic or a knockout setting. It is thus concluded that animal models that mimic the human development of advanced diabetic retinopathy are desperately needed for research on mechanisms and for drug development.

(e) *Systems Biology.* It has become clear – and chapters in this book reflect it – that diabetic retinopathy is more than a microvascular disease. Cell-cell communication under hyperglycemic conditions must be studied in tissue context including the impact of the neuroglia on vascular response to identify relevant signaling pathways addressable by therapeutics. On the cellular level, each glucose-induced abnormality is in a context with other molecules. The same can be viewed on the tissue level. The emerging field of systems biology is capable of analyzing the many simultaneously occurring events as complex, interconnected circuits. These circuits may have control (check) points amenable to biological interaction. The closer in vitro and in vivo systems will be modeled to diabetic retinopathy the better the answers will be provided with this technology.

Apart from these scientific areas which address current and future questions to be solved for an improved understanding of diabetic retinopathy, there are more urgent areas which have been identified as important. The technique of high throughput screening is a powerful tool to identify disease-relevant target molecules for treatment. However, the design of the model systems by which they are selected is highly critical. The adjustment on retinopathy is a challenging task, as is the identification of early biomarkers of retinopathy. Some biomarkers may help identify early functional or structural lesions in patients prone to progression to sight threatening stages. Others may indicate patients with fast progressing disease, while other biomarkers are sought which reflect relative protection over many years. A third group of markers in patients is essential that is also present in animals and which indicates early (nontransient) structural changes. These markers may also be useful to facilitate noninvasive imaging as the eye is the only organ in diabetes in which blood vessels can be visualized noninvasively.

If these and other activities will have led to the identification of putative therapies, patients with appropriate levels of the disease are essential for the mandatory clinical trials. The lag phase between target discovery and clinical application in routine patients is partly so long because of the paucity of existing collaborative networks that provide infrastructures for rapid outset of clinical trials. A positive exemption is the Diabetic Retinopathy Clinical Research Network (DRCR.net) and other networks which are currently developing.

References

1 Engerman R, Bloodworth JM Jr, Nelson S: Relationship of microvascular disease in diabetes to metabolic control. Diabetes 1977;26:760–769.

2 Wong TY, Liew G, Tapp RJ, Schmidt MI, Wang JJ, Mitchell P, Klein R, Klein BE, Zimmet P, Shaw J: Relation between fasting glucose and retinopathy for diagnosis of diabetes: three population-based cross-sectional studies. Lancet 2008;371:736–743.

3 Early Treatment Diabetic Retinopathy Study Research Group: Early photocoagulation for diabetic retinopathy. ETDRS report No. 9. Ophthalmology 1991;98:766–785.

4 Brownlee M: Biochemistry and molecular cell biology of diabetic complications. Nature 2001;414:813–820.

5 La Selva M, Beltramo E, Pagnozzi F, Bena E, Molinatti PA, Molinatti GM, Porta M: Thiamine corrects delayed replication and decreases production of lactate and advanced glycation end-products in bovine retinal and human umbilical vein endothelial cells cultured under high glucose conditions. Diabetologia 1996;39: 1263–1268.

6 Hammes HP, Du X, Edelstein D Taguchi T, Matsumura T, Ju Q, Lin J, Bierhaus A, Nawroth P, Hannak D, Neumaier M, Bergfeld R, Giardino I, Brownlee M: Benfotiamine blocks three major pathways of hyperglycemic damage and prevents experimental diabetic retinopathy. Nat Med 2003;9:294–299.

7 Berrone E, Beltramo E, Solimine C, Ape AU, Porta M: Regulation of intracellular glucose and polyol pathway by thiamine and benfotiamine in vascular cells cultured in high glucose. J Biol Chem 2006;281:9307–9313.

8 Babaei-Jadidi R, Karachalias N, Ahmed N, Battah S, Thornalley PJ: Prevention of incipient diabetic nephropathy by high-dose thiamine and benfotiamine. Diabetes 2003;52:2110–2120.

9 Donnelly R, Idris I, Forrester JV: Protein kinase C inhibition and diabetic retinopathy: a shot in the dark at translational research. Br J Ophthalmol 2004;88:145–151.

10 Chaturvedi N, Sjolie AK, Stephenson JM, Abrahamian H, Keipes M, Castellarin A, Rogulja-Pepeonik Z, Fuller JH: Effect of lisinopril on progression of retinopathy in normotensive people with type 1 diabetes. The EUCLID Study Group. EURODIAB Controlled Trial of Lisinopril in Insulin-Dependent Diabetes Mellitus. Lancet 1998;35:28–31.

11 Patel A, MacMahon S, Chalmers J, Neal B, Woodward M, Billot L, Harrap S, Poulter N, Marre M, Cooper M, Glasziou P, Grobbee DE, Hamet P, Heller S, Liu LS, Mancia G, Mogensen CE, Pan CY, Rodgers A, Williams B, ADVANCE Collaborative Group: Effects of a fixed combination of perindopril and indapamide on macrovascular and microvascular outcomes in patients with type 2 diabetes mellitus (the ADVANCE trial): a randomised controlled trial. Lancet 2007;370:829–840.

12 Beulens JW, Patel A, Vingerling JR, Cruickshank JK, Hughes AD, Stanton A, Lu J, McG Thom SA, Grobbee DE, Stolk RP, on behalf of the AdRem* project team and ADVANCE management committee: Effects of blood pressure lowering and intensive glucose control on the incidence and progression of retinopathy in patients with type 2 diabetes mellitus: a randomised controlled trial. Diabetologia 2009; Epub ahead of print; DOI 10.1007/s00125–009–1457-x.

13 Chaturvedi N, Porta M, Klein R, Orchard T, Fuller J, Parving HH, Bilous R, Sjølie AK, DIRECT Programme Study Group: Effect of candesartan on prevention (DIRECT-Prevent 1) and progression (DIRECT-Protect 1) of retinopathy in type 1 diabetes: randomised, placebo-controlled trials. Lancet 2008;372:1394–1402.

14 Sjølie AK, Klein R, Porta M, Orchard T, Fuller J, Parving HH, Bilous R, Chaturvedi N, DIRECT Programme Study Group: Effect of candesartan on progression and regression of retinopathy in type 2 diabetes (DIRECT-Protect 2): a randomised placebo-controlled trial. Lancet 2008;372:1385–1393.

15 Mauer M, Zinman B, Gardiner R, Suissa S, Sinaiko A, Strand T, Drummond K, Donnelly S, Goodyer P, Gubler MC, Klein R: Renal and retinal effects of enalapril and losartan in type 1 diabetes. N Engl J Med 2009;361:40–51.

16 Porta M, Bandello F: Diabetic retinopathy. A clinical update. Diabetologia 2002;45:1617–1634.

17 The DAMAD Study Group: Effect of aspirin alone and aspirin plus dipyridamole in early diabetic retinopathy. A multicentre randomized controlled clinical trial. Diabetes 1989;38:491–498.

18 The TIMAD Study Group: Ticlopidine treatment reduces the progression of nonproliferative diabetic retinopathy. Arch Ophthalmol 1990;108:1577–1583.

19 Early Treatment of Diabetic Retinopathy Study Group: Effects of aspirin treatment of diabetic retinopathy. ETDRS Report No. 8. Ophthalmology 1991;98:757–765.

20 Haritoglou C, Gerss J, Sauerland C, Kampik A, Ulbig MW for the CALDIRET study group: Effect of calcium dobesilate on occurrence of diabetic macular oedema (CALDIRET study): randomised, double-blind, placebo-controlled, multicentre trial. Lancet 2009;373:1364–1371.

21 Keech AC, Mitchell P, Summanen PA, O'Day J, Davis TM, Moffitt MS, Taskinen MR, Simes RJ, Tse D, Williamson E, Merrifield A, Laatikainen LT, d'Emden MC, Crimet DC, O'Connell RL, Colman PG, FIELD study investigators: Effect of fenofibrate on the need for laser treatment for diabetic retinopathy (FIELD study): a randomised controlled trial. Lancet 2007;370:1687–1697.

22 O'Doherty M, Dooley I, Hickey-Dwyer M: Interventions for diabetic macular oedema: a systematic review of the literature. Br J Ophthalmol 2008;92:1581–1590.

23 Hovind P, Tarnow L, Rossing K, Rossing P, Eising S, Larsen N, Binder C, Parving H-H: Decreasing incidence of severe diabetic microangiopathy in type 1 diabetes. Diabetes Care 2003;26:1258–1264.

24 Klein R, Knudtson MD, Lee KE, Gangnon R, Klein BEK: The Wisconsin Epidemiologic Study of Diabetic Retinopathy XXII. The twenty-five-year progression of retinopathy in persons with type 1 diabetes. Ophthalmology 2008;115:1859–1868.

25 The Diabetes Control and Complications Trial/Epidemiology of Diabetes Interventions and Complications (DCCT/EDIC) Research Group: Modern-day clinical course of type 1 diabetes mellitus after 30 years' duration. The Diabetes Control and Complications Trial/Epidemiology of Diabetes Interventions and Complications and Pittsburgh Epidemiology of Diabetes Complications Experience (1983–2005). Arch Intern Med 2009;169:1307–1316.

26 Zhang LY, Krzentowski G, Albert A, Lefevbre PJ: Risk of developing retinopathy in Diabetes Control and Complications Trial type 1 diabetic patients with good or poor metabolic control. Diabetes Care 2001;24:1275–1279.

27 Grant RW, Buse JB, Meigs JB, for the University HealthSystem Consortium (UHC) Diabetes Benchmarking Project Team: Quality of Diabetes Care in U.S. Academic Medical Centers. Low rates of medical regimen change. Diabetes Care 2005;28:337–442.

28 Prèvost G, Phan TM, Mounier-Venier C, Fontaine P: Control of cardiovascular risk factors in patients with type 2 diabetes and hypertension in a French national study (Phenomen). Diabetes Metab 2005;31:479–485.

29 De Berardis G, Pellegrini F, Franciosi M, Belfiglio M, Di Nardo B, Greenfield F, Kaplan SH, Rossi MCE, Sacco M, Tognoni G, Valentini M, Nicolucci A: Quality of care and outcomes in type 2 diabetic patients. A comparison between general practice and diabetes clinics. Diabetes Care 2005;28:2637–2643.

30 Gill GV, Woodward S, Pradhan S, Wallymahmed M, Groves T, English P, Wilding JP: Intensified treatment of type 2 diabetes. Positive effects on blood pressure but not glycaemic control. Q J Med 2003;96:833–836.

31 Saunders SA, Wallymahmed M, Macfarlane IA: Glycaemic control in a type 1 diabetes clinic for younger adults. Q Med J 2004;97:575–580.

32 Mathiesen ER, Kinsley B, Amiel SA, Heller S, McCance D, Duran S, Bellaire S, Raben A, on behalf of the Insulin Aspart Pregnancy Study Group: Maternal glycemic control and hypoglycemia in Type 1 diabetic pregnancy. A randomized trial of insulin aspart versus human insulin in 322 pregnant women. Diabetes Care 2007;30:771–776.

33 Ford ES, Little RR, Li C, Mokdad AH: Trends in A1c concentrations among U.S. adults with diagnosed diabetes from 1999 to 2004. Diabetes Care 2008;31:102–104.

34 The DCCT/EDIC Research Group: Retinopathy and nephropathy in patients with type 1 diabetes four years after a trial of intensive therapy. N Engl J Med 2000;342:381–389.

35 Caballero S, Sengupta N, Afzal A, Chang KH, Li Calzi S, Guberski DL, Kern TS, Grant MB: Ischemic vascular damage can be repaired by healthy, but not diabetic, endothelial progenitor cells. Diabetes 2007;56:960–967.

36 Uhlmann K, Kovacs P, Boettcher Y, Hammes HP, Paschke R: Genetics of diabetic retinopathy. Exp Clin Endocrinol Diabetes 2006;114:275–294.

37 The Diabetes Control and Complications Trial Research Group: Clustering of long-term complications in families with diabetes in the diabetes control and complications trial. Diabetes 1997;46:1829–1839.

38 Fraga MF, Ballestar E, Paz MF, Ropero S, Setien F, Ballestar ML, Heine-Suñer D, Cigudosa JC, Urioste M, Benitez J, Boix-Chornet M, Sanchez-Aguilera A, Ling C, Carlsson E, Poulsen P, Vaag A, Stephan Z, Spector TD, Wu YZ, Plass C, Esteller M: Epigenetic differences arise during the lifetime of monozygotic twins. Proc Natl Acad Sci USA 2005;102:10604–10609.

39 El-Osta A, Brasacchio D, Yao D, Pocai A, Jones PL, Roeder RG, Cooper ME, Brownlee M: Transient high glucose causes persistent epigenetic changes and altered gene expression during subsequent normoglycemia. J Exp Med 2008;205:2409–2417; erratum in J Exp Med 2008;205:2683.

Prof. Massimo Porta, MD, PhD
Department of Medicine, University of Turin
Corso Dogliotti 14
IT–10126 Turin (Italy)
Tel. +39 011 6632354, Fax +39 011 6634751, E-Mail massimo.porta@unito.it

Author Index

Subject Index